EMBARK Psychedelic Therapy for Depression

EMBARK Psychedelic Therapy for Depression

A New Approach for the Whole Person

BILL BRENNAN

ALEX BELSER

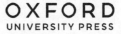

OXFORD
UNIVERSITY PRESS

OXFORD
UNIVERSITY PRESS

Oxford University Press is a department of the University of Oxford.
It furthers the University's objective of excellence in research, scholarship,
and education by publishing worldwide. Oxford is a registered trade mark of
Oxford University Press in the UK and in certain other countries.

Published in the United States of America by Oxford University Press
198 Madison Avenue, New York, NY 10016, United States of America.

Library of Congress Cataloging-in-Publication Data
Names: Brennan, Bill (Psychedelic psychologist), editor. |
Belser, Alex (Psychedelic psychologist), editor.
Title: EMBARK: psychedelic therapy for depression : a new approach for the
whole person / by Bill Brennan and Alex Belser.
Description: New York, NY : Oxford University Press, [2024] |
Includes bibliographical references and index. |
Identifiers: LCCN 2023048158 (print) | LCCN 2023048159 (ebook) |
ISBN 9780197762592 (paperback) | ISBN 9780197762615 (epub) |
ISBN 9780197762622
Subjects: LCSH: Depression, Mental—Chemotherapy. |
Hallucinogenic drugs—Therapeutic use. | Psychotherapy—Methodolody.
Classification: LCC RC537 .B7486 2024 (print) | LCC RC537 (ebook) |
DDC 616.85/27061—dc23/eng/20231214
LC record available at https://lccn.loc.gov/2023048158
LC ebook record available at https://lccn.loc.gov/2023048159

DOI: 10.1093/9780197762622.001.0001

Printed by Marquis Book Printing, Canada

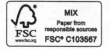

CONTENTS

LIST OF FIGURES

ACKNOWLEDGMENTS

In the last three years of developing EMBARK, we have perceived ourselves as weavers, braiding together time-honored threads of knowledge that have, by some twist of fate, found their way to our hands. It would be a distortion of the truth to propose that we, alone, wove these diverse strands into existence anew. These threads of wisdom have been gifted to us from a vast network of psychedelic teachers, guides, mentors, peers, companions, and participants. We express a deep sense of gratitude to the interconnected community from which this wisdom grows.

We begin by thanking the contributors to the book: first to our early codeveloper of the first EMBARK adaptation used in a clinical trial, Anthony Back, MD, who provided a training architecture and many helpful suggestions on how to organize a manual. Next is Jim Hopper, PhD, who believed in our model and our manuscript enough to give us a wealth of expert feedback that did not shy from pointing out the wonky bits. Many additional thanks go to Dee Dee Goldpaugh, LCSW, and Robin Brody, PsyD, for also bringing their clinical expertise to bear on this book.

We owe a debt of gratitude to our EMBARK team: Diane Hollman for finding the people and carrying our heart to the altar; Sarah Scheld, MA, for holding the sacred; Melissa Field for charting the way; Liz Galic, for being pretty amazing all around; Alex Kelman, PhD, for leading the EMBARK trainings and carrying us forward; Ashvani Gowan for making it work and getting it done; Michelle Selvaratnam for making all the connections; Robert Mino for getting our ducks in a row; Jason Brenzel for creating the EMBARK Open Access free online course; Sadé Kiani for making it visually beautiful; Leah Gibson for telling the story; Alexa Orban for being our media maven; and Sara Brittany Somerset, for sharing our message with the world.

With EMBARK, we placed a strong emphasis on ethics, guided by four care cornerstones. We would like to thank the faculty members who developed and taught the associated modules: First, NiCole T. Buchanan, PhD, helped us to expand the Culturally Competent Care cornerstone beyond mere JEDI (justice, equity, diversity and inclusion) platitudes. Second, Marcela Ot'alora G, MA, LPCC, established the trauma-informed care cornerstone for our work in psychedelics, drawing from her supervision in the treatment of PTSD. Third, Kylea Taylor, MFT, pushed us toward Ethically Rigorous Care in both ordinary and nonordinary consciousness. Lastly, Florie St. Aime, LCSW, fostered Collective Care, inviting elements of collective liberation to EMBARK.

We thank our additional EMBARK faculty: Dennis McKenna, PhD, our psychedelic polymath and guide to the "invisible landscape"; Manuela Mischke-Reeds,

MA, MFT, for teaching the Body-Aware domain; Adele Lafrance, PhD, for teaching the Affective-Cognitive domain; Jeffrey Guss, MD, for teaching the Relational domain and serving as a mentor and friend; Andrew Solomon, PhD, who helps us keep the noonday demon at bay; and Jordan Sloshower, MD, MSc, who reminds us of the sanctity of life, even in the face of great suffering.

We thank our trusted advisors: Stacia Butterfield, the guiding force behind our holotropic breathwork trainings, for her exceptional spirit; the pioneering duo Ingmar Gorman, PhD, and Elizabeth Nielson, PhD, who are training the next generations of psychedelic clinicians; Charlotte Harrison, who carved a path ahead, paving the way for us to follow; John Krystal, MD, who helped us see the big picture; Maurizio Fava, MD, who navigated us safely, steering us away from potential pitfalls in clinical trials; Tom Laughren, MD, who offered wise counsel through complex regulatory barriers; and Lynn Marie Morski, MD, JD, an ambassador for the potential of psychedelic medicine among doctors and clinicians worldwide. We give special thanks to our experienced clinical supervisors for the EMBARK programs, who guide our facilitators to do the real work: Dee Dee Goldpaugh, LCSW, Franklin King, MD, and Robert Krause, DNP APRN-BC. Finally, to Ladybird Morgan, RN, MSW, for her input on an earlier EMBARK manual and her stewardship of the clinical work on the trial that used it.

EMBARK would be merely an intellectual lark if many people had not stepped up to bring it to life. The creation of EMBARK would not have been possible without the generous financial support of Cybin throughout its creation, development, and piloting. We especially thank the following people: Doug Drysdale, for his leadership in calling for EMBARK to be "open-source . . . to support patients"; the founders of Cybin, Eric So, Paul Glavine, and John Kanakis, for seeing the importance of a meaningful therapy; Lori Challenger for corralling the Cybinauts to greater purpose; Brett Greene, who brought us into one of the strongest psychedelic science teams ever assembled, including the other founders of Adelia Therapeutics: Drs. Mike Palfreyman, Alex Nivorozhkin, Clint Canal, and Joshua Hartsel, for being brilliant nerds with big hearts; Allison House-Gecewicz, who makes it all happen; Angela Sorie, who kept our randomized controlled trials in New Jersey and Georgia from running off the rails; Aaron Bartlone for leading the charge; Dr. Amir Inamdar for helping us grow up and guiding our vision; and Drs. Sebastian Krempien and Pradeep Nathan for directing our research with psilocybin and DMT-based therapies. There were many people behind the scenes that built an infrastructure to hold the research with EMBARK: Naomi Morris; Timene Wilson; Lisa Salazar; Wayne Philip; David Wood; Erica Olson; Greg Cavers, Jeff Mason, and Drs. Amy Reichelt, Joan Krakowsky, Geoff Varty, and Michael Morgan. Thank you.

We thank the graduates of the EMBARK training, who are doing the work, facilitating psychedelic-assisted therapy with participants with depression and burnout.

Finally, we thank the participants who have embarked on this path with us. Thank you for helping us find the way together.

Bill Brennan: Thanking all the people whose impact on me made this book into what it is feels a bit like trying to pull the ocean through a straw, but I will try. The first note of appreciation goes to all the researchers and authors cited throughout this book, whose labor provided much of the knowledge woven into the EMBARK model.

Particular thanks are due to some of the critical and ethical voices in psychedelia to whom I have listened most deeply: Joseph Holcomb Adams, Adam Andros Aronovich, Camille Barton, Chaikuni, Elias Dakwar, Alicia Danforth, Neşe Devenot, David Dupuis, Jules Evans, Martin Fortier, Brenna Gebauer, Jennifer Jones, Daan Keiman, Franklin King, Emma Knighton, Elle Lancelotta, Shayla Love, Katherine MacLean, Olivia Marcus, Rebecca Martinez, Eilish Nagle, Tehseen Noorani, Laura Mae Northup, Rachel Petersen, Diana Quinn, Sara So, Kylea Taylor, and Rosalind Watts. Thank you sincerely for keeping me (and us all) focused on the harms that could come from every missed opportunity to develop this work wisely.

A round of posthumous appreciation is due to the two authors whose work did the most to kindle and nurture my early interest in psychedelics: Terence McKenna and Robert Anton Wilson, whose *Sex, Drugs, and Magic* provided a first glimpse of psychedelia to a D.A.R.E. teenager who was honestly just trying to read about sex and magic.

A very heartfelt thanks to my teachers, supervisors, and role models: Jacqueline Mattis, Ranger BlackSwan, Lane Gerber, Steen Halling, João da Mata, Margo Jackson, Almas Merchant, Lisa Lyons, Melissa Grace, Magdalena Pineda Casimiro, and others who may not appreciate the daylight of an acknowledgements section. Know that I will always carry every one of you into this work with me in an innermost way.

My tenderest love and appreciation go to those who have shared in this incredible work with me: the clients, trainees, supervisees, peers, mentors, healers, friends, and communities of practice that have filled in the closest circles around my heart. Nothing gives me more peace than knowing that we are the ones walking each other home.

That leaves only a most precious few. Charley Wininger, whose friendship and example have taught me so much of what I know about living and loving. Florie St. Aime, my closest coconspirator and a dear friend whose brilliance has lit the way through some of my darkest nights in this work. And my coauthor and beloved friend, Alex Belser. I remember when someone at a party in 2006 assumed we were brothers. All these years later, I think she might have been onto something.

And, finally, to my treasure of a partner, Samantha Barron. You have listened to me say the word "EMBARK" more times than anyone should ever have to. You have responded to my many requests for feedback with an expertise that has shifted the course of this book several times. But even these generosities are just dim reflections of the astonishing love that you have brought into my life. Thank you for bringing me closer to this world than I have ever been before.

Alex Belser: I am grateful to my teachers for their brilliance and generosity of spirit, especially my psychedelic teachers: Jeffrey Guss, MD, Annie and Michael

Mithoefer, MD, Bill Richards, PhD, Mary Cosimano, LMSW, Raquel Bennett, PhD, Bob Jesse, Robert Heffernan, Raquel Pallares, and many unnamed maestros who are deserving of our honor and respect. I thank my yoga teachers, Paul Manza and Hari Kaur, who helped me step into teaching for the first time. I thank Brian Joshin Byrnes for seeing me.

I have been so lucky to learn from a few great psychologists: Maria Lechich, PhD, Jillen Axelrod, PhD, and Jacob Ham, PhD. They taught me that I could be good enough.

Finally, my loved ones. This book would not have been possible without the care of Kelly Dungan, who invited the vision, and the support of James Mercer, who was steadfast against many odds. I have been held by the folx of the incomparable City Fae circle over many years (you know who you are). I thank Saajan Patel, Jessica Gieseke, and Tony Garcia for their friendship in dark times. I thank Ryan Hahn, who in 1998 first introduced me to psychedelics when he gave to me his dogeared copy of *LSD Psychotherapy*, which his friend had apparently "liberated" from a Tower Records.

I hold in my heart Tyler Armey, who is quietly wise and would not let me forget what really mattered. To my coauthor, Bill Brennan: it makes me smile to know you are in this world with all of us—we are in this together.

Lastly, I am grateful for Martin Devine, PhD and the thousand hours he spent with me. For what is it, if not a cure through love?

DISCLOSURE OF INTERESTS:

Bill Brennan and Alex Belser have received financial compensation from Cybin, Inc., during the time in which EMBARK was developed and when this book was written. Dr. Brennan is a paid consultant at Cybin. Dr. Belser was formerly Cybin's Chief Clinical Officer and is now a consultant. In the last 3 years, Fluence, Psychedelics Today, and Salt City Psychedelic Therapy & Research Dr. Brennan has also received compensation from Gilgamesh Pharmaceuticals, Fluence, Psychedelics Today, and Salt City Psychedelic Therapy & Research and Dr. Belser has received financial compensation as a teacher or lecturer from Harvard Medical School, New York University, Yale University, Karolinska Institute, the Integrative Psychiatry Institute, Adelia Therapeutics, Chacruna Institute, ATMA, Synthesis Institute, and the Embody Lab and has filed patents on the use of psychedelic compounds for the treatment of psychiatric indications.

AUTHORS' NOTE

Hello friends and colleagues.

As the authors of this book, we would like to take a moment to welcome you and to honor your interest in psychedelic therapy. You are joining a lineage of practitioners who have used psychedelic medicines in psychotherapeutic contexts for nearly a century. Since Western culture became aware of these medicines' therapeutic potential in the early twentieth century, they have inspired, moved, and often vexed us. They continue to challenge us as clinicians, theorists, and human beings.

We have developed EMBARK psychedelic therapy in the spirit of honoring the work of those who have come before us, of our teachers, and of our patients. It has been a heartfelt process of listening deeply and learning from our work as clinicians and supervisors in this field. Our hope is that the EMBARK approach may serve you well as you become stewards of this challenging and meaningful work.

INTRODUCTION: A New Approach for the Whole Person

Imagine that you are a newly certified psychedelic provider joining a group practice in psychedelic therapy.

In your first few weeks, you work with participants who have vastly different experiences. One participant expresses mystical insights, another spends the day shaking and trembling, a third makes peace with a deceased father, the fourth dives deep into grief and sobs for hours, and the last feels connected to their true self for the first time in their life but is not sure what to do about it.

When you and your colleagues gather for peer consultation, you are asked to reflect on these diverse and transformative journeys. How do you weave together the threads of these disparate experiences and discuss your approach to your role? As the therapist, how did you respond? How did you guide them? And why?

Welcome to the crux of the challenge of psychedelic therapy. How can we create a therapy approach that encompasses the varieties of psychedelic experience while retaining a coherent clinical structure?

THE DEVELOPMENT OF EMBARK

EMBARK Psychedelic Therapy for Depression: A New Approach for the Whole Person offers a thorough how-to guide for working therapeutically with psychedelic medicines to treat individuals struggling with depression. It is grounded in the EMBARK approach, a clinical framework for psychedelic-assisted therapy (PAT) that presents a compelling answer to many of the major questions facing the field at the moment. We feel that this book could not have come at a more critical time.

EMBARK Psychedelic Therapy Depression. Bill Brennan and Alex Belser, Oxford University Press. © Oxford University Press 2024. DOI: 10.1093/9780197762622.003.0001

A New Era of Psychedelic Medicines

Psychedelic medicines have been the subject of an ongoing explosion of re-search interest in the fields of psychotherapy, psychiatry, and drug development. Psychedelic research centers have been springing up at universities around the world like early-season tulips. The number of scientific publications about psyche-delic medicine continues to grow exponentially. Nearly overnight, the corporate landscape has gone from a zero to a multibillion-dollar industry. Leading med-ical journals, mainstream media outlets, and investors alike have begun to regard psilocybin and other psychedelic drugs as one of the next major developments in psychiatric care. The U.S. Food and Drug Administration has designated three psychedelic drug treatments as "breakthrough therapies," fast-tracking them on the path to becoming approved drug treatments.

Many psychotherapists and psychotherapists-in-training have turned their attention toward this emerging field. Given that this book has found its way to you, it is likely that you are one of them. While there are many different reasons for being drawn to psychedelic therapy, the allure is understandable. Many are likely drawn in by early research findings demonstrating promise in the treat-ment of a range of clinical presentations. Others may be excited by the prospect of facilitating the type of deeply meaningful experiences that psychedelic clin-ical trial participants have reported having. Others still may be drawn to the work by their own experiences of healing with these medicines and the profound experiences they engender.

This wave of professional interest has given rise to an emergent industry of psychedelic therapy training programs that has started to train scores of eager recruits. Their haste is understandable given the forecast by at least one influ-ential figure in the field that the number of psychedelic therapists required to meet clinical need during just the first year of approval will number in the tens of thousands (Hasty, 2022). For many aspiring practitioners, there is a deeply felt sense of urgency around getting their credentials in order before the floodgates are opened.

The Need for an Integrative Approach

However, this eagerness to start has unfolded against a backdrop of critical questions about the practice of psychedelic therapy:

- How does psychedelic treatment work?
- What is the role of a therapist in psychedelic treatment?
- What do we do to help a participant maximize their benefit from treatment?
- How do we orient ourselves to the unique ethical dimensions of psychedelic therapy?

- How do we apply our previous skills and training as therapists in this new modality?
- How do we support someone who is having a very difficult experience during (or after) a psychedelic medicine session?

Although psychedelic researchers are still very much grappling with these questions, we currently have a great deal of knowledge to help us navigate them in practice. Several dozen psychedelic clinical trials have been conducted, many with accompanying qualitative studies and mediation analyses that highlight what participants have found impactful. Decades of nonpsychedelic psychotherapy research have given us great insight into depression and how to treat it. Finally, the voices of senior psychedelic therapists, clinical trial participants, bioethicists, and others have given us their expert perspectives for consideration as we navigate the intricacies of psychedelic therapy.

However, what we found when we looked at prior models of psychedelic therapy (Brennan & Belser, 2022; see Chapter 2) was that they struggled to integrate these disparate strands of clinical knowledge into a coherent therapeutic framework. While each of them succeeded in holding an important piece of the whole picture, we found that they all lacked attention to one or more critical elements: a sufficient focus on ethics, an appreciation of the importance of the therapeutic relationship, or an understanding of the body as a site of healing. We also noticed that these prior models struggled to meaningfully integrate the potential added value of complementary evidence-based therapeutic approaches developed apart from psychedelics. They tended to either overlook their contributions entirely or incorporate them in a way that clashed with the uniqueness and complexity of psychedelic therapy.

We felt that the field was scaling up its training capacities without a therapeutic model that fully contended with all the most important facets of psychedelic therapy. We aimed to develop a new clinical approach that recognized the importance of each of these facets and put them into dialogue with the best contemporary clinical knowledge. Our intent was to create a model that provided a structure that is capable of continually integrating new findings as they arise.

The EMBARK Model: Our Response

The result of this creative process was the EMBARK model. EMBARK draws gratefully from the successes of earlier models while addressing the shortcomings we identified to present a coherent theoretical framework for psychedelic treatment and therapist training.

At its core, EMBARK is an integrative model that weaves together the most important facets of psychedelic treatment. It recognizes the diversity of experiences that can be elicited by psychedelic medicines and provides therapists with guidance on how to respond to the full spectrum.

EMBARK's holistic approach is reflected in its core structure. EMBARK is an acronym made up of its six "clinical domains," or parallel avenues by which treatment benefit could potentially arise for participants. Therapists are supported in working with psychedelic-induced phenomena in each domain, should they arise, so that they may contribute to positive treatment outcomes:

- **(E) Existential–Spiritual domain**: working with psychedelic-occasioned spiritual experiences so that they can support healing
- **(M) Mindfulness domain**: helping participants develop their ability to observe and respond more adaptively to their internal states
- **(B) Body-Aware domain**: framing the body as a doorway into deep healing
- **(A) Affective–Cognitive domain**: supporting participants in identifying, welcoming, and experiencing their emotional states and core beliefs more fully
- **(R) Relational domain**: inviting participants to attend to the importance of relationships in psychedelic treatment
- **(K) Keeping Momentum domain**: coaching participants to develop their intrinsic motivation for change into durable benefit

Built into this structure is the recognition that there are many possible trajectories of healing and that for any given participant, only a couple of these domains may become relevant.

What are the mechanisms of therapeutic change? Within each domain, EMBARK provides therapists with a conceptual model of mechanisms of therapeutic change. It also provides guidance on what interventions may best support these mechanisms. In this way, EMBARK facilitates a meaningful and orderly incorporation of nonpsychedelic evidence-based treatment (EBT) techniques, which allows the clinician to utilize their preexisting training and experience. The EMBARK approach to depression detailed in this book also provides therapists with practical instructions, suggested agendas, and example interventions for the preparation phase, the medicine sessions, and the integration phase of psychedelic treatment specifically tailored to depression.

In addition to its six clinical domains, EMBARK is built on "four care cornerstones." One of the most common deficits we found as we canvassed prior psychedelic therapies was an underappreciation of the ethical dimensions of psychedelic treatment. We wanted EMBARK to engage with ethical questions deeply and reflect our guiding belief that efficacious treatment is ethical treatment. The cornerstones consist of the following:

- **Trauma-Informed Care**: how can we recognize and attend to the unique ways that trauma manifests in psychedelic treatment?
- **Culturally Competent Care**: how can we integrate a focus on cultural factors into all elements of care?

- **Ethically Rigorous Care**: how can we minimize relational harm by responding appropriately to the unique ethical challenges of psychedelic therapy?
- **Collective Care**: how can we attend to the larger systemic challenges of participants' lives through all aspects of treatment?

Combined, these six clinical domains and four care cornerstones (sometimes referred to as 6 + 4) are the basic architecture of the EMBARK approach. See Chapter 2 for a full discussion.

EMBARK in Practice: Clinical Trials

We first developed EMBARK as a model that could be used across a range of psychedelic clinical trials exploring the use of different psychedelic substances to treat a variety of clinical indications. As such, we designed it to be adaptable to the purposes of any research group that wishes to use it as the therapeutic framework in their trial.

Toward this end, the EMBARK approach was created to be "transdiagnostic," meaning that its overarching structure (the 6 + 4) can be used as the basis for developing treatment approaches to many psychiatric diagnoses, such as major depressive disorder, generalized anxiety disorder, or alcohol use disorder. EMBARK was also designed as a "trans-drug model," meaning it can be thoughtfully adapted to be used with different psychedelic drugs, such as psilocybin and its analogs or N,N-dimethyltryptamine (DMT) and its analogs.

For each trial that uses the EMBARK model, a distinct manualized adaptation is authored. To do so, researchers can repopulate the six clinical domains with psychedelic phenomena occasioned by the drug being studied and aligning them with therapeutic mechanisms taken from the existing literature on treating the selected indication. The overarching structure provided by the model (the 6 + 4) serves as a framework for weaving together known best practices into a coherent, yet flexible and patient-centered, approach that fits the needs of each clinical trial. See Chapters 2 and 3 for more details on how these therapeutic mechanisms become a unified whole.

The results of a recent clinical trial, in which 79% of participants achieved full remission from depression, provide an emerging evidence-base for EMBARK. This book grew out of the treatment manual containing the EMBARK adaptation created for a double-blind, placebo-controlled randomized clinical trial that assessed the safety and tolerability of a psilocybin analogue, CYB003, developed by Cybin, in the treatment of major depressive disorder (MDD; ClinicalTrials. gov identifier NCT05385783). The interim results from this trial have been immensely positive. Participants who received a single 12 milligram dose of CYB003 in the context of EMBARK treatment showed rapid, robust, and highly statistically significant improvements in their depression symptoms compared to those who received placebo, with a -14.08 point between-group difference in reductions in depression scores (MADRS; $p = 0.0005$, Cohen's $d = 2.151$) three weeks after receiving the dose. Three weeks after a second 12 milligram dose, 79% of participants were in remission from depression. No treatment-related serious adverse events were observed. The EMBARK approach is also being tested in another randomized controlled trial. The first complete EMBARK adaptation was created for another trial led by Dr. Anthony Back at the University of Washington. The purpose of the trial was to assess the efficacy of psilocybin-assisted therapy with EMBARK in treating symptoms of depression and burnout suffered by healthcare clinicians as a result of frontline work in the COVID pandemic (ClinicalTrials.gov identifier NCT05163496). Final results are expected in 2024.

Over time, the CYB003-MDD manual grew into something that we thought could be of benefit to a broader audience. We developed it into the book you are currently reading as a way to open-source its approach to the clinical community for use in research and clinical contexts and to inform the development of psychedelic practitioner trainings.

ORIENTATION TO THIS BOOK

Intended Uses

Now that this book and the EMBARK approach it contains have been made widely available, we hope that it will be of value to different audiences for a variety of purposes, as a(n):

- **Instructional text about psychedelic therapy** for all those looking to delve into PAT, whether as part of a professional PAT training program, a university course, or self-directed study
- **Clinical handbook** for clinicians who administer psychedelic therapy in their professional practice in a jurisdiction where it is permitted
- **Treatment manual** for use in psychedelic clinical trials
- **Reference guide** for providers who do not directly provide psychedelic therapy but may work with patients who receive it from another provider

For readers who hope to conduct PAT treatment, we strongly recommend that they use this book as an adjunct to a PAT training program that includes additional didactic and experiential components (either in EMBARK or a comparable approach) and receive ongoing clinical supervision and/or peer consultation. PAT cannot be learned from any book alone, nor should it be conducted by a therapist practicing in professional isolation. Also, while readers who have not already undergone standard training as a psychotherapist will still learn a great deal about PAT from this book, they will likely lack the foundational skills and competency required to use this book as an instructional text for treating depression with PAT.

EMBARK Open Access: A Companion Resource

In the two clinical trials that have used EMBARK so far, therapists underwent an in-depth 75-hour training in the EMBARK curriculum or a comparable crossover training if they had previous experience in psychedelic therapy. Esteemed faculty, recognized as leaders in the field of psychedelic therapy, conducted the EMBARK training. It includes a series of 12 engaging, video-based training modules and accompanying exercises on the EMBARK model.

In line with our commitment to sharing our work with the research and clinical communities, we offer a free online foundational training program in the approach. EMBARK Open Access is the first free online course providing foundational facilitator training for psychedelic therapy. Upon completion of EMBARK Open Access, participants receive a record of completion, which may serve as a steppingstone to future training programs.

Cybin has made this course freely accessible online at https://embarkapproach. com. Over 3,000 clinicians enrolled in the first few months. The EMBARK Open Access program is an excellent companion resource to this book, allowing readers to further deepen their understanding of the approach.

Structure of This Book

EMBARK Psychedelic Therapy can be thought of in two halves. The first four chapters contain background information relevant to the conduct of psychedelic therapy. The second half of the book is more squarely focused on how to conduct a course of a course of treatment.

Chapter 1 begins with the basics. It presents a definition of what a psychedelic is and lays out some of the universal elements of PAT, such as the three-phase structure of treatment (preparation, medicine, and integration sessions), set and setting, and the importance of providing a therapeutic container. The chapter also provides a brief history of PAT in the Western world, from the early 20th century to the present day, to contextualize the current wave of research interest and offer a sense of how we got to where we are. The purpose of this chapter is to orient readers who have recently arrived in the field of psychedelic research.

Chapter 2 is where the EMBARK model gets its formal introduction. The chapter starts with a review of existing PAT models, with an emphasis on areas for improvement, and offers an in-depth rationale for the creation of EMBARK. It then provides a fuller discussion of the six EMBARK clinical domains, including the psychedelic-occasioned phenomena and research findings that informed their characterization. The four care cornerstones that undergird the ethical foundation of EMBARK are also outlined. General clinical considerations and guidance for therapists on how to attend to these cornerstones are provided. The chapter closes with a hypothetical case example that provides an over-the-shoulder look at how an EMBARK therapist conducts a course of PAT.

Chapter 3 is where the book narrows its focus to the EMBARK approach to treating depression. It opens with a description of 12 proposed mechanisms of therapeutic change presented across the 6 EMBARK domains. They frame the approach's understanding of the most common ways in which treatment benefit is likely to arise based on our prior understanding of depression and what is efficacious in its treatment. The chapter includes a description of how nonpsychedelic EBTs and other therapies influenced the development of these mechanisms and other aspects of the approach described in this book. It also includes a critique of the field's overreliance on neurobiological mechanisms in psychedelic therapy.

Chapter 4 addresses the question of what needs to be in place before treatment begins. It lays out the most critical considerations and treatment factors that should be attended to prior to initiating PAT. It discusses the importance of therapists' credentials, skills, personal growth, experiential training, personal psychedelic experiences, therapeutic presence, and commitment to receiving supervision, peer supervision, and support as a provider. The chapter also discusses the need for thorough screening of potential participants for medical and psychiatric conditions, contraindications with other medications, and general stability before treatment. It includes a section on the consideration of and controversies regarding the use of touch in PAT, exploring both historical and current perspectives. An "enhanced consent" process is recommended to ensure that participants understand the potential risks and benefits of the therapy. The chapter also addresses the setup of the physical space, the creation of appropriate music playlists, cultural factors, and considerations when involving other providers and the participant's family members.

Chapter 5 is where the specific treatment instructions begin. It outlines an approach to conducting the sessions that comprise the "preparation phase" of treatment, which consists of nondrug sessions that prepare the participant for the subsequent administration of a psychedelic medicine. It lists the key things that a therapist needs to do to prepare a participant and provides concrete instructions on how to conduct the sessions. It includes three suggested session agendas that offer a potential template and specific language examples for practitioners. The chapter concludes with a figure that contains "watch words" for the preparation phase that may be helpful as a mnemonic for recalling the information found in the chapter.

Chapter 6 of the book focuses on PAT "medicine sessions," in which the psychedelic medicine is administered. The chapter outlines your role in these sessions and provides a list of basic interventions that can be used to support a participant. It also offers guidance on how to support benefit within the six EMBARK domains during the medicine sessions. The chapter further discusses how to respond to common and challenging events that may arise during the psychedelic medicine session. The chapter concludes with a note on challenging experiences that could arise and advice for therapists in PAT clinical trials on what to do if a participant believes they received a placebo. Similar to Chapter 5, this chapter concludes with watch words to help with the retention and recall of chapter content.

Chapter 7 underscores the pivotal role of "integration sessions" in psychedelic therapy, nondrug sessions in which insights from medicine sessions are woven into the fabric of daily life. It presents the EMBARK model's flexible, participant-centric approach to integration. It provides guidelines for the therapist in selecting the most relevant integration goals for each participant. The chapter outlines a step-by-step process for integration and introduces the concept of three spheres of integration, which integrate the innovative idea of engaging with the macro-level dimensions of one's life as a therapeutic growth avenue. The chapter also provides guidance on handling disappointing medicine session experiences, responding to challenging events, and managing serious adverse outcomes. Like the last two chapters, Chapter 7 concludes with watch words.

Chapter 8 concludes the book with a reflection on the intense and meaningful journey of providing PAT. It points to future opportunities for EMBARK and those who wish to collaborate in its development. The chapter also presents a three-part vision for the field, including a shift from a treatment-focused approach to one that emphasizes a broader sense of well-being. It also discusses the important but overlooked role of community support and explores the question of what collective changes would best support the integration of PAT into our culture's approach to healing.

The book concludes with a series of appendices designed to support PAT practitioners. Appendix A focuses on self-care strategies for therapists, acknowledging the emotionally demanding nature of PAT. Appendix B offers a bullet-point summary of therapist aims from preparation through integration. Appendix C provides a quick reference or "cheat sheet" for working within the EMBARK domains. Appendix D presents a worksheet to help therapists tailor integration goals to each participant's unique experience.

Throughout the book, you will see quotations from participants, therapists, and scholars in the field. Quotations from Belser et al. (2017) and Swift and colleagues (2017; Belser is co-author) reflect the voices of participants in a clinical trial of psilocybin-assisted psychotherapy for depression and anxiety associated with a cancer diagnosis at New York University. Quotations from Brennan and colleagues (2021) are statements made by "underground" psychedelic practitioners in response to questions about how they have navigated the ethical dimensions of their relationships with clients. Finally, quotations from Swift and colleagues (2023; Belser is a co-author) come from religious leaders administered psilocybin at New York University and Johns Hopkins University. Participant identities are protected through deidentification and the use of pseudonyms.

We, the authors, sincerely wish you a fruitful and fulfilling journey through this book and throughout your work with participants.

An Overview of Psychedelic-Assisted Therapy

Although many of us think of psychedelics as dangerous drugs, it's time for a rethink. They are non-toxic, non-addictive, have very few side effects, and could potentially offer relief for people suffering from a range of psychological difficulties.

—Rosalind Watts, PhD

This chapter provides a basic understanding of what is meant by the term "psychedelic-assisted therapy." At first glance, this may seem like a deceptively simple thing to do. One could describe PAT as a form of psychotherapeutic intervention that is augmented by the introduction of a psychedelic substance, and this would be accurate. However, this answer raises a number of questions: What makes a substance "psychedelic?" How do we decide it is valuable in psychotherapy? What does it actually look like to put in practice? This introductory chapter is dedicated to addressing these foundational questions.

WHAT ARE "PSYCHEDELIC" SUBSTANCES?

LSD. Mescaline. Psilocybin. Most of us can likely rattle off the names of a few of the better-known psychedelics. Many of us may even have personal experiences with these substances, which inform our understanding of their characteristic features. But honing in on a concise definition of what makes psychedelic substances "psychedelic" can still be challenging. Internet searches and dictionary lookups offer little help, only underscoring the plurality of ways in which people have characterized these substances' effects on the human mind. Most definitions suggest that a psychedelic is a naturally occurring or synthetic substance that temporarily causes pronounced alterations in one's perception, cognition, emotion,

Embark Psychedelic Therapy for Depression. Bill Brennan and Alex Belser, Oxford University Press.
© Oxford University Press 2024. DOI: 10.1093/9780197762622.003.0002

and proprioception. However, this description is unsatisfying. It fails to truly capture the essence of what these substances do and differentiate them from other mind-altering substances, such as alcohol or oxycodone.

Instead, exploring the history behind the term "psychedelic" might provide a better starting point. It was coined by lysergic acid diethylamide (LSD) researcher Humphrey Osmond in 1957 as a replacement for a previous term: hallucinogen (which, notably, is still a widely used medical term for these substances). Osmond felt that this prior term placed too much emphasis on these substances' ability to induce hallucinations—a taxonomical red herring linked to early psychiatric attempts to understand psychedelics through the lens of psychotic hallucinations (Bonson, 2018). In a series of rhyming couplet correspondence with Aldous Huxley, Osmond created the replacement term, "psyche-delic," often translated as "mind manifesting." This new term shifted the focus from a substance that generated something fictitious to one that could reveal the hidden depths within ourselves and our surroundings.

The unique ability of psychedelics to manifest the mind distinguishes them from other consciousness-altering substances. Instead of suppressing or distracting, they have a higher likelihood of uncovering therapy-relevant content. PAT participants commonly experience a heightened awareness of preexisting material: a long-repressed emotion, a forgotten idea of oneself, a returned awareness of one's body, a spiritual presence in the background of their life. To reflect this, Stanislav Grof, a psychiatrist who administered LSD and other psychedelic medicines to thousands of participants, labelled psychedelics as "non-specific amplifiers of consciousness." This phrase has endured over time, even though each psychedelic substance has its own signature set of measurable amplifications (See Figure 1.1). As nonspecific amplifiers of consciousness, psychedelics often occasion highly personal significance and a sense of authentic self-revelation that makes these states of mind both unique and highly suitable for therapy.

While this pithy characterization of psychedelic effects may leave some seeking more precise explanations, a simple list is impossible. As substances that manifest the contents of the mind, their effects are as vast as our inner lives. The next chapter provides more detailed descriptions of common phenomena that a participant may experience. But for the purposes of working clinically with these substances, the most important takeaway about their effects is that they stem from a general, nonspecific ability to open the floodgates of the mind to a plethora of therapy-relevant content that is normally inaccessible.

VARIETIES OF PSYCHEDELIC COMPOUNDS

Which mind-altering substances warrant the term "psychedelic"? Currently, there is no clear consensus. For the ongoing wave of PAT research, the term psychedelic has been applied to a broad swath of substances with purported therapeutic efficacy, including MDMA and ketamine.

Psychedelic enthusiasts have proposed a variety of ways to classify these substances: by chemical structure (e.g., tryptamines, phenethylamines, ergolines,

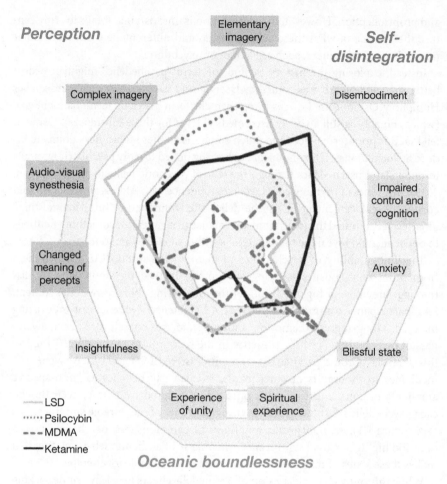

Figure 1.1. Unique Signatures of Psilocybin, LSD, MDMA and Ketamine. Reproduced from Rupp, 2017, with permission.

arylcyclohexylamines, N-methoxybenzyl [NBOMe] derivatives), by psycho-pharmacological mechanism (serotonergics, N-methyl-D-aspartate [NMDA] antagonists), or by source (plant medicine vs. synthetics). Here are a few high-level categories that are most commonly used in discourses about PAT:

Classic psychedelics. This category includes many of the most well-known members of the psychedelic family: LSD, dimethyltryptamine (DMT, the primary active component in ayahuasca, found in many other plants), mescaline (the primary active component in peyote and other cacti), 5-methoxy-dimethyltryptamine (5-MeO-DMT; found in psychedelic toad venom and several plants), and psilocybin (found in numerous species of mushrooms). They have all been used for the purposes of healing, divination, religious ritual, and/or hexing by Indigenous groups worldwide (though predominately in the western hemisphere) for centuries, if not millennia (Akers et al., 2011; Winkelman, 2019), and only became known to Western science during the late 19th and early 20th centuries.

Empathogens. The most well-known substance in this category is 3,4-methlyenedioxymethamphetamine, or MDMA, but it also includes MDA and dozens of other substances. MDMA is the primary expected ingredient in the street drugs Ecstasy and Molly, though these black-market versions notoriously contain many other adulterant substances. MDMA often gets swept up in the term "psychedelic medicine" despite its more accurate characterization as an "empathogen" (Nichols, 1986). Although MDMA was originally synthesized by Bayer Pharmaceuticals over a century ago, it was revived in the 1970s by Alexander Shulgin, who shared it with psychologists for its therapeutic potential. MDMA is a synthetic molecule that leads to dramatic temporary elevations of serotonin levels in the brain, as well as alterations to levels of oxytocin and prolactin, which together facilitate a subjective state of openness, relaxed psychological defenses, and feelings of profound mental acuity. Although the subjective effects of MDMA differ greatly from the classic psychedelics, the therapeutic approaches utilized are remarkably similar (Horton et al., 2021), which is perhaps unsurprising since they were derived in large part from earlier therapeutic work with LSD (Reiff et al., 2020). Some have even argued that MDMA and classic psychedelics may facilitate therapeutic outcomes through similar neural mechanisms (Bird et al., 2021).

NMDA antagonists. Drugs in this category are often called "dissociatives," but this name does not adequately reflect their therapeutic potential. The most widely known drug in this class, ketamine, has been used for decades for anesthesia and analgesic applications. In recent years a cottage industry of ketamine clinics have opened, using ketamine to treat depression, suicidality, and a host of other indications. Janssen, under Johnson & Johnson, developed an esketamine nasal spray (Spravato) that has been approved by the Food and Drug Administration (FDA) for treatment-resistant depression and suicidality. In therapeutic contexts that seek to leverage its subjectivity-altering effects, ketamine can be given in high doses that fit within a PAT paradigm or in lower doses that precipitate subtler alterations that facilitate more traditional therapeutic processes. Instead of acting on the serotonin system in the brain, ketamine works primarily on the glutamate system by way of its affinity for NMDA receptors. Ketamine's status as a psychedelic medicine is complicated by the fact that it is often administered via infusion at relatively low doses over multiple session administrations; this low-dosage strategy avoids inducing psychedelic effects. Although the majority of medical uses of ketamine are not psychedelic, per se, and although low-dose ketamine can be therapeutic, there are some clinics that offer ketamine in high enough doses to bring about a full psychedelic experience that can be well supported within a psychotherapeutic frame.

Applicability of This Book to Other Psychedelic Medicines

Although the approach found in this book was originally developed for CYB003, an analogue of psilocybin, much of it is likely to be helpful for practitioners working with other psychedelic medicines.

Applicability of EMBARK to Classic Psychedelics

The majority of the therapeutic approach outlined in this book is likely to be applicable to long-acting classic psychedelics other than psilocybin, such as LSD, due to the broad similarities in their effects and clinical considerations. However, we still advise obtaining drug-specific training when using novel substances clinically and would recommend a formal adaptation of the EMBARK model for new drugs to account for drug-specific properties. For example, when working with shorter-acting classic psychedelics, such as DMT, the approach may require adaptation, as many of the therapeutic interventions in this book are designed to be used with longer psychedelic windows (e.g., 3–8 hours). The therapeutic approach would have to be adapted to shorter-acting drugs, or those drugs would have to be administered in such a way as to facilitate a longer duration of drug effects (e.g., continual intravenous administration).

Applicability of EMBARK to MDMA-Assisted Therapy

One could also expand the circle of this book's applicability to include MDMA. Despite notable differences in their subjective effects, the therapeutic frameworks applied to MDMA and classic psychedelics are often similar, and researchers have begun to explore the possibility that these substances may be efficacious in treating the same indications. So, while clinicians are again strongly advised to seek substance-specific training before incorporating a psychedelic into their practice, much of *EMBARK Psychedelic Therapy* will serve as a supportive resource for the practice of MDMA-assisted therapy.

Applicability of EMBARK to Ketamine-Assisted Therapy

In the case of ketamine, the applicability of the EMBARK approach in this book is likely to depend on the dosage level. While clinicians who administer ketamine at subpsychedelic doses (e.g., 0.5 mg/kg intravenous [IV] infusion over 40 minutes) will find little value in this book, clinicians who administer moderate to higher doses of ketamine (e.g., 1.0–2.0 mg/kg intramuscular, 100 mg–300 mg sublingual lozenge) will find much to appreciate in the approach found in this book. Despite the substantial differences in psychedelic effects between ketamine and psilocybin, the detailed description in this book for creating a therapeutic framework for psychedelic experiences can be fruitfully applied to ketamine-assisted therapy. Our advice is to consider *EMBARK Psychedelic Therapy* as a secondary source of information on working therapeutically with ketamine, complementing a more ketamine-specific primary training resource.

A SHORT HISTORY OF PAT

For those who deeply believe in the promise of these sacred substances, in
medicine, in education, or in religion, it is a hopeful time.
                                        —Bill Richards, PhD (2015, p. 7)

Psychedelic substances have played a role in the healing lineages of diverse cultures worldwide throughout history, predating written records, as well as in the present day (see "What is Missing from this Story," below). However, it is only within the last 70 years or so that we have seen efforts to integrate psychedelics into Western culture's predominant institution of mental health healing: psychotherapy. Factor in nearly three decades of effective prohibition, and it is hard to escape the conclusion that PAT is still in its infancy or, arguably, early adolescence. Even at the crest of this current wave of resumed research interest, we are very much making the road by walking it.

As psychology and psychedelics began to cross paths, the early encounters primarily consisted of self-experimentation by researchers and academics. The earliest reports date back to 1895, mostly involving peyote or its primary active component, mescaline, which was isolated in 1897 (Rucker et al., 2018). Much of this self-experimentation was conducted by influential psychologists in the field, such as Heinrich Klüver and, famously, William James, who wrote about his nitrous oxide-occasioned mystical experiences in his seminal *The Varieties of Religious Experience* (1902/2003). For many, these substances were seen as potential tools for understanding psychosis and enhancing psychoanalytic treatment.

The Psychotomimetic Paradigm (1920s–1950s)

This early line of thinking was predicated on the idea of using psychedelic experiences to induce "model psychoses." Beginning in the 1920s, researchers who pursued this path dubbed these substances "psychotomimetics," which reflected the belief that they could mimic psychosis. Psychedelics were believed to replicate psychosis, potentially aiding in the understanding of its roots and suggesting novel treatments. They posited that model psychoses could be helpful in giving clinicians firsthand experience with psychosis in order to better empathize with schizophrenic patients (Friesen, 2022). Some even drew upon their experiences to argue for the existence of a not-yet-identified endogenous "psychotomimetic" chemical—a naturally occurring psychedelic molecule—in the brains of those who suffer from psychotic episodes.

These avenues of inquiry gradually petered out by the mid-1950s. One likely reason for this waning enthusiasm was a global diminution of the entire field of psychology's interest in understanding the nature of psychosis (Friesen, 2022). As psychoanalysis lost its influence and more medicalized approaches gained traction, a new paradigm emerged in which psychotic symptoms were to be eliminated by pharmacotherapy rather than understood analytically. In the current research, almost no one (with a few exceptions: Leptourgos et al., 2020; Mahmood et al., 2022) mentions the potential utility of using psychedelics as a phenomenological inroad into psychotic states.

Shift Toward PAT (1950s–1970)

Starting in 1949, the PAT paradigm began to take off, with psychedelics (particularly LSD) being studied in the treatment of a range of disorders, such as depression, anxiety, psychoneuroses, obsessive disorders, alcoholism, existential distress in those with cancer, and symptoms that would now be characterized as posttraumatic stress disorder (PTSD; Byock, 2018; Curtis et al., 2020). This research continued through the early 1960s, with roughly 1,000 papers and books published on the topic and over 40,000 patients treated (Grinspoon & Bakalar, 1981).

To gauge the level of enthusiasm and acceptance for psychedelic research at the time, it is worth noting that psychedelic research received significant funding from the National Institute of Mental Health (NIMH) in the 1950s and 1960s. A 50-year dry spell in federal funding followed. The spell was only broken recently in April 2021, when the NIMH funded Dr. Benjamin Kelmendi's research at Yale University into psilocybin treatment for OCD (Backman, 2022), and in October 2021, when it provided grant funding to Dr. Matthew Johnson's team's research using psilocybin-assisted treatment for smoking cessation (Johns Hopkins Medicine, 2021).

Research reports published in this era often presented resoundingly positive results. However, much of the research conducted during these years does not hold up by today's higher evidentiary standards. Early studies often suffered from critical flaws, such as absent or poorly designed controls, inconsistent application of treatment, lack of blinding, poor data reporting, lack of statistical and power analyses, poor outcome measure selection, and generally poor reporting of outcome data and adverse events (Rucker et al., 2018). Nevertheless, recent rigorous metanalyses of some of these studies (e.g., randomized controlled trials with blinding procedures) have found that there was good cause for excitement, particularly in the psychedelic treatment of depression and alcoholism (Krebs & Johansen, 2012; Rucker et al., 2016).

The Rising Tide of Regulations and Cultural Shifts: The Ebbing of PAT Research (1962–1970)

In 1962, the Kefauver–Harris Amendment to the Food Drug and Cosmetic Act raised the bar on how experimental research with novel drugs was to be conducted in humans (Bonson, 2018). This had two chilling effects on PAT research. The first was that Sandoz, a pharmaceutical company that held the patent for LSD and had previously distributed it freely to interested researchers, became more stringent in its distribution practices with LSD to protect its newly registered status with the FDA. Second, the researchers who continued to have access to psychedelic medicines were divided into two camps. The first bristled at the imposition of standards, such as randomized clinical trials and blinding procedures, that they considered ill-suited to psychedelic research. The other camp attempted to follow these new guidelines to the letter by administering psychedelic medicines as conventional psychiatric drugs, omitting the essential supportive therapeutic context (Oram, 2014), which led to disappointing and frequently null results. The field was at an impasse as to how they could maintain PAT's effectiveness within this new regulatory paradigm. The difficulty in meeting the escalating research standards of the field was one of the hurdles that led to the decline of this wave of PAT research (Dyck, 2005; 2008; Oram, 2014).

Another contributing factor to the cessation of this early wave of PAT research was the seismic shift in cultural attitudes about psychedelic substances. By the early 1960s, they had long since made their way into many corners of the growing countercultural pastiche in the United States and elsewhere. Many outside of these circles had come to associate psychedelics with a brand of dissidence they found threatening. Alarming (and, often, alarmist) media accounts featured stories of people who harmed themselves or others while under the influence of psychedelics. This perception was not entirely unwarranted, given the limited public knowledge about psychedelics, but it is evident in retrospect that a moral panic inspired by irresponsible media reporting played a role in swaying public sentiment.

In 1965, the U.S. Congress passed the Drug Abuse Control Amendments to the Food Drug and Cosmetic Act, which drastically reduced the amount of PAT research going on by limiting it to investigators who received special permissions from the U.S. FDA (Reiff et al., 2020). Under these amendments, PAT research slowed to a trickle. In 1970, President Nixon signed into law the Controlled Substances Act, which introduced a stifling degree of bureaucracy into PAT research that even the most tenacious researchers found impossible to surmount. The War on Drugs was in full swing, and this early era of psychedelic research effectively ended (Bonson, 2018). Two final nails were put in its coffin in 1975 when the NIMH officially ceased funding psychedelic research and when the monstrous CIA mind-control experiments known as MK-ULTRA came to light. These CIA experiments, which used psychedelics in all manner of bone-chilling human rights abuses, became public knowledge, cementing the connection between these substances and wickedness in the public imagination for years to come (Bonson, 2018).

Underground Networks (1970–2006 and Present)

However, while psychedelic therapy had lost its place in legally sanctioned research settings, it still found other places to thrive. An underground network of PAT practitioners arose to carry the torch during the decades of prohibition, which stretched from 1970 to 2006, when PAT clinical trials research reentered academia. During these years, underground trainings took place in which hundreds of therapists learned approaches drawn from the earlier clinical trials and applied them to the treatment of thousands of participants worldwide (Passie, 2018; Sessa & Fischer, 2015; Stolaroff, 2004). These underground communities of practice became incubators in which longstanding PAT protocols were updated. Some of these innovations were found to be helpful enough to incorporate into PAT approaches used in recent clinical trials (Passie, 2018; Söderberg, 2023). Other mutations pushed past the bounds of clinical wisdom and, unchecked by any system of oversight, gave rise to abusive interventions that have done harm to participants (Goldhill, 2020; Passie, 2018).

The Founding of Psychedelic Advocacy and Research Organizations (1986–Present)

Another spark during these dark ages for PAT was the founding of organizations that would advocate and provide funding for a second wave of clinical research. They built organizations, such as the Multidisciplinary Association for Psychedelic Studies (MAPS), the Heffter Institute, the Beckley Foundation, and the Council on Spiritual Practices, without which there may not have been a psychedelic resurgence. They found funders and connected the right people to lay the financial, research, and regulatory groundwork for a resumption of PAT research.

The Resurgence of Psychedelic Research (2006–Present)

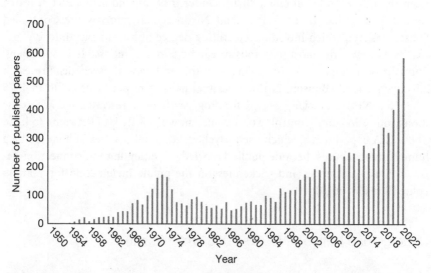

Figure 1.2. Number of Papers About Psychedelic Therapy Published Per Year from 1952 to 2022. *Source*: As reported on PubMed (https://pubmed.ncbi.nlm.nih.gov as of 13 December 2022) by searching for "psychedelic therapies" (Mastinu et al., 2023, with permission)

Today, we can witness the results of these organizations' efforts. Since 2006, the results of dozens of PAT clinical trials have been published in peer-reviewed journals, the vast majority highlighting the therapeutic potential of these substances. Some of the most notable findings include:

- Several studies in which psilocybin-assisted therapy durably reduced depressive symptoms for weeks or often months after the end of treatment (Carhart-Harris et al., 2016; 2018a; 2021; Davis et al., 2021; Goodwin et al., 2022; Sloshower et al., 2023; von Rotz et al., 2022)

- Several studies in which problem drinking behavior associated with alcohol use disorder was reduced by psychotherapy combined with psilocybin (Bogenschutz et al., 2015; 2022) or MDMA (Sessa et al., 2021)
- A study in which participants markedly reduced their tobacco consumption after psilocybin-assisted therapy (Johnson et al., 2014)
- A handful of studies that found PAT with LSD, psilocybin, or MDMA to be effective in reducing anxiety and depression due to a life-threatening illness (Gasser et al., 2014; Grob et al., 2011; Griffiths et al., 2016; Ross et al., 2016; Wolfson et al., 2020)
- A multisite trial with 96 participants that found that MDMA significantly reduced PTSD symptoms (Mitchell et al., 2021)
- A trial that paired MDMA with conjoint therapy and found a similar reduction in PTSD symptoms (Monson et al., 2020)
- Several clinical trials in which ayahuasca was administered to participants in a supportive milieu that found that it reduced their depression (Palhano-Fontes et al., 2019; Sanches et al., 2016)
- One clinical trial in which psilocybin-assisted therapy reduced OCD symptoms in participants for whom other treatments had failed (Moreno et al., 2006)
- A trial in which psilocybin administered along with group therapy was found to be helpful in reducing AIDS-related demoralization (Anderson et al., 2020a)
- An MDMA-assisted therapy trial that found improvements in eating disorder symptoms (Brewerton et al., 2022)
- A trial that found reductions in autistic adults' social anxiety after MDMA-assisted psychotherapy (Danforth et al., 2018)
- Twenty-nine separate studies that, taken together, show strong support for ketamine's ability to acutely treat depressive symptoms, suicidality, and substance use disorders (Walsh et al., 2022)
- Encouraging results from clinical trials and case studies that demonstrate promise for ketamine's ability to treat symptoms of PTSD (Ragnhildstveit et al., 2023)
- A plethora of ongoing clinical trials investigating all of these substances plus others in the treatment of COVID-related burnout, body dysmorphic disorder, anxiety disorders, autism spectrum disorder, and more (Rush et al., 2022)

While these studies point toward new ways of treating mental health conditions, the evidence base substantiating the efficacy of PAT is still in its formative stage. The field has yet to overcome some significant methodological obstacles: difficulties with blinding, small sample sizes, researcher effects, insufficient reporting of detail on associated therapeutic interventions, and inadequate reporting of adverse events (Breeksema et al., 2022a; Brennan et al., 2023; de Laportalière et al., 2023;

Muthukumaraswamy et al., 2021, 2022; van Elk & Fried, 2023). Nevertheless, compared to conventional treatments, these clinical trials often result in large-magnitude effect sizes and strong response and remission rates. The published literature is expanding exponentially, as shown in Figure 1.2. The future of PAT research appears promising.

What Is Missing From This Story?

Before ending this summary of the research that has brought us to the present day, it is important to strike a note of circumspection. So often, the story of PAT research gets told as the triumphant three-act play presented in the previous section—and with good reason. There is much to celebrate and honor in the groundbreaking clinical work and advocacy that has brought us here. But, like any story, it is only part of a larger mosaic of stories that embody the full reality. To make a good-faith contribution to this field, both we—the authors—and you—the readers of this book—must engage critically with it. This will be encouraged throughout *EMBARK Psychedelic Therapy*. Let's consider a few pieces missing from the narrative so far to broaden our lens on the approach detailed throughout the rest of this book.

MARGINALIZATION OF INDIGENOUS PERSPECTIVES AND LINEAGES

The resurgence of Western psychedelic research and practice has led to increasing concerns from many Indigenous Nations regarding cultural appropriation, lack of recognition of the sacred cultural positioning of these medicines, exclusionary practices in research and praxis, and patenting of traditional medicines. Indigenous voices and leadership have been notably absent from the Western psychedelic field currently widely represented by Westerners.

—Yuria Celidwen, PhD, and colleagues (2023, p. 1)

First, this way of telling the story of psychedelics sidelines the contributions of roups that, for centuries, have developed and practiced approaches to healing with these substances that fall outside the bounds of clinical research. Were it not for many Indigenous communities holding these substances sacred for long before European colonialists arrived, Western clinicians and scientists may never have come to know the value of psilocybin, ayahuasca, mescaline, ibogaine, and other plant-based psychedelics. How best to respect these groups' primacy, to ensure that their voices are heard and amplified, and to duly value and reward their dedication to these plant medicines is still a question the field of PAT has not fully answered (Celidwen et al., 2023; George et al., 2020; Leite,

2021; Negrin, 2020). Some have put forth initiatives that would share the profits of this psychedelic revolution in medicine and develop true partnerships with Indigenous groups so that they can contribute to the direction that psychedelics take in Western cultures (Sharma, 2021). Others have argued that there can be no true reciprocity until the historical and ongoing relationships of dominance and exploitation between these groups and Western cultures are addressed in their entirety and redrawn into a new global paradigm (Phelps, 2022). We, as a field and as individual PAT practitioners, need to continue to engage deeply with this often-overlooked part of the story, lest the psychedelic renaissance becomes just another point along a long line of extractive colonial events (Williams et al., 2022).

ETHICAL PRINCIPLES OF TRADITIONAL INDIGENOUS MEDICINE

In response to the marginalization of Indigenous perspectives in psychedelic medicine, a group of Indigenous practitioners, activists, scholars, lawyers, and human rights defenders (Celidwen et al., 2023) came together to develop a set of ethical guidelines and suggested ethical actions for PAT researchers and practitioners. They point to cultural appropriation, lack of recognition of the sacred cultural positioning of these medicines, exclusionary practices in research and praxis, and patenting of traditional medicines. They present eight ethical principles as a way to correct the course we are currently on: reverence, respect, responsibility, relevance, regulation, reparation, restoration, and reconciliation. Their full report is an essential read for PAT practitioners (Celidwen et al., 2023).

WESTERN UNDERGROUND PSYCHEDELIC PRACTICES

Other communities and subcultures within the Western world have also brought psychedelic substances into their own sacred, nonclinical practices (Partridge, 2018). For decades, small groups of psychedelic users have built underground communities around the intentional and reverent consumption of these substances. Some of this community-building has served to strengthen the resolve and the solidarity of collectives that have organized against injustices committed toward themselves and their neighbors (Lovato, 2022). Other groups have drawn on their psychedelic experiences as catalysts evolving into environmentalist groups that have fought to preserve our ecosystems (Greer, 2022). Some groups have used psychedelics to simply connect with other group members in a deeper way as an antidote to the isolation that so many of us feel. These include the LGBTQ+ MDMA rave scene of the 1990s as well as radical queer psilocybin group rituals on Beltane. Like Indigenous communities, these groups have often not had a seat at the table when decisions are being made as to how psychedelics will be integrated into the broader culture (Miceli McMillan & Jordens, 2022), despite having had a formative influence on how psychedelics are used therapeutically and the harm reduction protocols used in clinical settings (Söderberg, 2023). They often worry that advancing a clinical, medicalized approach to psychedelics will benefit only financially gainful uses of psychedelics while leaving them in the legal jeopardy of the underground (Noorani, 2020). Their piece of the story is another to keep in mind as practitioners to remain humble and ensure that our clinical framing leaves room in the world for other thoughtful uses of these remarkably flexible substances (Beiner, 2021).

Systemic Psychedelic Harms Perpetrated Against LGBTQ+, BIPOC, Incarcerated, and Other Oppressed Groups

Another omission from the story is a reckoning with the systemic harms that have been done to members of marginalized or oppressed social groups in PAT research contexts. For instance, leaders in the psychedelic community have been complicit in the systemic oppression of queer people. Throughout the first wave of research (1950s through early 1970s), PAT practitioners used psychedelics in conversion therapy, an unethical and harmful practice (Belser, 2019; Belser & Keating, 2022; Cavnar, 2018). Timothy Leary claimed LSD was a "specific cure for homosexuality" (Belser & Keating, 2022). Ram Dass (formerly Dr. Richard Alpert) published two case reports in which he used conversion therapy to coerce his gay male clients to have sexual relationships with women (Ens, 2022). Psychedelic conversion therapy programs were normative and were documented during the 1950s and 1960s in institutions such as Hollywood Hospital, where Cary Grant was treated (Belser & Keating, 2022). Lesbian and bisexual women in the United Kingdom were treated with LSD to "overcome their sexuality" (Carr & Spandler, 2019). Psychedelic shock therapies of up to 800 micrograms of LSD (eight times a standard dose) were used against teenage gay boys in France (Dubus, 2022). Masters and Houston, authors of the canonical text, *The Varieties of Psychedelic Experience*, even claimed their treatment with mescaline led to the "heterosexualization" of homosexual patients (1966). The profession of psychology has unfortunately used psychoanalytic language and theories to legitimize these harmful practices (Davidson, 2022). Many homophobic and transphobic practices continue to this day in psychedelic retreat centers, churches, clinic forms, and treatment practices. For example, the conventional male–female therapy dyad used in PAT (and still "typically" used in current submissions to the FDA) instantiates the gender binary and marginalizes trans and nonbinary clinicians. The psychedelic community has continued a policy of erasure and has thus far failed to acknowledge its own history of psychedelic conversion therapy and the harms it caused.

Other first-wave researchers conducted studies in incarcerated populations, who were disproportionately People of Color, using coercive treatment incentives such as sentence reductions or the provision of illicit drugs to addicted prisoners

(Strauss et al., 2022). In addition to these unethical recruitment procedures, much of this research was conducted without adequate informed consent or safety provisions. Advocates for culturally inclusive and socially responsible PAT research have highlighted the continuing legacy of racial discrimination in PAT, such as the dramatic underrepresentation of people of color in PAT trial participant pools (Fogg et al., 2021; Herzberg & Butler, 2019; Michaels et al., 2018), which has significant implications for the field's developing ability to serve underserved communities (Smith et al., 2022). When this part of the broader story gets erased from our collective memory, we run the risk of ignoring the continuing impact of historical oppressions on our practices, making PAT less inclusive and accessible than most of us would like it to be (Thrul & Garcia-Romeu, 2021).

HARMFUL BOUNDARY TRANSGRESSIONS IN PAT

Finally, the story of PAT remains incomplete without a discussion of the field's history of harmful boundary transgressions. Under the influence of a psychedelic, participants become uniquely vulnerable, suggestible, and incapable of advocating for themselves. Tragically, there has been a steady stream of PAT practitioners in the underground and in research settings (Goldhill, 2020; Passie, 2018) alike who have taken this opportunity to gratify themselves—sexually or otherwise—at the expense of those under their care.

Some advocates in the field express deep concern that this vulnerable state, inherent to the psychedelic experience, will continue to pose a risk as PAT expands. Responses to this concern are being developed by a number of actors in the field. Still, the impact of their efforts remains to be seen, and relational harm reduction will require a concerted and collective effort. It remains incumbent upon us as PAT practitioners to attend to this legacy in our own work and prepare ourselves for the unique ethical challenges of working with nonordinary states of consciousness.

Where Are We in the Story?

It is reasonable to suggest that, as of this writing, the story of PAT is entering its most exciting chapter. Recent research has given us a glimpse of the tremendous potential it may hold to improve the well-being of millions. At the same time, the field has also grown irreversibly aware of the critical questions and potential pitfalls it has ahead of it. Psychedelic therapy has the opportunity to become a major force for beneficence, as long as it can conjure up a fitting answer to the questions and challenges it faces. The EMBARK model was put forth in this spirit.

Chapter 2 will discuss how EMBARK's clinical domains and ethical care cornerstones reflect this commitment. But first, this chapter will conclude with an orientation to some of the fundamental, universal components of PAT.

COMMON ELEMENTS OF PAT

Psilocybin can offer a means to reconnect to our true nature—our authentic self—and thereby help us find meaning in our lives.

—Mary Cosimano, LMSW

Three-Phase Treatment Structure

In all clinical trials so far, psychedelic medicines have been administered within a tripartite treatment structure that consists of preparation sessions, medicine sessions, and integration sessions. We draw from recent reviews (Brennan & Belser, 2022; Brennan et al., 2023; Horton et al., 2021) to summarize the common elements of each phase.

PREPARATION SESSIONS: COMMON ELEMENTS

In preparation sessions, therapists work toward a series of aims intended to prepare a participant to receive benefit from their upcoming medicine session. This has generally included several key components: (a) building rapport and learning about the participant's lived experience, (b) providing psychoeducation about treatment and the potential effects of the psychedelic medicine to be administered, addressing any fears, questions, or concerns, (c) helping the participant learn to attend to their internal experience, (d) encouraging an attitude of approaching challenging psychological content that may arise, (e) ensuring that the participant has a sense of how to regulate themselves in moments of distress via breathing or other self-regulation techniques, (f) defining the participant's intentions for treatment, (g) creating agreements around the use of therapist–participant touch during session, and (h) continually screening for any conditions that would contraindicate further treatment. Often, therapists give the participant suggestions for at-home preparation, such as developing a mindfulness practice or continuing their psychoeducation via an app (e.g., Goodwin et al., 2022).

The length, quantity, timing, and content of preparation sessions have varied across research groups, though each preparation phase has generally consisted of 1–4 sessions that are 60–90 minutes in length and may occur at an approximately weekly frequency before and after medicine sessions. In the first wave of PAT research and in underground contexts, practitioners often incorporate more preparation sessions. Typically, a "sandwich schedule" is used, in which the last preparation and first integration sessions are scheduled to occur on the days immediately before and after the medicine session for proximal.

MEDICINE SESSIONS: COMMON ELEMENTS

During a medicine session, sometimes called a medication session, a dosing session, or a study drug administration session, a participant is supported as they undergo an inner-directed experience of the psychedelic medicine. Generally, the therapist's role is to foster a context of safety, noninterference, and as-needed support that facilitates this process. The participant is invited in this session to engage openly with any content that arises for them in a manner characterized by acceptance and receptivity, to the extent that is available to them.

During a medicine session, therapists tend to be significantly less directive than they were in preparation sessions, instead favoring a stance of responsiveness to participant needs. A medicine session may begin with a check-in with the participant and/or any exercises that may prepare them for the day, such as a relaxation practice or a brief refresher course on the self-regulation skills they practiced during the preparation phase. These sessions last as long as the effects of the medicine, plus the amount of time before it takes effect and the time it takes the participant to become settled at the end. Depending on the substance being used, a session may take anywhere between 1 and 12 hours. For psilocybin, session length is ordinarily 6–7 hours, and for MDMA, it is typically 5–6 hours, although the medicine session length is often 8 hours in clinical trials to account for booster doses and to ensure participant safety before concluding the session. Ketamine-assisted therapy sessions are typically 2.5–4 hours.

In this book, we use the term "medicine sessions" to refer to these sessions. For researchers, given that placebo or another drug may be administered, they may choose to refer to them as "experimental sessions" or "study drug administration sessions" instead. Many researchers refer to it as a "dosing session," but we tend to avoid this nomenclature due to its implicit suggestion that the participant is passively "getting dosed," which may discount their agency.

INTEGRATION SESSIONS: COMMON ELEMENTS

Integration sessions, sometimes called debriefing sessions, offer the participant a space to describe their psychedelic experience, reflect, make meaning, and plan posttreatment practices that support ongoing benefit. Generally, the integration phase consists of 1–4 sessions that are 60–90 minutes in length. Therapists may also incorporate outside interventions from other modalities pertinent to the participant's diagnosis in order to bring added benefit. Ensuring participant stability and safety is crucial during this phase, with careful monitoring for any destabilization and addressing of feelings of neglect or abandonment. Appropriate linkages to continued care and peer support networks may be supportive for a participant.

MULTIPLE-DOSE TREATMENT DESIGNS

Treatment designs can vary in terms of how many iterations of each phase are included. The simplest base case consists of a preparation phase, a medicine session, and then an integration phase. Adding a second medicine session or third medicine session introduces additional integration phases (e.g., see Figure 1.3). In this design, integration sessions between medicine sessions may include hybrid elements of preparation. If multiple medicine sessions are included, the amount of time to schedule before readministering the psychedelic medicine is another important consideration. Some clinical trials have waited three to five weeks, while

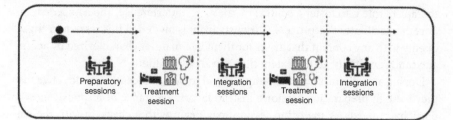

Figure 1.3. Example of a Treatment Design With Two Medicine Sessions.

others in nonresearch contexts have recommended longer. Considerations for designing a treatment that fits the needs of each participant will be discussed in Chapter 4.

Therapist Dyads

> *They were—they were so exceptional in their care of me through the therapy sessions, and we developed a very close bond. I felt very comfortable with them. I felt I was in very good hands, and I wanted to share the things that were pertinent to our communal intent that we had spoken to.*
> —Mike (Belser et al., 2017; Swift et al., 2017)

To date, participants in PAT trials have typically been attended to by a therapist dyad. Both therapists have typically been present for all phases of treatment, though some research groups have begun to hold preparation sessions with only one therapist, while both are present during the remainder of treatment (e.g., Goodwin et al., 2022).

The practice of having therapist dyads was pioneered by early PAT researchers Betty Eisner and Sydney Cohen (1958) and was originally thought to improve treatment outcomes by potentiating the process, possibly by providing a broader range of opportunities for relational phenomena such as transference. The dyad approach was incorporated by the current wave of PAT research as a protective factor against therapist sexual abuse of participants (Harlow, 2013, quoted in Passie, 2018; see Belser & Keating, 2022 for a discussion of this problematic rationale). The dyad was subsequently found to have added benefits, including more safety in emergencies, enabling one therapist to take a break during long sessions, and an enhanced ability to cope with challenging transference (Passie, 2018). The insistence on a male–female therapist dyad found in PAT research has been criticized as upholding a gender binary and inherently excluding people who do not identify as cisgender male or female (Belser & Keating, 2022).

However, it is worth noting that underground PAT practitioners typically work as individuals, and there are ongoing conversations in the field as to whether a two-therapist dyad model will be financially feasible. The practice of having a cotherapist may come to be seen as less essential as time goes on.

Set and Setting

I had expectations that it was going to be wild and interesting and kind of fun and maybe a bit scary, but I was very confident in my guides. That I felt well prepared and really confident that whatever transpired, whatever happened, that I was fine, I would be safe and well taken care of.
— Presbyterian Minister (Swift et al., 2023)

Given the "mind manifesting" and "amplifying" aspects of psychedelic experiences, all PAT approaches center the concept of "set and setting."

"Set" refers to the mindset with which a participant arrives that will implicitly frame their experience with the psychedelic medicine. It consists of acute, treatment-related factors, such as their hopes, anxieties, fears, expectations, fantasies, attitudes, and beliefs about the medicine, the treatment, therapy in general, and their ability to receive its benefits. It also includes more enduring characteristics of the participant, such as their personality, trauma history, temperament, interpersonal style, and so on.

"Setting" refers to elements of the environment in which the medicine session takes place. It includes physical elements, such as decor, lighting, cleanliness, music, scents, and any evidence of care or lack of care put into these elements. Many aspects of the therapist—their actions, words, quality, or presence—are part of the setting and can influence set, so attentiveness to both is crucial.

In PAT, participants experiencing psychedelic effects are uniquely sensitive to these extra-pharmacological factors to an extent without precedent. Unlike traditional pharmacotherapy, the therapeutic outcomes are highly influenced by the interplay between the participant's mindset and the therapeutic environment. Therefore, cultivating an optimal set and setting is an essential component of a well-supported PAT treatment.

The Importance of Providing a Therapeutic Container

It's not just the psilocybin sessions [but] it's that human connection, and the support that comes with that human connection, that ultimately leads to success at the end of the day.
— Participant (Noorani et al., 2018)

Within the field of psychedelic medicine, an ongoing debate has arisen. It centers around how much nondrug therapeutic support is necessary. Do psychedelics need to be administered with robust therapeutic support, or is a basic safety protocol sufficient to ensure participant safety, maximize clinical efficacy, and extend the durability of treatment benefits?

Systemic pressures to make PAT more affordable to insurance payors and participants paying out-of-pocket have led some actors in the field to experiment with reducing or eliminating the nondrug therapeutic component of PAT

(Brennan et al., 2023). This fits well within the logic of the existing medical system and conventional pharmacotherapies. Psychedelic treatments are relatively expensive compared to genericized selective serotonin reuptake inhibitors (SSRIs), the current first-line treatment standard, raising the question of whether paying for the therapy associated with PAT is worth it. In pharmacoeconomic modeling, payors may determine that paying the premium for psychedelic therapy is only warranted if the effect sizes and durability continue to prove substantially better than conventional treatments. In other words, psychedelics may have to demonstrate not just noninferiority to existing treatments, but substantial superiority. Unfortunately, there is reason to believe that a continued shift toward minimal therapeutic framing may ultimately undermine the strong efficacy psychedelic medicines have shown in clinical trials to date.

A strong consensus among leading experts from both the first wave and the present wave of PAT research has emerged that psychedelic medicines are most beneficially administered within a context of supportive therapeutic care (Carhart-Harris et al., 2018c; Carhart-Harris & Nutt, 2017; Eisner, 1964; Fischer, 2015; Garcia-Romeu & Richards, 2018; Greer & Tolbert, 1998; Griffiths et al., 2011; Grinspoon & Doblin, 2001; Grof, 1980; Gukasyan & Nayak, 2022; Guss, 2022; Johnson et al., 2008; Leary et al., 1963; Stolaroff, 2004; Thal et al., 2021; Watts, 2022). As such, nearly all psychedelic clinical trials in the current wave of research have included some form of psychological support during medicine sessions and various forms of talk therapy during preparation and integration sessions (Horton et al., 2021).

While nobody has yet to conduct the set of research studies that would be required to definitively generate evidence for the importance of therapeutic support, here is a rationale for it based on the evidence we currently have:

- Therapeutic alliance has been found to impact treatment outcomes (Murphy et al., 2022).
  - In a clinical trial that used psilocybin to treat moderate to severe depression, a strong therapeutic alliance predicted greater presession rapport, greater emotional breakthrough during medicine sessions, and greater reductions in depressive symptoms at six weeks.
  - Emotional breakthrough during the first psilocybin session also predicted increased therapeutic alliance leading into the second session.
  - This stronger alliance predicted a reduction in depressive symptoms at six weeks posttreatment, suggesting that alliance is a determinant of durability.
- High-support conditions have been found to lead to better outcomes than standard support conditions (Griffiths et al., 2018).
  - A study of healthy participants compared a "high-support" versus a "standard-support" condition, both with a high dose of psilocybin.
  - The high-support group, which received 35 hours of support over 6 months, demonstrated significantly higher scores on measures of

altruistic/positive social effects, positive behavior changes, spirituality, engagement in reflective practices, and enduring personal significance of psilocybin experiences compared to the standard-support groups, which only got 7 hours of support.
- These results indicate that the amount of nondrug support provided alongside psilocybin administration can influence positive outcomes associated with psilocybin.
- A historical comparison of four comparable 1960s psychedelic studies with and without therapeutic support found that greater support predicted better outcomes.
  - Oram (2014) compared clinical trials investigating LSD treatments for alcoholism funded by the National Institute of Mental Health in the 1960s.
  - Studies with minimal or no therapeutic support generated null results: only limited and transient effects of LSD on alcoholism (Ditman et al., 1969; Hollister et al., 1969).
  - In contrast, the only study that included robust therapeutic support (e.g., 20 hours of preparation) demonstrated significant improvements in problem drinking behavior at 6 months compared to the control group (Kurland et al., 1971).
- Other findings in support of the impact of relational elements in psychedelic treatment have been reported.
  - A naturalistic study found that relational components of participant experiences in psychedelic retreats, such as preceremony rapport, perceived emotional support, and instances of self-disclosure, contributed to feelings of togetherness and shared humanity (communitas) during ceremonies and retreats. These experiences of communitas in turn predicted greater psychological well-being and social connectedness at four weeks postretreat (Kettner et al., 2021).
  - Another study found that psychedelic retreat-goers' evaluations of the retreat setting, which includes the perceived quality of their relationship to others present during psychedelic experiences, predicted higher well-being scores two weeks after the experience (Haijen et al., 2018).
- Clinical trial participants have also made their preference for more therapeutic support known as well. Several qualitative studies of participant experiences have found that the vast majority report that the therapeutic care and support they received from their therapists was a crucial element in the success of their treatment (Lafrance et al., 2017; Noorani et al., 2018; Watts et al., 2017).
- The authors of a recent review of the neuroscientific research on psychedelic treatment reported that psychedelics have the ability to leave the brain in a "neuroplastic" state of facilitated social and emotional learning for days or weeks after treatment, suggesting that postmedicine

integration sessions can leverage a critical learning window (Calder & Hasler, 2022). They state:

> *Therapeutic interventions combined with [SSRI] antidepressants, which also modestly promote neuroplasticity, have been shown to be more effective than either intervention alone, and the same is likely true of psychedelics. Enhanced neuroplasticity, coupled with a psychedelic experience in a safe setting and accompanying therapy, could ultimately generate a therapeutic effect that is more than the sum of its parts. (p. 5)*

- Appropriate therapeutic support may also enhance participant safety.
  - Breeksema and colleagues (2022) recently reviewed the adverse events that have arisen in modern PAT trials, such as suicidality, self-harm, and exacerbation of symptoms. They concluded that "treatment designs that reduce or minimize positive contextual components (e.g., time spent preparing participants, number of therapists, strength of the therapeutic relationship, time spent providing aftercare and integration) may increase the incidence of adverse events" (p. 14).

Overall, this research underscores the crucial role of therapy as a fundamental component of psychedelic treatment, supporting the rationale for its inclusion to maximize clinical efficacy, durability of benefits, and participant safety.

Psychedelic Therapy Versus Psychedelic Support

Another debate around the elements of nondrug therapeutic support in PAT centers on what to call it. In this book, we use "psychedelic-assisted therapy (PAT)" and "psychedelic therapy" interchangeably. Some approaches favor the language of "psychedelic-assisted psychotherapy (PAP)"—a term reserved for therapy administered by a licensed psychotherapist—and others use the phrase "psychological support" provided by facilitators and practitioners, often in collaboration with a licensed psychotherapist (as discussed in Chapter 4: "Therapeutic Credentials and Skills"). It is important to note that EMBARK can be applied in each of these contexts, depending on the protocol and the practitioner using it.

An additional note on nomenclature: we refer to the individuals undergoing treatment as "participants," although other providers might use the term "client" or "patient."

Introduction to the EMBARK Approach

> *If psychedelics are ever to be integrated into modern clinical medicine, the usage protocols are as important as the medicines themselves. [The] EMBARK program, which incorporates a multi-dimensional approach to therapies that enable them to be tailored to a variety of patient needs . . . is setting high standards for the future of psychedelic therapy.*
> —Dennis J. McKenna, PhD

This chapter provides a thorough introduction to the EMBARK model. It begins by laying out the rationale for the model's creation and describing the key elements of its structure (the 6 + 4: six clinical domains and four care cornerstones). It concludes with an illustration of how these elements come together to form a unified approach to psychedelic treatment. Our intent is that the reader come away with a clear understanding of both the spirit of EMBARK and what it looks like to conduct psychedelic therapy within its approach.

EMBARK'S RATIONALE

An Assessment of Prior Psychedelic Therapy Models

To begin the process of developing EMBARK, we assessed the strengths and shortcomings of existing PAT models. We canvassed the published literature and assessed a range of combination therapies that used MDMA or classic psychedelics and had been demonstrated to be safe and efficacious in initial clinical trials (see Table 2.1 for an up-to-date version of the list we used). Many of them were very thoughtful, elegant models that provided rich insight into how to support participants and that we gratefully wove into what we were developing.

EMBARK Psychedelic Therapy for Depression. Bill Brennan and Alex Belser, Oxford University Press.
© Oxford University Press 2024. DOI: 10.1093/9780197762622.003.0003

Table 2.1. CLINICAL TRIALS OF PSYCHEDELIC MEDICINES
FOR PSYCHIATRIC INDICATIONS

Pub. year	First author	Drug	Indication
2006	Moreno	Psilocybin	Obsessive-compulsive disorder
2008	Bouso	MDMA	Posttraumatic stress disorder
2011	Grob	Psilocybin	Anxiety in context of advanced-stage cancer
2011	Mithoefer	MDMA	Posttraumatic stress disorder
2013	Oehen	MDMA	Posttraumatic stress disorder
2014	Gasser	LSD	Anxiety due to life-threatening illness
2014	Johnson	Psilocybin	Tobacco addiction
2015	Bogenschutz	Psilocybin	Alcohol use disorder
2016	Carhart-Harris	Psilocybin	Treatment-resistant depression
2016	Griffiths	Psilocybin	Psychiatric diagnoses with anxiety or mood symptoms in context of life-threatening cancer
2016	Ross	Psilocybin	Anxiety disorders in context of life-threatening cancer
2016	Sanches	Ayahuasca	MDD
2018	Danforth	MDMA	Social anxiety in the context of autism
2018	Mithoefer	MDMA	Posttraumatic stress disorder
2018	Ot'alora	MDMA	Posttraumatic stress disorder
2019	Palhano-Fontes	Ayahuasca	Treatment-resistant depression
2020a	Anderson	Psilocybin	AIDS-related demoralization
2020	Monson	MDMA	Posttraumatic stress disorder
2020	Wolfson	MDMA	Anxiety due to life-threatening illness
2021	Carhart-Harris	Psilocybin	MDD
2021	Davis	Psilocybin	MDD
2021	Dos Santos	Ayahuasca	Social anxiety disorder
2020	Jardim	MDMA	Posttraumatic stress disorder
2021	Mitchell	MDMA	Posttraumatic stress disorder
2021	Sessa	MDMA	Alcohol use disorder
2022	Bogenschutz	Psilocybin	Alcohol use disorder
2022	D'Souza	DMT	MDD
2022	Goodwin	Psilocybin	Treatment-resistant depression
2023	Goodwin	Psilocybin	Treatment-resistant depression
2023	Holze	LSD	Anxiety disorders, or significant anxiety in context of life-threatening illness
2023	Shnayder	Psilocybin	MDD in context of cancer
2023	Schneier	Psilocybin	SSRI-resistant body dysmorphic disorder
2023	Sloshower	Psilocybin	MDD
2022	von Rotz	Psilocybin	MDD

NOTE: Adapted from Brennan et al., 2023.

Still, we found that each of them overlooked one or more key aspects of psychedelic treatment, which could lead them to underprepare the therapists trained in these approaches. This section will present a brief description of these missing elements before moving into a discussion of how EMBARK was designed to fill in the gaps.

LACK OF ATTENTIVENESS TO THE BODY

In psychedelic clinical trials, many participants have indicated that shifts in their embodied experience were a critical feature in how therapeutic benefit arose for them (Belser et al., 2017; Bogenschutz et al., 2018; Watts et al., 2017). Some reported enhanced interoceptive awareness, somatic synesthetic experiences, or alterations to their sense of self as embodied beings (Belser et al., 2017). Others located undesirable emotions (e.g., grief, shame, resentment) or physical illness (e.g., cancer, sequelae of problem drinking) in specific places in their bodies and sometimes reported subsequent "purgative," "purifying" (Watts et al., 2017, p. 550), or "washing" (Belser et al., 2017, p. 17) experiences that they felt led to improvements in these conditions. Many describe a new, healthier relationship with the body.

In our review, we found that many of the models (with some exceptions, e.g., Mithoefer et al., 2017) neglected the importance of the body in psychedelic healing. Instead, they mirrored many psychotherapies in their focus on therapeutic changes that unfold at the level of the brain or mind. This may be an inappropriate way to frame the actions of psychedelic medicines, given that many PAT trial participants report that their experiences involve the body.

Despite a trend toward embodiment as a broad interpretative framework in the social and behavioral sciences (Csordas & Hardwood, 1994; Gibbs, 2005; Niedenthal et al., 2005), many earlier PAT approaches were missing an embodied dimension in their frameworks for understanding treatment benefit. They have tended to overlook the body as a site of wisdom and healing, even when their participants did not.

LACK OF FOCUS ON THE THERAPIST–PARTICIPANT RELATIONSHIP

In psychedelic clinical trials, participants have reported that the therapeutic alliance was an important determinant of their improvement (see "The Importance of Providing a Therapeutic Container" in Chapter 1). In our review of prior approaches, we found that many therapies did not sufficiently attend to the relational aspects of psychedelic work. Namely, they did not give adequate attention to the healing potential of the therapist–participant relationship in their notions of how healing unfolds in PAT.

This is a loss because, as noted by the creators of one of the models that served as an exception (Mithoefer et al., 2017), the unique relationship dynamics that arise in a PAT medicine session may offer unparalleled opportunities for relational repatterning: reconfiguring deeply entrenched maladaptive ways of relating to others that may contribute to the participant's presenting symptoms. To obtain such benefits requires more than the basic instructions found in many models that focus on how to build rapport and provide a basic level of safety. It would require thoughtful, well-developed clinical guidelines on how to work with the therapist–participant relationship as a fundamental part of the healing process.

LACK OF A THERAPEUTIC FRAMEWORK FOR RELIGIOUS, SPIRITUAL, AND MYSTICAL EXPERIENCES

Despite the widespread association between religious, spiritual, and mystical experiences (RSMEs) and PAT recognized by researchers and laypeople alike, prior PAT models generally offered limited guidance to therapists on how to help a participant prepare for or integrate such experiences. This is a worrisome blind spot, considering that between 66 and 86% of trial participants have reported that their medicine session experiences were among the most spiritually meaningful in their lives (Hartogsohn, 2018), with many reporting that elements of RSME were integral to their healing process. We observed that most prior models focused their attention elsewhere, with only a handful of them offering a therapeutic framework for engaging with spiritual or mystical content.

INSUFFICIENT FOCUS ON ETHICS

A long line of experts has held that PAT is home to a unique set of ethical challenges (Anderson et al., 2020b; Brennan et al., 2021; Devenot et al., 2022a; Harlow, 2013, as cited in Passie, 2018, p. 12; Northrup, 2019; Taylor, 2017). Therapists who enter the field will likely encounter ethical situations that they have never encountered before in their traditional clinical practice. They will work with participants in dramatically heightened states of vulnerability, suggestibility, and impaired autonomy. It is unacceptable to expect that a therapist's prior conventional training in clinical ethics will prepare them adequately for navigating these new challenges. There is an increased risk of iatrogenic harm that must be attended to.

We also felt that it is insufficient to frame ethics in a way that is ancillary to a model of clinical work. Because of the heightened stakes in PAT, ethics need to be woven into every aspect of treatment, and PAT models should reflect that. For the most part, we did not find this when we surveyed the field. Prior PAT models typically delimited ethics as a list of specific proscribed behaviors or a single standalone module in their associated training program or deferred to standard professional codes of ethics.

In addition, the discourses on ethics have tended to focus solely on the prevention of relational boundary transgressions (e.g., therapist sexual abuse, other harmful forms of relationships). As crucial as this is, we believe it is only a fraction of the broader ethical landscape. The therapeutic experiences elicited by psychedelic medicines engage the cultural, societal, and structural dimensions of healing and well-being. As such, we felt that the ethical foundation of a PAT model should be comprehensive enough to provide a space for practitioners to attend to these factors as well. In sum, we concluded from our assessment that existing approaches to PAT had yet to give ethical considerations their full due, in terms of both the depth and the breadth of analysis required to do so.

LIMITED CONCEPTUALIZATION OF THE ROLE OF THE THERAPIST

We also found that some prior PAT models conceived of the role of the therapist or facilitator as providing only basic support and safety to the participant. We felt that this limited sense of the therapist's role was not reflective of the full reality of what therapists are called upon to do in medicine sessions to ensure treatment efficacy. Our experience has convinced us that, even if a PAT model conceives of therapists as only playing a supportive role, they will still face a range of challenging clinical situations that call for a skillful clinical response. We were concerned that these models' more limited perspective would underprepare therapists to respond safely and supportively to these situations.

LACK OF GUIDANCE ON HOW TO INCORPORATE THE THERAPIST'S PRIOR SKILLS AND INTERVENTIONS

Furthermore, the lack of therapist guidance provided by these "basic support" models may also compel therapists to respond to the participant by using their own interventions and ideas about what is appropriate in psychedelic therapy. While we appreciate the latitude this could give them to draw from their experience and clinical wisdom, we worried (as have others; Johnson, 2020) that doing so in an ungoverned way may at times lead to the introduction of inappropriate, or even harmful, interventions. After all, what works in a traditional therapy context may not always be appropriate in a psychedelic therapy context. This lack of scaffolding could also pose a problem for research standardization in clinical trials, as it leaves the therapeutic approach largely undefined (McNamee et al., 2023).

LIMITED CONCEPTUALIZATION OF CHANGE MECHANISMS

Understanding the "how" of psychedelic therapy efficacy is crucial: how exactly does psychedelic therapy "work?" In our review, we noticed that models providing little guidance on therapist interventions also tended to be vague about mechanisms of change. In other words, they often did not explain how a medicine session experience could result in a participant becoming less depressed, essentially treating the process as a "black box" (Belser, 2018).

While this openness to interpretation could potentially empower participants to draw their own conclusions about what was helpful about their treatment, we were concerned that it could often lead to participants feeling undersupported by their therapists when seeking help to understand their treatment experiences. These models could leave therapists without a theoretical basis to support a participant in determining what would be helpful to take away from their treatment. Consider a scenario where a participant's medicine session triggers new, confusing physical feelings. They might be paired with a therapist who, without an interpretive framework, is unable to help them reframe this disconcerting experience into something that could be seen as expected and perhaps beneficial.

CHALLENGES ASSOCIATED WITH INCORPORATING NONPSYCHEDELIC EBTs

In recent years, some PAT researchers have responded to these last three critiques by looking to the existing psychotherapy literature and creating models that incorporate a nonpsychedelic EBT (e.g., cognitive-behavioral therapy (CBT), acceptance and commitment therapy (ACT), motivational interviewing) as a framework for developing a preset roster of interventions and a unified theory of therapeutic change. At first glance, these models provide compelling responses to concerns about other models' limited conceptualization of the therapist's role, lack of guidance on interventions, and limited conceptualization of change mechanisms (Guss et al., 2020). However, our assessment found that these models, in their adoption of a single, preexisting EBT with no prior relationship to psychedelic medicines, raised new concerns.

Overdetermination of change mechanisms. We believe any good psychedelic therapy should be able to accommodate the varieties of psychedelic experience. As noted in Chapter 1, psychedelics produce remarkably variable experiences: participants have reported experiences that are spiritual, existential, emotional, relational, cognitive, visual, or embodied (Belser et al., 2017; Malone et al., 2018; Masters & Houston, 1966; Miceli McMillen & Jordens, 2022; Nielson et al., 2018; Watts et al., 2017). The benefits that they have drawn from treatment have resulted from experiences within each of these domains.

There are many potential clinical trajectories that could arise from this broad range of experiences: one depressed participant may have a mystical experience that alleviates their sense of meaninglessness; another might feel a sense of social connectedness that lifts the spell of their isolation; another depressed participant may have an experience that shifts their understanding of their rigid identity; and yet another may reconnect with their body in a way that joyfully rekindles a lost interest in enjoyment in life. Since pre-existing EBTs were not created for PAT and were imported from outside the field, they are more likely to fail to attend to the variety of ways in which benefits arise in PAT treatment (Bathje et al., 2022).

In PAT, no single nonpsychedelic EBT can accommodate the diverse range of experiences. Adopting an EBT's theory of change narrows the understanding of PAT and limits its potential benefits for participants and for therapists. Incorporating a single EBT restricts how participants may interpret their suffering, identity, and hopes. For example, a depressed participant undergoing PAT treatment based in an ACT approach may feel pressured to shift the focus of their integration sessions away from the relational or spiritual dimensions of their medicine session experience, which may be most meaningful for them, in favor of exploring its impact on aspects of psychological flexibility.

If a therapist attempts to fit a participant's experience into an EBT's predetermined framing, this may also create friction between them and the participant, which could degrade the therapeutic alliance and negatively impact treatment. The participant may even feel disempowered, in that their right to autonomy of meaning-making was taken away from them, which may contribute to feelings of shame and/or give rise to a therapist–participant dynamic that exacerbates existing relational trauma.

Exclusion of therapist's prior skills and interventions. Therapists working within PAT models that incorporate a single EBT will have to learn how to work within the language and toolbox of the chosen EBT. For those who are not familiar with this approach, this will require them to set aside their favored clinical background and work with an unfamiliar approach. This will present various challenges.

To begin, it will require them to undergo additional training. After that, they will still likely take a while to gain comfort and familiarity working in this new approach. As they attempt to "stick with the script" of the new EBT, the therapists will likely not be doing their best clinical work for some time, which poses a significant threat to treatment efficacy in time-limited clinical trial settings. Their discomfort with the newly acquired approach might also be registered by participants in a way that undermines their confidence in the treatment and degrades the therapeutic alliance. Additionally, if the therapists revert to their preferred ways of working to avoid these challenges, they will do so at the expense of treatment fidelity—they will no longer be working as the model tells them to.

Questions of efficacy. PAT models that adopt existing EBT frameworks and interventions have been suggested to enhance efficacy in PAT (Sloshower et al., 2020). Some leaders in the field have even argued that among competing therapeutic approaches, CBT-based psychedelic therapies should be the "default" as they "have the strongest rationale" and "provide the best starting point in terms of safety and efficacy," in part because they are supported by evidence from nonpsychedelic studies (Yaden et al., 2022, p. 1).

We agree with our colleagues that when selecting a therapy approach, it is important to work from evidence with a coherent rationale. However, we note that in the field of psychedelic research, nobody has yet compared therapeutic frameworks, conducted dismantling studies, or piloted head-to-head comparisons between CBT-based psychedelic therapies and other competing approaches such as ACT, MDMA-assisted therapy (MDMA-AT), or EMBARK, for example. Without these data, when surveying the psychotherapy options, we caution that it may be too soon to name any particular approach as the gold standard (Ozcubukcu, 2022). It remains to be seen whether existing EBTs' claims to efficacy will translate to a psychedelic context or whether the EBT is the determinant of treatment benefit. Since most EBTs have not yet have been rigorously assessed in psychedelic contexts, there remain problems of generalizability, adaption, validation, and replication. Any assertion of added efficacy based on prior evidence should thus be considered carefully.

EMBARK'S INNOVATIONS

A Broad, Multifactorial Lens on Therapeutic Processes and Outcomes

In creating EMBARK, we sought to learn from prior models, senior teachers in the field, and leading evidence to support what participants were telling us about what was happening for them. We also sought to avoid the shortcomings of prior models, including the agnosticism of basic support models as well as the constrictive

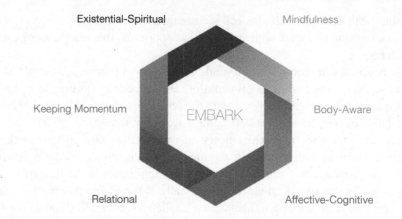

Figure 2.1. EMBARK's Six Clinical Domains

overdetermination of EBT-inclusive models. The EMBARK approach takes as its starting point the variety of experiences engendered by psychedelic medicines. The model prepares therapists to support each person uniquely in a participant-centered approach across the full spectrum of possible clinical trajectories.

The word *EMBARK* is an acronym of the six clinical domains:

1. Existential–Spiritual
2. Mindfulness
3. Body-Aware
4. Affective–Cognitive
5. Relational
6. Keeping Momentum

Figure 2.1 provides a visual schema of the six domains. Each of these domains represents a parallel avenue by which benefit may arise and anticipates events that commonly arise in PAT sessions. For each domain, the EMBARK approach provides indication-specific mechanisms of change, specific actions that a therapist can take in support of these mechanisms throughout all three phases of treatment, and suggestions for how these events may drive related integration goals.

An Approach for the Whole Person

For most people, one or two of the six domains will emerge over the course of treatment as clinically relevant to their experience. The flexibility of the model is intended to support individuals in their journey of self-discovery and growth across all dimensions of their being. In its integration of existential, spiritual, mindful, somatic, affective, cognitive, relational, and relapse-prevention elements, EMBARK is an approach for the whole person.

The nature of these six clinical domains and how they come together as a unified whole will be discussed later in this chapter. For now, the most important thing to understand is that they represent EMBARK's commitment to the idea that the potential benefits of PAT are multiple—that there are "many roads" and not "one way." We believe that a structured approach to working with this multiplicity supports optimal treatment benefit.

Structured Curation of Elements From Several Evidence-Based Therapies

EMBARK's modular structure allows for the curated incorporation of helpful elements from several EBTs without becoming overly reliant on one. For example, the EMBARK approach to depression incorporates mechanisms of change and suggested interventions from a variety of EBTs that are used to treat depression: emotion-focused therapy, ACT, CBT for depression, short-term dynamic psychotherapy, and so on. These depression-alleviating mechanisms are combined with our understanding of how PAT works to create a range of domain-specific mechanisms of change within each EMBARK domain. These domain-specific mechanisms are then thoughtfully woven together into a unified treatment approach that retains the model's plural, heterogenous lens on how treatment benefits may arise. In other words, it draws from existing EBTs without becoming wedded to a single theory of change.

An Invitation for Therapists to Use Their Prior Skills in a Structured Way

We acknowledge that experienced psychotherapists arrive already possessing deep clinical skills, a host of practiced techniques, and years of experience in the consulting room. EMBARK's six-domain structure and its "plug and play" relationship with EBTs encourages therapists to utilize their preexisting skill sets in a way that is flexible yet sufficiently structured. EMBARK encourages therapists to use the interventions with which they are most comfortable and experienced, provided they meet specific criteria outlined in this manual. By inviting therapists to work within their comfort zone, EMBARK aims to enable them to show up more confidently and comfortably with participants, which may facilitate the therapeutic alliances they build.

The guidelines laid out for interventions in Chapters 5–7 define the scope of possible interventions, ensuring their alignment with treatment goals and providing therapists with a clear understanding of their intended objectives. For example, if a participant would benefit from the application of a soothing technique during a medicine session, therapists can use a technique from a range of modalities— somatic experiencing, a CBT approach, a mindfulness-based approach—as long as it meets the needs of the moment and aligns with the guidelines provided for this intervention. This eases the burden on therapists to become proficient in novel interventions and allows them to draw on the broad skill sets they bring to PAT in a way that is thoughtfully delimited. Having clearly defined aims and guidelines also facilitates the operationalization of what needs to be accomplished in sessions for the purposes of standardization in research settings.

A Transdiagnostic and Trans-Drug Model: Adaptable to a Range of Clinical Indications and Psychedelic Medicines

EMBARK is conceived as a general, transdiagnostic approach to PAT that can be adapted to the specific clinical indication being treated in any given setting. The version of EMBARK detailed in this book is tailored specifically for use in treating MDD (though it is applicable more generally to other manifestations of depression). An EMBARK approach to treating, say, generalized anxiety disorder, would contain a different set of treatment goals and interventions that draw their influence from a different set of EBTs that have specific efficacy in treating that indication. EMBARK's six domains are designed to remain relevant to any clinical indication, enabling a range of mechanisms and interventions from various incorporated therapies to coexist in a clear, meaningful, theoretically coherent, and pragmatically useful fashion. In this way, EMBARK's structure can be thought of as a kind of "meta-model" that forms the basis for the construction of many indication-specific models, such as the one in this manual.

Attending to Previously Overlooked Factors: Somatics, Relationships, Spiritual Experiences, and Ethics

EMBARK devotes an unprecedented degree of attention to some of the treatment elements discussed earlier: existential and spiritual phenomena, embodied phenomena as a catalyst for healing, relational aspects of treatment, and ethical considerations. The first three elements are infused into EMBARK via its "Existential–Spiritual," "Body-Aware," and "Relational" domains, respectively. EMBARK's commitment to the ethical dimensions of PAT is represented by its four ethical care cornerstones. These components of the approach are discussed in more detail in the following sections of this chapter.

EMBARK'S SIX CLINICAL DOMAINS

This section includes a description of each of EMBARK's six clinical domains. The specific interventions and mechanisms or therapeutic change associated with these domains will come in later chapters of this book. The current chapter is meant to introduce, define, and demarcate these six sets of psychedelic phenomena into the domains that will serve as the structure for everything else to come.

Existential–Spiritual

> *What's the point of my existence? Why am I even here? Like there's no point*
> *of doing any of this because my existence is meaningless . . . That hasn't*
> *happened since this experience. Not once. The buzz of anxiety is gone.*
>   —Unitarian Universalist Minister (Swift et al., 2023)

Psychedelic medicines catalyze profound encounters with mystical or spiritual content (Breeksema et al., 2020; Griffiths et al., 2006; Podrebarac et al., 2021) and existential concerns, such as mortality (Swift et al., 2017), alienation (Watts et al., 2017), or questions of meaning in life (Belser et al., 2017; Ross et al., 2016, 2021). This is perhaps not surprising, given the historical and current use of psychedelic plants and fungi in the religious practices of many cultures worldwide (Schultes et al., 2001). Participants in PAT trials often speak of these existential–spiritual phenomena as sacred and consider them essential curative elements in their treatment (Belser et al., 2017; Bogenschutz et al., 2015; Griffiths et al., 2006; Johnson et al., 2014; Podrebarac et al., 2021).

One particular subset of these phenomena—mystical experiences—has garnered significant research attention in PAT trials to date. In PAT research, this set of phenomena is usually measured with the Mystical Experiences Questionnaire (MEQ; Barrett et al., 2015; MacLean et al., 2012), which operationalizes mystical experiences along the following set of factors: positive mood, transcendence of time and space, ineffability, and other mystical qualities, such as an internal sense of unity, an external sense of unity, a noetic quality, and a sense of sacredness. Another tool often used to assess mystical experience is the oceanic boundlessness dimension of the Altered States Questionnaire (ASC; Studerus et al., 2010), which includes subfactors such as insightfulness, blissful state, experiences of unity, and spiritual experience.

These mystical experiences often co-occur with a psychedelic phenomenon commonly known as ego dissolution. This refers to a diminution or total loss of one's sense of personal identity, which can be experienced positively as a type of mystical phenomenon (e.g., oceanic boundlessness, experiences of unity) or negatively as an anxiety-producing experience (Nour et al., 2016). The terms "ego dissolution" and "ego death" have become common parlance in popular media discussions of PAT. In practice, it remains an often misapplied term that stands in for a range of alterations to one's sense of being as a separate, coherent "self" (Devenot et al., 2022a).

The potency of participants' mystical experiences has been found to predict a range of treatment benefits (Kangaslampi, 2023; Ko et al., 2022), such as reductions in depressive symptoms (Davis et al., 2021; Roseman et al., 2018), increased motivation to stop problematic cocaine use (Dakwar et al., 2014), decreases in cancer-related depression and anxiety (Griffiths et al., 2016; Ross et al., 2016), greater success with nicotine cessation (Garcia-Romeu et al., 2015; Johnson et al., 2014), and other positive changes in psychological functioning (Griffiths et al., 2018). Other research has found that these experiences often lead study participants to durably shift their metaphysical beliefs away from materialism and toward a worldview in which living and nonliving beings are ascribed consciousness (Nayak & Griffiths, 2022) and that this shift correlates with antidepressant outcomes (Timmerman et al., 2021).

We have yet to develop a clear, agreed upon sense of how mystical experiences exert their therapeutic effects (Breeksema & van Elk, 2021; Jylkkä, 2021; Roseman et al., 2018; Sanders & Zijlmans, 2021), but there has been a consensus across both waves of PAT research that mystical phenomena are a definitional feature of psychedelic medicines and the benefits they can bring (Johnson et al., 2019).

Sometimes a participant will have a very powerful spiritual experience on psilocybin but will minimize their experience, saying something discounting like, "Well, it was important to me, but I didn't have a complete mystical experience like I heard about on that podcast." As psychedelic practitioners and researchers, it is important to challenge our conception of mystical experiences and broaden the dialogue. The spiritual diversity of participant accounts suggests that mysticism is a multifaceted phenomenon, rather than a singular, totemic experience.

Importantly, EMBARK's existential–spiritual domain refers to a broader range of phenomena than just one construction of mystical experience. Existential themes and spirituality both comprise a huge continent within the human experience, and there exist a huge variety of experiences that could fall within their borders. The experiences that most commonly arise in psychedelic medicine sessions are listed here, with credit to the qualitative work of many authors (for review, see Breeksema et al., 2020; Belser et al., 2017; Griffiths et al., 2019; Podrebarac et al., 2021):

- Sense of oceanic boundlessness
- Sense of ineffability, or inability to apply words to what one is experiencing
- Experience of transcending time and/or space
- Sense of the underlying perfection of all things
- Sense of deep, nonconceptual knowing, or receiving wisdom that cannot be put into words
- Sense of having specific insights into the nature of reality
- Sense of the universal interconnectedness of humans (and perhaps non-human beings)
- Broadening of one's perspective on life to include a "bigger picture" perspective
- Fear of losing one's grip on oneself and/or ceasing to exist
- Reevaluation of one's relationship to mortality and/or thoughts about the afterlife
- Deeply felt encounters with the meaningfulness of existence (or lack thereof)
- Sense of encountering a divine or demonic presence
- Sense of merging with a divine presence or the whole of reality

- Sense of encountering or being guided by outside entities (e.g., spirits, saints, ancestors)
- Sense that nature or reality has its own pervasive intelligence
- Sense that inanimate objects are alive during the session (and perhaps always)
- Sense of traveling to other planes of existence, often "more real" than ordinary reality
- Experience of thought processes rife with mythic, archetypal, or symbolic content
- Sense of remembering events from past lives

As is probably clear, many of these phenomena are outside the bounds of what you may be used to working with in your standard practice. More than the phenomena in the other five domains, existential–spiritual phenomena sharply diverge from everyday life and traditional psychotherapy. When they arise in our participants, they should continually awaken us to the profundity and sacredness that we are asked to hold space for as PAT practitioners. The existential–spiritual domain of EMBARK serves as a place in the model to honor that demand.

Mindfulness

OK, so you didn't get the biggest slice of cheese in life, but it's OK. It helps me cope a little bit better. I don't get overwhelmed—my anxiety attacks that I had practically every night are somewhat nonexistent. I do get it, to some extent a little bit now and then, but I really found a way to kind of talk myself through it, like, "it's OK; whatever you're feeling right now, it's not the end of the world and you'll deal with it." So, since then, that holds kind of like a little tool kit and just knowing or feeling what life is about and hey, this isn't a big deal. Relax, it's OK.

—Mary (Belser et al., 2017; Swift et al., 2017)

When it's used in psychotherapy, mindfulness is typically defined as the practice of maintaining a more neutral, nonreactive awareness of the present moment, particularly of one's own thoughts, feelings, embodied sensations, and impulses. It is often accompanied by a sense of calm, compassion, and helpful distance from what is observed. Mindfulness-based therapies often develop a person's capacity for cultivating this state to give them more choice in how they respond to internal and external stimuli through behavior and reactive emotions.

Many PAT trial participants have reported shifts in their internal experience that reflect a similar kind of distant, nonreactive awareness. The psychedelic medicine they have taken often gives them an opportunity to take a step back and observe the workings of their mind from a kind of observer consciousness. Some have described this shift as a kind of "mental freedom" or an escape from "the prison of the mind" (Watts & Luoma, 2020, p. 95). Others have framed it as a greater sense of sovereignty in relating to what is occurring in their own mind (Bogenschutz et al., 2018), greater self-compassion (Agin-Liebes, 2019), or a disruption of their habitual sense of self (Belser et al., 2017; Roseman et al., 2018).

Some other medicine session events that fit within this domain include:

- Transcendence of rigid, maladaptive ideas about oneself
- Sense of coming into one's "core" or "true" self, which differs from ideas about oneself
- An ability to feel and offer compassion toward wounded "parts" of oneself from one's "core" or "true" self
- Experiences of general self-compassion
- Insight into ordinarily nonconscious mental processes associated with habits of suffering
- Experiences of being able to "let go" of suffering associated with habitual mental behavior
- Disruption of ruminative thought processes

What these spontaneously arising experiences have in common is that they align with many of the benefits ascribed to the cultivation of mindfulness in other psychotherapies. In essence, these experiences reflect participants' movement toward becoming better able to attend to themselves, recognize their symptomatic internal states, and respond to them with greater self-compassion and self-regulation. In support of this, some clinical trial participants have reported the following enduring posttreatment shifts as a result of these phenomena:

- Greater psychological flexibility (Watts & Luoma, 2020)
- A stance of greater equanimity toward challenging emotions and beliefs about oneself (Watts et al., 2017; Wolff et al., 2020)
- "Cognitive defusion," or coming into a less fixed sense of self that is less identified with negative beliefs about oneself (Watts & Luoma, 2020)
- Increased ability to recognize and name internal states (van der Kolk et al., 2023)

This domain shares a good deal of conceptual overlap with the notion of psychological flexibility that has been emphasized by other PAT models. These approaches have placed these mindfulness-related phenomena at the center of their theories of therapeutic change. For example, Watts and Luoma (2020) have developed the accept, connect, embody (ACE) model of PAT, which views the development of psychological flexibility as a primary therapeutic outcome. To support participants in reaching this goal, they draw from ACT, which posits cognitive defusion and a flexible experience of the self (self-as-context) as treatment goals. Similarly, the *Yale Manual for Psilocybin-Assisted Therapy of Depression* (Guss et al., 2020) draws heavily from ACT, the hexaflex model of psychological flexibility, and elements of mindfulness-based cognitive therapy, such as self-transcendence. EMBARK's Mindfulness domain honors and incorporates these perspectives and holds these mindfulness-adjacent outcomes as an important constitutive element of PAT treatment.

Body-Aware

[The experience] felt moving on a corporal level— on a very corporal level. Like, you don't understand it strictly in your head. You understand it as a being, as a body, as a full body.
— Caleb (Belser et al., 2017; Swift et al., 2017)

Embodied phenomena have not received much attention in PAT research to date (Belser et al., 2017) and thus represent an underexplored source of contribution to therapeutic outcomes. The inattention to these phenomena in clinical research on PAT may be a reflection of the effort to characterize PAT within the institutional bounds of Western psychiatry, a field that is more exclusively concerned with the mind. When the body is evoked, it is usually as the site of unwanted symptoms, medication side effects, or adverse treatment events.

Instead, the body is more productively thought of as an integral part of how healing unfolds in PAT (Harris, 2023; Ho et al., 2020). Subjective reports from PAT clinical trial participants have suggested that embodied phenomena have played an important part of the healing that occurs in their medicine sessions (Belser et al., 2017; Watts et al., 2017). They have reported that their body is engaged in a variety of ways including, but not limited to:

- Altered proprioception and interoception
- Heightened sensitivity to embodied events
- Fluctuations in perceived body temperature
- Tension and pain with no organic cause
- Cathartic discharge through trembling, shaking, movement, facial expression, or vocalizing
- Dissociation and numbness
- Sense of being extremely energized
- Erotic or sexual sensations
- Embodied feelings of great calm or tranquility
- Embodied feelings of spaciousness or constriction
- Various forms of alterations in breathing that are related to therapeutic material
- Psychologically meaningful movements or adjustments in posture or position
- Experiences of locating undesirable material (e.g., grief, shame, resentment, anger) or physical illness (e.g., cancer, sequelae of problem drinking) in one's lived experience of their body
- Gagging, dry-heaving, or vomiting, often experienced by the participant as positive, purgative, or cleansing
- Sensations of energy running through conduits in the body

- Sense that something in the body is relaxing or "releasing" in a therapeutically meaningful way
- Sense of being in conversation with a part or the whole of one's body
- Renegotiation of one's relationship to the body

There are few EBTs that provide support in conceptualizing or responding to these phenomena, though several innovative somatic psychotherapy approaches have offered suggestions, including sensorimotor psychotherapy (Ogden & Fisher, 2015), hakomi (Weiss et al., 2015), and the trauma-resiliency model (Grabbe & Miller-Karas, 2017). Several of these approaches provide a frame for understanding some of these embodied events as processes by which trauma is healed. There is also extensive precedent in indigenous approaches to working with embodied phenomena induced by psychedelic medicines, particularly medicines like ayahuasca that are purgative in nature (Fotiou & Gearin, 2019). The contributions of these models will be discussed throughout this book as they become relevant.

Even so, there is no single model that captures the full breadth of embodied healing phenomena that can arise during a PAT medicine session. Generally, the phenomena in this domain arise spontaneously and lead to therapeutic benefit when a participant tunes into them in a receptive approach that is sometimes referred to as "listening to the wisdom of the body." This stance involves a kind of subtle sensing of and feeling into embodied experiences that encourage the participant to stay present to their unfolding at the level of the body rather than rushing to interpret them or turn them into a source of cognitive meaning (Harris, 2023). EMBARK's Body-Aware domain holds a space in the model for guidance on how to help participants engage in such a process.

Affective–Cognitive

> I had a very strong feeling of self-hatred. Like, really strong. It hurt. But almost immediately at the same time, I felt like that was ridiculous and like, "Why would you hate yourself? You're wonderful. It makes no sense." . . . I was both shocked that I hated myself more than I was aware that I did, but then there was an immediate relief.
>
> —Erin (Belser et al., 2017; Swift et al., 2017)

Medicine sessions often give rise to dramatic shifts in a participant's emotions (Belser et al., 2017; Breeksema et al., 2020; Watts et al., 2017). PAT trial participants routinely report that they experience a high degree of emotionality that is ordinarily unavailable to them. They may feel intensified versions of feelings they often feel, as well as feelings to which they do not normally have access. These include the full gamut of wanted and unwanted feelings, including bliss, love, despair, fear, grief, and many others. The strength of these emotions may lead a participant to feel that they are unbearable, or it may make them feel like a liberating form of catharsis. They may feel like both at the same time, since many of the affective experiences found in this domain reflect novel mixtures of previously separate experiences, as seen in the quote that opens this section.

These intense experiences of affect often come coupled with potent confrontations with one's maladaptive beliefs about oneself or the world (Bogenschutz et al., 2018). These confrontations are often more candid, direct, and unavoidable than they would normally be for a participant. Often, participants are surprised by the arising of these beliefs, experiencing them as both shocking and immediately recognizable as intimately and innately "theirs." Uncovering or encountering these beliefs brings them into one's lived experience, which may lead to them being transformed into a more adaptive belief during the medicine session or sometime after.

Affective–Cognitive phenomena that may arise in a medicine session include:

- Strong, full-range emotional openings
- Emotional distress, fear, or panic
- Emotionally resonant internal visual phenomena
- Insights into the motives and emotions driving one's behaviors
- Challenging confrontations with one's beliefs about self or the world
- Emotionally evocative "autobiographical review," or vivid recall of personal memories
- Shifts in the felt meanings ascribed to past events
- Feelings of forgiveness toward self and others
- Feelings of immense gratitude

When working with depressed participants, the following specific affective–cognitive phenomena might arise:

- Anger, either that which the participant can embody and express or that which they experience as present but blocked
- Maladaptive feelings about the self, such as shame, guilt, failure, or inadequacy
- Maladaptive beliefs about the self (e.g., "I'm incomplete." or "I'm worthless.")
- Desirable emotions, such as joy or love, which may seem hard to embody or express
- Personal grief
- Cultural grief
- Challenges with grieving, such as a sense of being "blocked" in one's ability to grieve or a sense that one is grieving excessively

Engaging more openly with these emotions and beliefs during a medicine session has become a widely accepted practice among PAT models. Participants are typically invited to experience, embody, and express them during a medicine session. This practice mirrors that found in several nonpsychedelic EBTs, such as ACT's emphasis on acceptance of emotions (Hayes et al., 2012) and emotion-focused therapy's emphasis on entering into maladaptive states toward the end of transforming them (Greenberg & Watson, 2006). The ACE model of PAT (Watts & Luoma, 2020) centers on a similar approach to emotions and core beliefs. The Affective–Cognitive domain of EMBARK follows suit in its recognition of the importance of welcoming and working with these phenomena in PAT.

Relational

[My therapists] were the best to speak to. They're just so . . . amazing to have them just be there. Obviously the first, in the beginning of the session, I felt that whole panic. But once I got past that, and to have them both there and to share that with them . . . they were absolutely amazing. I felt so . . . I didn't feel judged; I felt so open to speak to them and tell them my life, and not feel like, "Oh my god; what will they think of me?"

—Mary (Belser et al., 2017; Swift et al., 2017)

Relational elements of PAT represent another domain of potential therapeutic effect that has received insufficient attention from researchers and existing PAT models to date (Aronovich, 2020; Barnes, 2022; Barnes & Briggs, 2021; Kettner et al., 2021). The therapeutic opportunities presented by the relationship between the participant and the therapist have been largely overlooked in favor of a focus on the benefits that may arise from the participant's internally focused experience of the medicine. This has led some (Barnes, 2022; Barnes & Briggs, 2021) to consider dominant approaches to PAT to be "one-person psychologies," in contrast to those that contend more intentionally with the relationships between the two (or three) people in the room.

Although most PAT approaches to date emphasize an inward-focused approach in which the participant wears headphones and an eye mask during medicine sessions (Horton et al., 2021), many participants elect to emerge and engage interpersonally for at least part of the session. Their altered state gives rise to altered interpersonal dynamics with the therapist, which include amplified versions of those found in traditional psychotherapy, including transferences, projections, or enactments of traumatic dynamics. As in talk therapy, the appearance of these phenomena represents an opportunity for clinical gain if handled skillfully or rupture and harm if handled poorly.

Some specific relational phenomena that may arise in a medicine session include:

- Dramatic alterations of the meanings ascribed to the relationship by the participant
- Significant increases or decreases in the participant's trust of you

- Heightened participant suggestibility
- Heightened participant vulnerability to relational harm
- Heightened participant sensitivity to your words, actions, and presence
- Ascription of great power, skill, or wisdom to you by the participant
- Intensification of the participant's usual attachment style or other relational behavior
- Enactments of relational dynamics from the participant's past, including traumatic relationship dynamics
- Participant engagement in greater boundary-testing, possibly as part of an enactment
- Participant requests for greater or lesser care or connection from you
- Shifts in participants' expectations of your role
- Greater potential for boundary transgressions
- Greater potential for therapist interventions to elicit beneficial relational repatterning
- Reevaluating or recognizing the current value of relationships with loved ones
- Deeply felt desire to repair one's relationships with loved ones
- Feelings of openness and/or emotional empathy that persist after the session
- Apparent regression to a younger developmental state, often with the interpersonal needs and communicative abilities of this developmental age

Notably, many of the terms found on this list (e.g., transference, regression, enactment) have their origins in psychoanalytic and psychodynamic schools of psychotherapy. This is likely the result of several factors, including the theoretical leanings of early PAT therapists who originally framed these phenomena and the richer language for describing the appearance of complex modes of relating found in these schools of clinical thought. Nonetheless, you are encouraged to reframe any of these phenomena in the clinical language with which you are most comfortable. Mithoefer and colleagues (2017) have suggested the term "working with the multiplicity of the psyche" (p. 68) as a more universal framework for understanding how different aspects of a participant's psyche may arise in a medicine session and exert a greater than usual influence on how they interact with you.

Foundational to this domain is a recognition of the participant's social world and its relationship to their well-being. Relational challenges are a transdiagnostic feature of most psychiatric indications, typically serving as both a contributing factor to and a consequence of one's struggles. When a participant arrives to treatment, they are bringing this social world with them into their medicine sessions.

Even if they do not engage in any of the aforementioned relational dynamics with you, healing in this domain may still occur by way of internal phenomena that draw upon the participant's social world. PAT trial participants have exhibited increased openness and emotional empathy after a medicine session (Carhart-Harris et al., 2018b; Pokorny et al., 2017), which will likely have significant consequences for their relational life. They also may have experiences of love, forgiveness, grief, anger, boundary-setting, or compassion toward their loved ones, whether alive or no longer so, that mark the beginning of a shift toward healing these important relationships. Finally, even when there is little to no active engagement with you, your mere presence in the room can have significant relational meaning for the participant. The Relational domain in EMBARK represents all of the ways in which the therapist–participant relationship and other relationships that become salient during treatment can contribute to healing.

Keeping Momentum

It makes you question everything about yourself, figure out what you want to change, what you want to keep the same, what is good, what is bad. You know how to really integrate things in your life, and I think it has a very lasting effect.
—Victor (Belser et al., 2017; Swift et al., 2017)

The end of a course of PAT treatment is, in some ways, only the beginning. To obtain enduring benefit from treatment, every participant must put in the work of making life changes—new habits, new behaviors, changes to the contexts around them—inspired by what arose in their medicine session. They need to seize whatever sparks of motivation for and commitment to making changes that have arisen and, with your support, turn them into a workable plan of action that will support continued improvements and prevent a relapse into depression.

Maintaining posttreatment progress is a crucial aspect of ensuring sustained benefits in any of EMBARK's six domains. The most profound and lasting benefits from a mystical experience or an emotional revelation often emerge when they are perceived as the initiation of a more spiritually or emotionally aligned lifestyle. This domain is a throughline in EMBARK for cultivating the kind of motivation for change that will drive outcomes in all other domains. It signifies the continuous therapeutic effort from the first screening until posttermination toward generating the necessary momentum to make and maintain posttreatment changes.

Much of the work in the Keeping Momentum domain involves capturing lightning in a bottle by building upon the momentum that arises in a medicine session to propel change work during integration. This momentum arises through a range of medicine session phenomena (Bathje et al., 2021; Belser et al., 2017; Bogenschutz et al., 2018; Gasser et al., 2015; Griffiths et al., 2018; Malone et al., 2018; Nielson et al., 2018; Watts et al., 2017; Watts & Luoma, 2020):

- Feelings of strong motivation to make changes
- Increased sense of self-efficacy for making changes
- Feelings of readiness and commitment to make changes
- Increased hope and optimism

- A sense of renewal or having a clean slate
- Insights into what has driven problematic habits
- A desire to change problematic habits
- Shifts in identity that may inspire changes in behavior
- Revisions to one's life priorities
- Updates to one's values
- Reconnection to one's existing values
- Recognition of one's strengths or virtues and the possibilities for action these provide
- Increased tendency toward prosocial behaviors
- Reduced cravings (for participants with substance use disorders)
- A desire to change one's career path
- A desire to take action to improve our collective well-being

From a relapse prevention perspective, an important part of keeping momentum is encouraging the participant to prepare and plan for stressors and hardships in integration and beyond. An occasional low-energy week is to be expected when one struggles with depression, but it does not have to result in a full-blown depressive episode. In other words, setbacks are inevitable, but full relapses can often be prevented with enough momentum.

A Note on Phenomena that Involve Multiple Domains

EMBARK's six domains are meant to serve as a helpful rubric for understanding participant experiences and how to support them. However, they should not be applied inflexibly as rigidly demarcated categories. Frequently, participants will have experiences during a medicine session that evoke more than one domain, such as an embodied spiritual experience or an emotional opening that occurs within a relational moment with a therapist. In such cases, you are encouraged to draw from this book's guidance for each of the relevant domains and to blend it in a way that·befits your assessment of how to best support the participant.

EMBARK'S FOUR CARE CORNERSTONES

The EMBARK psychedelic therapy model rests upon four cornerstones of ethical care: Trauma-Informed Care, Culturally Competent Care, Ethically Rigorous care, and Collective Care. Together, they represent EMBARK's building on the premise that efficacious treatment is ethical treatment. These cornerstones are woven into all levels of any EMBARK approach, from conceptualization of the indication to specific techniques in treatment. Figure 2.2 provides a visual schema of EMBARK's four care cornerstones. This section will briefly introduce the cornerstones and provide an overview of why each is important in PAT.

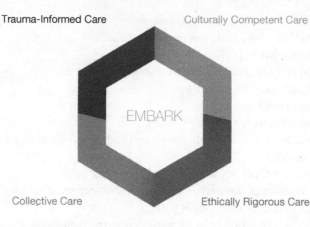

Trauma-Informed Care   Culturally Competent Care

EMBARK

Collective Care   Ethically Rigorous Care

Figure 2.2. EMBARK's Four Care Cornerstones

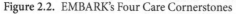

Importantly, the instructions provided throughout this book on how to work in alignment with these four ethical cornerstones should not be seen as sufficient for attaining expertise in any of them. It would be impossible for any written text to convey the full degree of competence and skill required. To conduct PAT in a way that truly encompasses these cornerstones, you are strongly encouraged to seek additional training and supervision in a setting that honors each of them.

Trauma-Informed Care

You know safety is 100% important because you cannot resolve trauma if you do not feel safe, because safety is part of the trauma. So really feeling like the people holding space are doing it in a very adept way. I can just relax into that and I'm safe.

—Participant (Lafrance et al., 2017)

The approach in this book aims to respond proactively to the well-documented prevalence of trauma in the populations you are likely to treat and the crucial importance of attending to its presence throughout treatment. It rests on the notion that, even if no trauma history is noted during screening, one should still work in a way that assumes its presence and prepares to encounter it with every participant.

By trauma, we refer to both (a) a history of exposure to death, threatened death, actual or threatened serious injury, or actual or threatened sexual violence (sometimes colloquially referred to as "big T" trauma) and (b) events that are not necessarily life-threatening but can still pose serious emotional challenges, such as a history of emotional abuse, types of neglect, bullying, serious illness, financial hardships, regular exposure to oppressive cultural dynamics (e.g., racism, homophobia), divorce, and other conflicts that may lead to emotional distress and behavioral changes ("small t" trauma). Throughout this book, instructions are provided for recognizing and responding to the unique and complex ways in which trauma manifests in PAT.

This section presents a brief overview of some of the main themes of trauma-informed care that will show up in later chapters.

Importance of relationship. A helpful basis for the provision of trauma-informed care is provided by SAMHSA's (Substance Abuse and Mental Health Services Administration, 2014) six key principles: safety; trustworthiness and transparency; peer support; collaboration and mutuality; empowerment, voice, and choice; and cultural, historical, and gender issues. You should continually work to build and maintain a therapeutic relationship founded on attentiveness to these six principles and ensure that your chosen interventions do not infringe upon them.

This and other forms of attentiveness to the therapeutic relationship are the heart of providing trauma-informed care. Much of the suffering that results from traumatic experience hinges on the enduring experiences of disempowerment and disconnection to which they give rise (Herman, 1998). You should thus take great care to ensure that your relationship with a participant is one that fosters empowerment and connection every step of the way.

Empowerment. Empowering the participant entails recognizing when they are stepping into their autonomy, supporting them in doing so, and celebrating this with them. This could take many forms. They may decline a suggestion you make about how to act during a medicine session. They may reject your interpretation of their medicine session experience. They may express a wish to collaborate more actively in treatment planning. It is up to you to recognize when a step into autonomy and empowerment is occurring and to respond appropriately.

For starters, you should avoid imposing any of the recommended interventions in this book on a participant in an authoritarian way that undermines their movement toward empowerment (unless there is an immediate risk to their safety). For this reason, you will find that the instructions throughout the book are couched in phrases like "explore with the participant . . . ," "collaboratively determine . . . ," and "consider suggesting . . . ."

Restoring the ability to connect. Participants with trauma are also likely to use their relationship with you as an opportunity to restore their disrupted ability to connect with someone. It is thus essential that you work with them to ensure that the therapeutic relationship is one in which they feel maximally safe to do this, as they are likely to be sensitive to any sign of potential risk. Your attentiveness to factors such as your therapeutic presence or your reactions to the participant can help you to avoid eliciting feelings of fear, shame, or disempowerment that may undermine their attempts to connect with you. This attentiveness should begin from the first point of contact with a participant and continue up to the point at which they have transitioned into the follow-up care you have helped them to arrange for themselves.

Shame. Shame is often deeply intertwined with PAT participants' traumatic experiences and will likely appear as an important element for many. Psychedelic medicines frequently facilitate the emergence and processing of shame-laden memories, emotions, and core beliefs (Mathai et al., 2023). Participants may wrestle directly with questions of self-worth, intrinsic goodness, or lovability. Others may embody and live out their shame during a medicine session by acting in ways that are congruent with the image of themselves it presents. In any event, it is essential to offer them an empathic, non-judgmental presence that implicitly holds their inherent goodness for them as they engage with their shame. This is particularly important in PAT medicine sessions, in which participants' sensitivity to real and perceived therapist endorsements of their shame may be heightened (Brennan et al., 2021). With appropriate support, many participants are likely to move through their shame to a place of increased self-acceptance and self-compassion (Healy et al., 2021).

Supporting participants who become dysregulated. Participants in a psychedelic medicine session may feel capable of revisiting their trauma in an undefended way that involves a strong connection to their embodied and sensory memories of traumatic events (Weiss et al., 2023). This drive toward open exploration brings both the possibility of great healing and the risk of moving too fast, jumping over one's self-protective capacities, and becoming highly dysregulated, or losing the ability to modulate one's emotional and embodied experience. Supporting a participant who becomes dysregulated while revisiting traumatic memories requires skillful discernment about when to encourage someone to remain open to challenging material and when to invite them to check in with their defenses and receive permission from all parts of themselves before rushing forward into a harmful degree of activation.

At times, participants who have taken a psychedelic medicine demonstrate an increased capacity for titrating the amount of trauma processing they deal with and a greater ability to self-regulate as they do so. Other participants will require additional support to self-regulate.

Because they are likely to be focused internally as they approach dysregulation, it can be challenging for you to know when they are getting there. While not foolproof, it can be helpful to watch for cues that a participant is becoming hyper-aroused (e.g., scared eyes, alterations in breathing, irritability, hyper-vigilance). As always, involve the participant collaboratively in determining what they may need, and seek their input as to how their experience is impacting them.

Sometimes a participant may appear to become hypo-aroused during this exploration (e.g., dissociating, shutting down, feeling the effects of the medicine less, getting sleepy). Although they (and you) may find this frustrating insofar as it seems like a less potent experience, give them permission to be where they are and let go of any ideas about where they "should" be. This movement away from emotional intensity may reflect an automatic, self-protective means of avoiding the harm of excessive arousal. Consider that a new, helpful focus for the session might be attending to how it is for them to be in this state and seeing what they can learn about it. Try to bracket any frustration or corrective impulse you might hold about this kind of response and be cautious about defining it for yourself or the participant in the language of "resistance."

Sometimes, PAT is conceptualized as a more aggressive procedure in which a participant is broken down with high doses of drug, forceful physical interventions, and/or disorienting stimuli; it has even been conceived historically as a shock therapy (Dubus, 2022). But these types of approaches are likely to be, at best, unnecessary for bringing benefit and, at worst, very harmful to participants. Throughout this book, you will be instructed to lean more into supporting and working with participants' defenses or dissociation rather than trying to overcome them. To reference an oft-cited saying from internal family systems, we advise that you "respect the protectors."

FORMS OF EMOTIONAL SELF-REGULATION

When working with participants who carry trauma, part of your role will be to support and strengthen their capacity for emotional self-regulation. The following three forms of self-regulation are often helpful capacities to focus on. Practices that can increase participants' access to them are found throughout this book.

Titration: Titration is the process of breaking down overwhelming or intense emotional experiences into smaller, more manageable parts. It involves focusing on a smaller aspect or component of the emotional experience rather than trying to tackle the entire overwhelming feeling at once. This allows individuals to gradually process and regulate their emotions in a more controlled manner.

Resourcing: Resourcing involves identifying and utilizing internal and external sources of support and resilience to help individuals regulate their emotions during times of distress. These resources may include positive memories, images, or sensations; supportive relationships; grounding techniques; self-soothing strategies; or other tools that individuals find helpful in managing their emotions effectively.

Pendulation: Pendulation, also known as "pendulating attention," is a process of shifting attention between distressing or activating experiences and more resourceful or neutral experiences. By oscillating between distress and a safe, neutral state, individuals can regulate their emotions and gradually build tolerance and resilience in navigating challenging emotional states.

Enactments. Occasionally a participant might act through an old relational pattern with you, often to an amplified extent, as part of what is sometimes called an enactment. This is likely to occur in a way that is outside of their awareness, and it may vary in how perceptible it is to you, as it may or may not involve overt behaviors. Such enactments provide an opportunity for harm and retraumatization if mishandled. Consistently attending to the possibility that you and the participant are engaged in an enactment together is another key element of trauma-informed care. While this book is not a substitute for receiving training in how to recognize and respond to enactments, instructions on how to attend and respond to them are offered throughout the book (see "Relational: Medicine Session" in Chapter 6).

Enactments are generally thought to be coconstructed—that is, they will often draw upon your own psychological material and lead you to respond in a way that may not be guided by your best clinical judgment. This serves as another way in which engaging in your own continual process of personal development (i.e., becoming aware of and processing your personal material) and professional consultation and supervision can serve your work with participants (see Chapter 4 for more on this topic). Developing your ability to respond appropriately and ethically to enactments is essential because, even though they are the result of a complex, bidirectional interplay between your material and that of the participant, the responsibility to minimize any harmful behavior that results is always yours.

Aftercare. Finally, it is important to note that trauma-informed care does not stop at the end of treatment. PAT treatment can be a disruptive, unsettling experience, particularly for participants who revisited a past trauma during a medicine session. They may reach the end of treatment while still experiencing sequalae of trauma, and for some people, terminations can activate feelings of abandonment. As such, this book presents some guidance on how to support participants who require more care than a few integration sessions.

As noted earlier, merely reading this book does not provide sufficient training in how to work in a trauma-informed way. Working with trauma presents significant challenges that require a degree of training that is beyond the scope of this or any book. We advise you to seek such training in order to minimize the likelihood of doing additional harm to participants who carry trauma.

Trauma-Informed Care is a cornerstone of EMBARK, especially because of the alterations in consciousness that psychedelic medicines induce. These altered states can bring forth deeply buried or previously unrecognized traumatic experiences, making participants particularly vulnerable and raising the potential for unintended harms. Recognizing trauma's pervasive influence, a trauma-informed approach in PAT is critical, as it fosters an environment of safety, empowerment, and healing.

Culturally Competent Care

> *Early research on the use of psychedelics to treat trauma has focused primarily on combat veterans, a vast majority of whom are men. Without careful attention paid to make psychedelic therapy safe and inviting for women and people who are genderqueer or transgender, norms which make it safer for cisgendered men to participate in such healing will only intensify.*
> —Betty Aldworth (2019, p. 55)

The field of mental health has reached a consensus that the ability to provide care to people who differ from the therapist in terms of race, culture, gender, sexual orientation, class, age, disability status, immigration status, and other social locations is an essential part of delivering effective treatment. However, training therapists to consider these factors when treating those who are culturally different has lagged behind this realization.

This has been particularly true in clinical trials of PAT, which have received much scrutiny for not recognizing the importance of cultural considerations, particularly racial and gender inclusivity in clinical trial participant pools (Fogg et al., 2021; George et al., 2020; Herzberg & Butler, 2019; Michaels et al., 2018; Stauffer et al., 2022; Williams et al., 2020). While a truly comprehensive response to these concerns would entail structural and cultural changes in the field of PAT research that go beyond therapist training, this book includes suggestions on how to minimize iatrogenic harm caused by culturally incompetent treatment by helping therapists to engage in culturally attuned ways that avoid replicating oppressive dynamics in the therapist–participant relationship.

The approach found throughout this book is akin to a form of cultural competence that is often referred to as "cultural humility." This newer term rejects the notion that therapists should possess authoritative knowledge about the cultures from which their participants come and bring that knowledge to bear in therapy as a kind of expertise. This kind of expert approach has been increasingly criticized (Lekas et al., 2020) for its tendency to encourage stereotyped, homogenized cultural knowledge that is inappropriately tied to dynamic, intersectional people, thereby re-creating oppressive dynamics in the therapist–participant relationship.

Instead, cultural humility emphasizes the inherent complexity of people's cultural identities and encourages an approach to difference that emphasizes ongoing self-reflection about one's biases and appreciation of participants' expertise about their own lived experience. Therapists aim to be continually reflective of how cultural differences in the therapeutic relationship might be impacting what is occurring and regularly invite input from participants about how they would like to shift their care accordingly. This approach is also more in sync with a trauma-informed approach to care due to its emphasis on participant empowerment. It also makes the most sense coming from the authors of this book, who as a cisgender White man and a cisgender White straight-passing queer man, have spent more time learning cultural humility than acting as experts on others' cultures.

In our clinical practice and training, we make a concerted effort to decenter whiteness and other dominant identities. By doing so, we aim to dismantle the systemic biases that exist within mental health care and create an inclusive and equitable therapeutic environment. This involves actively acknowledging and addressing the privileges and biases associated with these dominant identities.

The culturally competent approach in this book prompts you to consider and discuss the impact of cultural factors at many points throughout treatment. For instance, you are asked to reflect on cultural differences in the ways in which participants experience and communicate their depression. Differences here can have a significant impact on how a participant experiences their symptoms and how they present them to you. For example, some cultures may emphasize somatic or spiritual dimensions of their suffering, and you will need to work in a way that is congruent with their lived experience rather than imposing your own perspective.

Additionally, differing cultural ideas and attitudes about depression may also impact the extent to which a participant feels comfortable seeking help. For instance, Black Americans' depression is stigmatized by the dominant culture in various ways, which leads them to seek help less readily and underreport their symptoms (Dean et al., 2022; Yu et al., 2022). Some participants may show up to treatment less willing to "complain" or ask for what they need, and it is your responsibility to hold the possibility that this is happening and respond thoughtfully.

Participants may even present to treatment with a stance toward you that appears to be pathological paranoia, particularly during medicine sessions. However, this may in fact reflect an adaptive cautiousness about medical treatment born of their prior experiences of medical racism, a real phenomenon in which doctors provide inadequate or even harmful care to people from racial minority groups. Also, consider the possibility that Participants of Color may come to treatment with attitudes about mind-altering substances informed by the racist policies and outcomes favored by the War on Drugs, which may have led them to equate any substance use with the mass incarceration of members of their community.

Culture may also impact participants' attitudes toward having a therapist physically close to them, the amount of touch with which they are comfortable, their feelings about your instructions to "surrender" to the effects of the medicine, their relationship to emotional expression, or their discomfort with other aspects of treatment, such as anything that physically restrains them (e.g., headphones, eye mask).

Given that psychedelic experiences are heavily influenced by a participant's set and setting, the content of a participant's internal experience during a medicine session may reflect elements of their culture. Participants from cultural backgrounds that emphasize the importance of familial connections may experience types of intergenerational or ancestral healing that are not commonly considered due to our field's ethnocentric bias toward Western individualism. Participants from different cultures may also process their own personal traumas using different signifiers. One person might close their eyes and see threatening visions of snakes, while another might see dogs. An oceanic vision of water may mean oneness to some and danger to others.

Finally, consider that when treatment ends, a participant's cultural and social location (e.g., race, class) may impact their prognosis, as they may be reentering various forms of oppression that impact their well-being. These are some, but not all, of the concerns that you should keep in mind when aspiring to work in a culturally humble way that avoids replicating oppressions in PAT treatment in order to make this work safe and accessible for all.

Still, it is important to emphasize again the importance of seeking additional training in order to work in a culturally humble manner. Becoming a therapist who is truly competent in this regard requires a lifelong dedication to learning and growing one's self-awareness so that preconceptions can be more and more effectively bracketed. We encourage readers to explore additional supports for this process, including professional training, dedicated support groups, and guided self-reflective practices.

We would also like to acknowledge that the provision of culturally competent care, while crucial, does not obviate the continued need for cultural adaptations of PAT (Williams et al., 2020). The homogeneity of participant pools in many psychedelic studies (Davis et al., 2020) has undermined the generalizability of the therapy protocols used in these studies and the outcomes they have elicited to a diverse range of potential participants. Greater inclusivity in all aspects of PAT research is still needed in order to create approaches that are responsive to the needs of participants across a broader spectrum of social locations.

Ethically Rigorous Care

> *My own kind of psychological issues, personal issues or whatever, I am responsible for keeping an eye on all of that and ensuring that my blind spots, my needs and desires, whatever, are not infiltrating the relationship in an unconscious way.*
>
> —Psychedelic guide (Brennan et al., 2021)

The relational ethical challenges found in PAT are either unique to psychedelic work or they are meaningful intensifications of challenges found in traditional psychotherapy. As a result, even having completed standard ethics trainings, therapists are likely to enter this work lacking the training and expertise required to respond to these challenges in a way that prevents relational harm to participants. This book includes attentiveness to the unique relational risks (Anderson et al., 2020b; Brennan et al., 2021; Harlow, 2013, as cited in Passie, 2018, p. 12; Johnson, 2020; McNamee et al., 2023; Northrup, 2019; Taylor, 2017) that arise when psychedelic medicines are introduced into a therapeutic relationship, including:

Suggestibility. After taking a psychedelic medicine, participants enter a state of heightened suggestibility for the duration of its effects (Carhart-Harris et al., 2015; Dupuis, 2021; Dupuis & Veissière, 2022; Sjoberg & Hollister, 1965). They become less able to use their discernment about incoming information, which renders them more easily influenced by your instructions and suggestions. This creates an exaggerated power dynamic to which you must remain exquisitely attentive when making interpretations or suggesting activities.

Touch. Historically, touch-based interventions have been considered an integral component of PAT medicine sessions (Eisner, 1967; Grof, 1980; Martin, 1964). The use of supportive touch has been considered a helpful resource for some participants, though it also introduces a novel source of risk of harm (Devenot et al., 2022b; McNamee et al., 2023). The use of touch is particularly complicated given a participant's suggestible state, in which their autonomy is impaired and they are unable to consent to interventions that were not previously agreed upon. The important topic of touch will be covered in its own section in Chapter 4.

Amplified therapist–participant dynamics. Therapist–participant interactions under the influence of a psychedelic medicine tend to contain a heightened frequency and intensity of relational phenomena such as transferences, projections, and enactments (Brennan et al., 2021). In other words, the dynamics found in PAT treatment are more likely than those in traditional talk therapy to be influenced by the participant's past experiences in relationships, which could set the stage for harmful transgressions.

As discussed earlier in the "Trauma-Informed Care" section, these enactments of past relationships may include traumatic dynamics. In addition, other past relational dynamics that did not involve abuse or violence, such as those around unmet developmental needs for love or validation from caregivers, can also be embedded in the therapeutic relationship. While these phenomena are present in traditional therapy, they may be more likely to arise in PAT, perhaps because psychedelic experiences elicit and amplify these challenging dynamics. Simultaneously, the course of psychedelic therapy is often much shorter than ongoing therapy, so the clinical "runway" is compressed for working through such therapist–participant dynamics, which creates a greater risk of unskillful and thus potentially harmful interactions. See "Relational: Medicine Session" in Chapter 6 for further discussion.

Dynamics that could foster harmful dependency. This particular dynamic deserves special mention. If a participant travels to a difficult emotional place during a medicine session and you are present as their only lifeline, this may create the conditions for them to develop a strong sense of dependency on you. This could lead to significant distress and deterioration when treatment (and your relationship with them) comes to an end (McNamee et al., 2023). This risk of harm should be attended to throughout treatment through clarifying expectations and favoring interventions that support participant autonomy over dependence.

Challenges to one's professional role. A participant under the influence of a psychedelic medicine may experience a loosened sense of identity, role, and interpersonal boundaries. While in this state, they may invite you to take on a more flexible professional stance than that to which you are accustomed. They may encourage you to be more "human" (i.e., less formal or distant) during the session. They may ask you personal questions. They may exhibit a kind of radical openness that you may feel inspired to match. If you respond unthoughtfully to such events, it may confuse the relational frame of the treatment and cause relational harm to the participant, such as encouraging unrealistic expectations of the relationship.

Minimizing relational harm in the face of these and other challenges requires a range of added considerations that are woven throughout this book. However, we again emphasize the importance of additional ethical development beyond the contents of this book, including further training in psychotherapeutic ethics, further training in PAT-specific ethics, ongoing clinical supervision, peer consultation, and a range of other activities that support you in your own personal development (see Chapter 4 for further discussion).

> **ETHICS: DON'T GO IT ALONE**
>
> While *EMBARK Psychedelic Therapy* offers a fair amount of guidance on how individual PAT practitioners can practice ethically, this is only one part of what it means to provide ethically rigorous care. A truly comprehensive approach to minimizing relational harm must include preventative measures at other levels of care beyond the scope of this book, such as organizational and cultural levels. Still, there is much you can do as a practitioner to contribute to this broader vision of how to protect participants:
>
> - Avoid working in isolation
> - Ensure that you are working within an accountability structure that your participants know how to access
> - Participate in regular supervision or peer consultation groups. EMBARK faculty member and PAT ethics expert Kylea Taylor recommends finding or creating a group that supports you in being vulnerable with your peers and developing your self-awareness (Taylor, 2024).
> - Avoid organizational dynamics that favor unaccountability (e.g., hierarchical dynamics where those who accrue power are beyond reproach)

Collective Care

> *There could be a workshop after a retreat, giving you a different perspective. Exploring broader perspectives of what it means to be happy and healthy, the intrinsic relationship between individual health and the health of communities, societies, cultures and environments. Not only this individualistic, neoliberal tendency to put all the weight and responsibility on the individual—"change your lifestyle, make better personal choices, heal your trauma."*
>
> —Adam Aronovich (quoted in Evans, 2023a)

The underlying causes of the struggles and symptoms that bring PAT participants into treatment are not entirely locatable in the personal and biological conditions of their lives. The fields of medicine and psychology have become increasingly attentive to the fact that these micro-level conditions are heavily influenced by the macro-level or structural conditions of the society in which participants live. These societal factors include discrimination built into governing institutions (e.g., legal systems, policing), inequities in access to resources (e.g., housing, medical care, work, social services), structural deficits in community cohesion and mutual support, and systemic inattentiveness to those with increased needs (e.g., those with disabilities, the elderly).

Collective care means supporting the well-being of participants in a durable and maximally effective way by expanding the focus of therapeutic work beyond the individual to the systems and structures in which they are embedded.

In the EMBARK model, we strive to avoid an overly individual, pathologizing approach to conceptualizing and addressing a participant's struggles. For example, a participant named "Ksenia" presents with low mood, lack of motivation, difficulty concentrating, and feelings of worthlessness. The therapist diagnoses Ksenia with major depressive disorder and considers individual factors in the etiology and treatment of the depression. However, if the therapist does not consider the broader systemic or structural factors impacting the client, they might miss crucial elements contributing to the client's depression. Ksenia may be facing chronic job insecurity or financial stress, or perhaps she's dealing with the impact of ongoing discrimination based on her race, sexual orientation, or gender identity. In this case, the therapist's narrow focus on individual factors—interpreting the depression as a disorder rooted solely within the individual—ignores the influence of these larger systemic stressors. Ksenia's depressive symptoms might not be simply an individual pathology but could also be a reasonable response to ongoing external pressures and injustices. By acknowledging these systemic pressures, the therapist can help Ksenia understand her depression within a broader context, reducing feelings of personal blame and shame, and mobilize an expanded set of resources for intervention.

This expanded focus should be present throughout the work, including in codetermining the most supportive actions both you and the participant can take after the end of treatment. For some participants whose depression has roots in the collective conditions they face, this may entail their participation in collective organizing toward bringing about changes in these shared conditions. You are also asked to consider, as part of your support of the participants with whom you work, engaging in your own form of action that supports this type of collective-level change.

This more collective notion of working toward wellness may seem at odds with psychedelic healing practices. However, if one were to look at the spectrum of ways in which psychedelics have been used for healing across time and space, it would become clear that this approach is more the norm than the aberration. Western psychology is unique in its hyper-individualistic focus on the question of how to support wellness (Davies, 2021; Prilleltensky, 1994; St. Aime, in press). If PAT inherits this bias, it is to its own detriment (Brennan, 2020; Davies et al., 2023). Many indigenous forms of psychedelic healing, such as the various *vegetalista* traditions in the Peruvian Amazon (Marcus, 2022), see wellness as something that hinges less on something that is purely inside the participant and more on the myriad relationships they have with the world around them (Katz, 2017). Others have used psychedelic substances for perceived collective benefit as part of rituals or the divination of information that is of benefit to the entire community.

While EMBARK is still very much based in a Western psychological framework, it incorporates a modicum of collective focus in its clinical approach by asking therapists to attend to structural factors during treatment and inviting them to broaden their role and become more holistic advocates for the participants they have committed to serve (see "Integration—Spheres of Integration" in Chapter 7).

THE IMPORTANCE OF STRUCTURAL COMPETENCE

Failing to attend to the structural factors that influence patients can lead us to miss the bigger picture of their suffering and may reduce our ability to provide meaningful support. Figure 2.3 is adapted from Neff and colleagues (2020). The shaded box reflects the most apparent aspects of a patient's presentation, while the solid arrows represent the sequence of life events that led up to their seeking treatment, and the dotted arrows represent the influence of "macro" or structural factors on this trajectory.

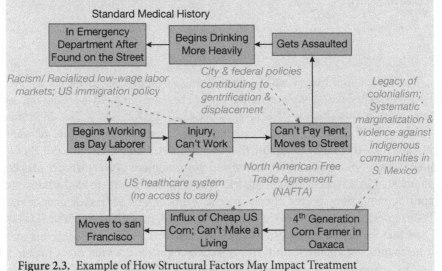

Figure 2.3. Example of How Structural Factors May Impact Treatment

HOW EMBARK'S COMPONENTS COME TOGETHER

To summarize, EMBARK has six clinical domains and four care cornerstones. The domains are: Existential–Spiritual, Mindfulness, Body-Aware, Affective–Cognitive, Relational, and Keeping Momentum. The four cornerstones of care are Trauma-Informed Care, Culturally Competent Care, Ethically Rigorous Care, and Collective Care. Together, this 6 + 4 design is the clinical architecture of EMBARK.

The following figure visually summarizes how this architecture forms the basis for each EMBARK adaptation for a specific drug applied to a specific clinical indication:

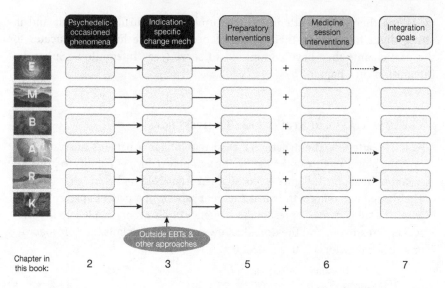

Each adaptation begins with a consideration of the phenomena occasioned by the psychedelic substance being used. They are grouped by domain, as they were in this chapter ("EMBARK's Six Clinical Domains"). The clinicians adapting EMBARK then review existing EBTs, other approaches, and relevant literature for the indication being treated. They determine which known therapeutic change mechanisms associated with the treatment of this disorder may be augmented by effects of the psychedelic medicine and use them as the basis for crafting indication-specific change mechanisms for this EMBARK adaptation. For example, a research team treating generalized anxiety disorder with LSD may posit that the drug could facilitate cognitive restructuring and develop this into a mechanism of change within the Affective-cognitive domain. See Chapter 3 for the change mechanisms associated with the EMBARK approach found in this book.

These putative change mechanisms across the six clinical domains then serve as the basis for the therapeutic approach throughout all three phases of treatments. In essence, therapists work with the participant to create the conditions of maximal likelihood that these mechanisms result from the participant's experience with the psychedelic medicine. Importantly, it is not expected that all mechanisms will come into play for each participant. Instead, each unique course of treatment will likely favor one or a few of these mechanisms. The mechanisms that arise as important for a participant are not willfully selected by either them or their therapist. They arise out of the mostly unpredictable interplay between the participant's unique psychological makeup and the effects of the psychedelic substance they have taken.

Accordingly, therapists and participants alike maintain a degree of agnosticism about the path that a course of treatment will take during the preparation phase and medicine session. Their work with a participant in preparation and medicine sessions is largely focused on preparing them to potentially benefit from any one (or a few) of the full range of change mechanisms. This work is reflected in the therapist aims found throughout Chapters 5 & 6.

Once the medicine session happens, this agnosticism is put aside. The integration phase begins with the therapist and participant using the medicine session as the basis for deciding which change mechanisms came into play and how to best support their continued unfolding. This will differ greatly for participants, and these differences can be meaningfully structured around the six EMBARK domains. Some may have a medicine session experience that emphasized the E, A, and R domains, while another may favor M and B. Participants and their therapists can then work toward the integration goals within the domains that arose as a way to focus the rest of their treatment in the place that is most relevant for them. Every EMBARK adaptation should thus include a full stable of integration goals across all six domains that align with the respective change mechanisms. See Chapter 7 for the integration goals found in this book's approach.

Navigating an Example Course of Treatment

With all of its domains and cornerstones and treatment goals and therapist aims, EMBARK can seem like a lot to learn. However, EMBARK-trained therapists who have put the approach into action in real-world settings have found it to be more streamlined and common-sense than it initially appeared. They report that the 6 + 4 slip into the background of their clinical thinking, like a helpful mnemonic structure rather than a checklist that requires diligent attention. This section will weave a fictional, yet representative story about a course of EMBARK treatment that will hopefully provide a sense of how the model works in practice.

A participant named "Tuấn", who has been diagnosed with MDD, is scheduled to come in for his first preparation session two weeks from now to start his journey through a course of PAT treatment that includes one medicine session in a local clinic. His therapist, Sandra, uses this window of time to go through the considerations in Chapter 4 ("Considerations Prior to Meeting with a Participant"). Meanwhile, Tuấn is going through his medical and psychological screening, which indicates that he is an appropriate candidate for PAT.

PREPARATION SESSIONS
Just prior to the first preparation session, Sandra reviews the chapter on preparation (Chapter 5), which provides her with support in conducting preparation sessions. It contains therapist aims to complete before the end of the preparation phase in order to create a container that is safe and facilitative of therapeutic benefit. Most of aims are basic ones that Sandra would do anyway as a therapist, but they include some PAT-specific interventions, such as working on skills that will support Tuấn in his medicine session. At this point in the treatment, neither

Sandra nor Tuấn are expected to have any sense of which of the six EMBARK clinical domains might emerge as most important to his treatment. So, Sandra goes into preparation with the overarching intention of setting Tuấn up to benefit from any of them. Sandra makes a printout for herself of Appendices B and C, which serve as cheat sheets that support her throughout treatment. Appendix B reminds her of all the therapist aims she needs to accomplish in each phase of treatment, and Appendix C serves as a general reminder of how she can support healing across the six EMBARK clinical domains.

However, the part of the manual Sandra treats as her North Star for the first preparation session is the agenda provided in the chapter on preparation (Chapter 5). It lays out a suggested, ready-made plan for the session that incorporates some of the therapist aims. Still, she finds it helpful to spend time reviewing the section of Chapter 5 titled "Working Within the EMBARK Clinical Domains," since it gives her a deeper sense of what the agenda is asking her to do and includes ethical considerations based on EMBARK's four care cornerstones.

The first preparation session goes well. Both parties feel good about the prospect of continuing treatment together. Although Sandra does a lot of listening to Tuấn during this session, she also does some educating about the treatment and answering whatever questions Tuấn has. Sandra keeps in mind that, because her role in preparation is to lay the groundwork for the full range of outcomes that Tuấn might experience during later phases of treatment, it requires her to be a bit more focused on skill-building and psychoeducation than she will be during the medicine or integration sessions, where she will shift into following Tuấn and what arises for him a lot more.

During the second preparation session, Sandra checks in with Tuấn to see if he has learned any self-regulation practices in previous courses of therapy. It turns out that he learned a technique known as square breathing, which they discuss and practice together as a resource that either of them can call upon should Tuấn need to ground himself at any point during treatment.

Next, Sandra guides Tuấn through a basic somatic awareness practice as a way to strengthen his ability to attend to his internal experience during the medicine session. The manual provides an example script that can be used, but Sandra prefers to use one with which she is more comfortable. She sees her orientation as primarily cognitive-behavioral and leads a weekly DBT skills group. Given what she's learned about Tuấn's history and level of functioning, she decides to incorporate a somatic awareness practice that she has found to be effective in her work with other participants. Before the session, she ensures that this substitution is okay to do by reviewing the guidelines for this aim set out in the chapter on preparation (Chapter 5). She determines that her exercise fits those guidelines, so she uses it rather than the example provided in the agenda.

The third preparation session goes smoothly as well. In this session, Sandra is asked to help Tuấn understand the importance of moving toward challenging feelings with self-compassion. She decides to discuss this topic with Tuấn using the language of DBT, since that is most familiar to her. Again, she checks the preparation guidelines and ensures that her approach falls within them.

Sandra and Tuấn also spend some time in this session checking in to see how Tuấn currently feels about his connection with Sandra going into the medicine session together. Tuấn names that he sometimes wonders if Sandra is judging him. Sandra welcomes this disclosure. They work through it together until Tuấn feels that it has been processed to the point where he can notice it and explore it with curiosity, either in his internal experience or out loud with Sandra, if it arises during the medicine session.

MEDICINE SESSION

The medicine session is just a few days away. Sandra returns to Chapter 4 to go over some of the considerations that pertain most to the medicine session. She prepares the space and develops a playlist. She gives special attention to the sections on the development of therapeutic presence. She assesses whether anything might be impeding her ability to provide an appropriate presence and takes steps to address this using some of the suggestions in Appendix A.

Sandra reviews the chapter on medicine sessions (Chapter 6). She refers to the agenda for a list of specific steps she can take to start the session. She also reviews the "Working Within the EMBARK Domains" section for a broad understanding of her role in supporting benefit. Sandra also takes time to review the sections on basic interventions and responding to common/challenging events that may arise. These sections provide specific, concrete advice on what to do while Tuấn is experiencing the effects of the medicine.

During the medicine session, Tuấn has a powerful experience. After experiencing some initial nausea, he spends a good deal of time silently folding his hands in front of his face in a pose that looks like prayer. During this time, Sandra refrains from interfering while remaining quietly present to what is unfolding for Tuấn. She begins to think to herself that something spiritual is unfolding for Tuấn and notes that she will explore this possibility with him during his first integration session. In the meantime, she recalls the guidance provided for working in the E domain in the "Working Within the EMBARK Domains" section of the chapter on medicine sessions (Chapter 6) and uses it to support the maintenance of a therapeutic container that facilitates fruitful spiritual experiences, in case that is what is happening for Tuấn.

Later in the medicine session, Tuấn starts crying. The crying gradually turns to sobs that continue for 20 minutes. Sandra thinks back to the guidance provided in the section on responding to common events in the chapter on medicine sessions (Chapter 6) and decides to offer support to Tuấn. He appreciates this and takes her hand, though he makes it clear that he does not want to discuss the content of what he is going through. Sandra respects this and provides him with a supportive presence as he continues to sob for another 10 minutes or so. In her mind, Sandra is realizing that his strong emotional opening likely falls within the Affective–Cognitive domain, and his acceptance of support from her falls within the Relational domain. She tries to recall the guidelines provided for working within these two domains in the chapter on medicine sessions (Chapter 6) and puts this information in dialogue with her spontaneously arising sense of how to work with Tuấn. She also notes that it may be worth exploring integration goals in these domains (as well as the E domain) during the integration phase. The medicine session ends, Tuấn is deemed safe to go home with the support of his designated support person, and all parties leave.

Sandra takes down some written notes that will help her remember the important elements of what occurred. She notes that the E, A, and R domains may be salient. She looks at Appendix D, a worksheet for selecting from suggested integration aims, to check if she overlooked any events that would suggest other domains and determines that she has not. Sandra engages in her go-to self-care practices after a long day of supporting Tuấn.

INTEGRATION SESSIONS

Prior to meeting with Tuấn for the first integration session, Sandra reviews the chapter on integration (Chapter 7). She meets with Tuấn for the first integration session and invites him to discuss whatever feels most important to him from the medicine session. He talks about his strong emotional opening, telling Sandra that this was the first time he ever felt like he got the chance to grieve the end of his first marriage, which he also felt allowed him to forgive himself for a lot that happened in that relationship. With his consent, Sandra helps Tuấn explore this self-forgiveness with an eye toward how it has impacted his depressive symptoms. She highlights the courage he displayed in his willingness to engage with such a challenging source of grief and invites him to explore how he could draw from this experience to find similar ways to make room for hard feelings in his day-to-day life.

When Sandra feels it makes sense clinically, she brings up the handholding. She asks Tuấn about what it was like to have someone present with him during that moment of grief. This serves as a springboard for an exploration of his difficulty in accepting support from others. They both agree that this would be another important area, in addition to the areas of self-forgiveness and learning to approach challenging emotions, that they could work on further during the remaining integration sessions.

Sandra realizes that Tuấn hasn't said anything about the seemingly spiritual moment he had earlier in the session. Without using any leading questions, she asks him what was happening for him as he lay still with his hands folded in front of him. He reports that he was navigating some very challenging nausea during that moment and needed to stay focused on his breathing so that he wouldn't vomit. Sandra realizes that her assumptions were incorrect and pivots away from the E domain and toward the integration aims found in the B domain. Tuấn is invited to discuss this moment of nausea, but he does not feel that it was a very significant moment for his treatment. Sandra appreciates this and refrains from pursuing it further.

In the remaining two integration sessions, Sandra draws from the suggestions in the "Suggested Integration Goals" section of the chapter on integration (Chapter 7) in order to support Tuấn in moving toward the goals in the A and R domains that he feels follow naturally from his medicine session experience.

The discussions between her and Tuấn explore the new opportunities for healing and growth that feel like natural evolutions of his experience. Collaboratively, they discuss new habits and practices he would like to take on to sustain these opportunities, as well as any new ways of engaging with the contexts around him—personal relationships, his workplace, and so on—that may also support his continued healing and growth.

During integration, they collaboratively assess what, if any, forms of posttreatment support would be most helpful for Tuấn. He decides he would like to begin working with a weekly therapist on the grief he got in touch with during his medicine session. Sandra provides him with referrals and helps him set up a first appointment with a therapist he feels good about. They share a heartfelt acknowledgement of the brief, yet profound healing journey they went on together and bid each other farewell.

3

EMBARK Mechanisms of Change in the Treatment of Depression

*Antonin Artaud wrote on one of his drawings, "Never real and always true,"
and that is how depression feels. You know that it is not real, that you are
someone else, and yet you know that it is absolutely true.*

—ANDREW SOLOMON, PhD

How might a depressed participant benefit from a course of psychedelic therapy?
This chapter details how the EMBARK model approaches the treatment of
depression.

This chapter introduces the 12 suggested mechanisms of change that structure
the EMBARK approach to treating depression. All but one are based on therapeutic mechanisms drawn from existing, nonpsychedelic therapies used to treat
depression, while the 12th (mystical experience) is a commonly observed mediator of antidepressant outcomes in PAT research. These 12 mechanisms were
selected for their relevance to commonly observed outcomes of PAT treatment
for depression and their ability to meaningfully map onto and inform therapeutic
responses to the common psychedelic treatment events detailed in the last chapter.
The EBTs and other therapies that informed these 12 mechanisms are described in
a later section of this chapter ("Outside Therapies Used in this Manual").

Importantly, these suggested mechanisms should not be seen as the full gamut
of ways in which benefit may arise in PAT. Psychedelic therapy is a new modality
that may introduce mechanisms of its own that we have yet to conceptualize.
You are very likely to find at some point in your practice that a participant is
benefitting from treatment in a way that does not fall into any of the 12 suggested
mechanisms. When this happens, refrain from trying to corral them into these
12 mechanisms or any a priori sense of what their experience means. These
suggested mechanisms are just that—suggestions. A later section in this chapter
("Other Potentially Beneficial Participant Experiences") discusses some common

EMBARK Psychedelic Therapy for Depression. Bill Brennan and Alex Belser, Oxford University Press.
© Oxford University Press 2024. DOI: 10.1093/9780197762622.003.0004

participant experiences that may lead to benefit but do not map onto any existing EBT's mechanism of change.

While this chapter should not be seen as a comprehensive roll call of all of the ways in which benefits could arise in PAT, it provides a suggested set of lenses for conceptualizing benefit in PAT treatment. These lenses were designed to connect with existing psychotherapeutic theories of change and thereby offer opportunities for you to use the prior therapeutic skills, knowledge, and interventions you bring into this work.

A HOLISTIC VIEW OF DEPRESSION

Clinically significant depression impacts the lives of millions. In 2020, approximately 21 million adults in the United States experienced a major depressive episode (Substance Abuse and Mental Health Services Administration [SAMHSA], 2020). Major depressive disorder (MDD) is the leading cause of disability in Americans between the age of 15 and 44 (SAMHSA, 2020). Its prevalence has increased since 2005 (Proudman et al., 2021). Existing interventions are ineffective for a substantial subset of those afflicted (Cuijpers et al., 2020). Considering the limitations of existing treatments, might we find hope in the emerging field of psychedelic-assisted therapy (PAT)?

Psilocybin-assisted therapy has shown preliminary efficacy in treating both MDD and treatment-resistant depression (TRD) (Carhart-Harris et al., 2021; Davis et al., 2021; von Rotz et al., 2022), as well as depressive symptoms related to a cancer diagnosis (Griffiths et al., 2016; Ross et al., 2016). These studies show large effect sizes and impressive rates of response and remission compared to conventional antidepressant treatments.

The EMBARK approach in this manual was developed for use in a clinical trial investigating the treatment of MDD. However, its applicability is not limited to people who meet specific criteria for this diagnosis. Depression is more usefully conceptualized as a set of symptoms that often cluster together—anhedonia, lack of motivation, decreased energy, poor self-concept, sleep disturbances, and so on—and that can be present in the absence of a formal diagnosis or coexist with a range of other diagnoses. The field is moving toward transdiagnostic approaches with the advent of the research domain criteria (RDoC) framework, a research initiative by the National Institute of Mental Health (NIMH), and efforts such as the Unified Protocol in CBT treatment, which can be applied transdiagnostically to different disorders and problems (Farchione et al., 2012). The approach in this book (and PAT in general; Kelly et al., 2021) may lead to improvements in symptoms in a way that transcends any specific diagnostic category.

We invite you to apply the treatment approach in this book in a way that is responsive to the specific symptoms and struggles of the participant with whom you are working. Depression is a multifaceted disruption of functioning that may impact many aspects of a participant's life, such as their beliefs about themselves, their interpersonal relationships, their emotional self-regulation capacities, and their lived sense of their body. It is also a disorder with a complicated etiological picture, as there are likely many constellations of genetic, developmental, and cultural factors that could contribute to one becoming depressed. The diversity and complexity of depressive presentations require a flexible, participant-centered approach.

The deeply personal nature of psychedelic experiences makes PAT an approach well suited to meet this need. If the participant is properly prepared, the experience brought about by administering psilocybin to them may open up trajectories of healing that are matched to their unique experience of depression. It is generally believed that PAT brings about therapeutic outcomes not by exerting a stereotyped set of effects on every individual but by opening the door for that person's innate healing wisdom to—in a context of skillful therapeutic support—go where it needs to go and do what it needs to do. For some, the work of therapy will be about feeling and understanding long-avoided emotions. For others, the process may center around reconnecting with spirit. Others still might find what they need by connecting with you from within the open and vulnerable state that the medicine puts them in.

In EMBARK, you are asked to engage participants collaboratively and flexibly in a broad range of ways that responds to the diverse, multifaceted nature of depression. Prominent MDMA-assisted psychotherapy researcher Michael Mithoefer (2018) summarized this by saying that "the therapist must strive to allow and encourage each patient to create a new therapy for themselves." To do this, therapists take a stance characterized by flexibility, responsiveness, adaptiveness, and respect for participants' autonomy and wisdom about what is best for them.

The EMBARK model was created to support these precise qualities. Its six clinical domains allow for a diversity of possible ways to conceptualize and support each participant's unique therapeutic path.

SUGGESTED MECHANISMS OF CHANGE WITHIN EACH CLINICAL DOMAIN

The 12 suggested mechanisms of change include the following:

Existential–Spiritual	• Mystical experiences
	• Spiritual self-development
Mindfulness	• Freedom from rumination
	• A more flexible identity
	• Greater compassion for oneself
Body-Aware	• Embodiment and enlivenment
	• Somatic trauma processing
Affective–Cognitive	• Transforming emotions and updating core beliefs
	• Increased acceptance of emotions
Relational	• Relational repatterning
	• Increased interpersonal connectedness
Keeping Momentum	• Building motivation for beneficial new habits and other life changes

Do not be alarmed by the quantity (12) of these possible mechanisms and what this might imply for your role in supporting them. As noted earlier, each individual's course of treatment will lead them down their own unique path, which will likely only include a small number (one to four) of these mechanisms. A participant will almost never require active support across all of these mechanisms.

In a course of treatment, the specific mechanisms are not selected at the start. In fact, they are not "selected" at all, either by you or by the participant—they are emergent during the course of treatment. The mechanisms can be recognized and worked with collaboratively. Your aim, in part, is to support the participant in receiving benefit in the ways associated with those specific mechanisms. The rest of this manual has been designed to provide a streamlined and user-friendly way of doing just that.

Existential–Spiritual Mechanisms of Change

> *[The psilocybin] just opens you up and it connects you . . . everything is interwoven, and that's a big relief . . . I think it does help you accept death because you don't feel alone, you don't feel like you're going to, I don't know, go off into nothingness. That's the number one thing—you're just not alone.*
> —Erin (Belser et al., 2017; Swift et al., 2017)

MYSTICAL EXPERIENCES
Many individuals who undergo PAT report having profound mystical or spiritual experiences as described in the previous chapter. To date, several clinical trials that have found evidence for the efficacy of psilocybin in treating either treatment-resistant depression or cancer-related depression also discovered that the antidepressant benefit was mediated by the intensity of the mystical phenomena that were elicited during the medicine session (Carhart-Harris et al., 2018a; Griffiths et al., 2016; Roseman et al., 2018; Ross et al., 2016). Roseman and colleagues (2018) examined this further and found that two dimensions of the Altered States Questionnaire (ASQ), "oceanic boundlessness" and "dread of ego dissolution," were found to be more predictive of positive treatment outcomes than other ASQ dimensions that captured perceptual effects.

The exact mechanism of therapeutic benefit is not entirely understood, but it is proposed that these experiences may lead to significant shifts in perspective and values, reduced egocentrism, improved self-efficacy, and increased openness, which can all contribute to psychological well-being. Although there is no way to guarantee the occurrence of a mystical experience, you can provide a therapeutic context in which your participant is more likely to experience a profound religious, spiritual, or mystical experience by incorporating emerging best practice guidelines (such as those in this book). Preparedness for psychedelic medicine sessions been found to be associated with beneficial mystical experiences (McAlpine et al., 2023).

Be wary of chalking up clinical benefit to any single mechanism: in one study of cancer-related distress, only 13% of the variability in depression was explained by the mediating influence of the mystical experience. That means that 87% of depression improvement was attributable to other unknown mechanisms (Griffiths et al., 2016).

Summary: Participants may experience profound mystical experiences that come in a variety of forms. Such experiences can profoundly change their worldview about the nature of reality and may have a variety of downstream effects. You can help participants prepare for and integrate these experiences by not neglecting spiritual counseling work in the session.

Associated EBTs and other clinical approaches: Spiritually, existentially, religiously, and theologically-integrated (SERT) psychotherapy approaches (Palitsky et al., 2023), spiritual guidance (Miller et al., 2008), also known as spiritual evocation (Miller, 2004)

SPIRITUAL SELF-DEVELOPMENT

In previous studies, many participants—often a majority—evaluated their psychedelic medicine session experiences as spiritually significant events (e.g., Griffiths et al., 2006). When Griffiths and colleagues (2018) provided their participants with support in cultivating ongoing spiritual practices, both before and after the psilocybin session, this enhanced the beneficial outcomes they obtained from treatment, such as positive behavior changes and prosocial attitudes, beyond those of a group that did not receive this added support. As such, you are invited to collaboratively work with a PAT participant who comes away from their medicine session with a desire to cultivate some element of their spiritual life—a new practice, a deepened faith—as an important part of the integration phase of treatment.

Summary: PAT participants may wish to develop their spiritual life posttreatment. This may support positive outcomes. Support them in doing so, particularly in ways that bring other people into the process with them.

Associated EBTs and other clinical approaches: SERT-integrated psychotherapy approaches (Palitsky et al., 2023), spiritual guidance (Miller et al., 2008), also known as spiritual evocation (Miller, 2004)

Mindfulness Mechanisms of Change

> *The other piece of it that's changed was just this connection with this place that I can go to in myself and find peace and comfort. That when I'm feeling anxious I can tap into through meditation, going back and listening to the music again, you know, it's like, you can't take that away from me now. It's there. So, I am changed by this. And in pretty significant ways.*
> —Brenda (Belser et al., 2017; Swift et al., 2017)

There are three proposed mechanisms within the M domain. They can often be found over the course of PAT in individuals who report feeling more mindful and less automatized. Benefits seem to begin when the participant steps out of their habitual mental processes and ordinary sense of self in order to take a more "bird's eye" or "witness consciousness" perspective. These mechanisms have been conceptualized using different terminology as aspects of "psychological flexibility" by Watts and Luoma (2020).

FREEDOM FROM RUMINATION

Rumination is a symptom present in many people's experiences of depression. Nolen-Hoeksema and colleagues (1997) define rumination as "passively and repetitively focusing on one's symptoms of distress and the circumstances surrounding these symptoms" (p. 855). Engaging in this behavior can augment depression in a number of ways. Rumination can promote avoidance of more constructive forms of problem-solving and strengthen negative self-beliefs. Through these and other mechanisms, rumination can both maintain depression and trigger relapses for individuals in remission. Disrupting this habitual behavior has therefore been proposed as an efficacious way of treating depression (Watkins, 2016).

Previous clinical trials where psilocybin-assisted therapy was given to individuals suffering from depression revealed its efficacy in offering a state of "mental freedom"—an escape from automated mental behaviors, or the "prison of the mind" (Watts & Luoma, 2020, p. 95). In place of these old habits, they discovered an enhanced mindfulness and a newfound capability to exert control over their mental activities and to limit the extent of their engagement in ruminative processes. Remarkably, these impacts were seen to persist for several weeks or even months following a session. If you notice that a participant experiences this break in this habitual mental behavior, it may be beneficial to work with them to use this window of newfound freedom to develop an enduring ability to minimize or interrupt rumination.

Summary: Rumination keeps people depressed and can drag them back into depression when they are feeling better. Psychedelic medicines may pause ruminative processes long enough for the participant to work with you on building skills to stop it from coming back.

Associated EBTs and other clinical approaches: Rumination-focused cognitive-behavioral therapy, mindfulness-based cognitive therapy, acceptance and commitment therapy, other mindfulness-based approaches

A MORE FLEXIBLE IDENTITY

Many who suffer from depression have a fixed, negative perception of themselves that is maintained by the habitual arising of self-critical beliefs (e.g., "I am a failure."). Because these beliefs arise automatically, they can become one's lens for interpreting the world and may come to feel like the inescapable truth of who one is. The strength of this overidentification may make it feel impossible for these individuals to "step outside" of these beliefs. They become a maladaptive, inflexible sense of self that serves to anchor the individual in their depression.

In mindfulness-based interventions, one key objective is often to foster a sense of detachment or nonidentification with one's thoughts and emotions. This is often referred to as developing an "observer" or "witness" perspective. It involves fostering an awareness of one's thoughts and emotions without judgment or resistance, which can lead to a more flexible, less rigid sense of self.

PAT treatment with psilocybin has been found to facilitate similar beneficial outcomes. In several studies (Belser et al., 2017; Watts et al., 2017; Watts & Luoma, 2020), participants have reported experiences of becoming more able to break out of their fixed identity and take a more flexible perspective on who they are. They became more able to identify with an expanded sense of self that was "bigger" than their habitual, self-critical self.

The psychedelic experience of breaking out of a fixed identity and taking on a more flexible perspective mirrors this concept in mindfulness and meditation. This maps onto key concepts in several psychotherapeutic approaches, such as "unblending" in internal family systems, "cognitive defusion" in ACT, and identifying and challenging core beliefs or schemas in CBT. If this experience arises for a participant during their medicine session, work with them during the integration phase to sustain this flexible sense of self and the distance from distressing self-beliefs that it provides.

Summary: People with MDD develop a rigid, negative sense of who they are. Psychedelic medicines may lift them out of this momentarily and give them a broader, less "stuck," less self-critical perspective on themselves, which can be durably sustained by supportive practices.

Associated EBTs and other clinical approaches: Mindfulness-based cognitive therapy, ACT, CBT for depression, other mindfulness-based approaches, internal family systems

GREATER COMPASSION FOR ONESELF

An added benefit that often follows the adoption of a more flexible identity is a greater ability to be self-compassionate. For some, it feels as if loosening the grip of the habitual, self-critical self allows other deeper, wiser parts of the self to come to the fore and provide self-compassion—often toward the self-critical parts of the psyche that have become relaxed (Watts & Luoma, 2020). This increased capacity for self-compassion has been found to occur in psychedelic-assisted psychotherapy with psilocybin (Agin-Liebes, 2020) and MDMA (van der Kolk et al., 2023). If worked with during the integration phase, these experiences can be developed into an enduring resource in a participant's struggles with depression.

Summary: Once a participant has broken free from their rigid, depressive identity with the aid of a psychedelic medicine, they may discover an ability to be compassionate toward the wounded, reactive, and self-critical parts within themselves. If this ability is sustained with appropriate practices, it can be an antidepressive resource going forward.

Associated EBTs and other clinical approaches: ACT, emotion-focused therapy (EFT), compassion-focused therapy, mindfulness-based approaches, internal family systems.

Body-Aware Mechanisms of Change

> *My fear just coalesced and I mentally saw it, it was right here, and it was a big black thing right there under my ribcage . . . my fear was there and I, I just was overcome with anger with rage, with rage that this thing was fucking me up and I screamed get the fuck out! Just get out, I evicted, I ejected the fear, and it was gone . . . The fear was gone.*
>
> —Edna (Belser et al., 2017; Swift et al., 2017)

EMBODIMENT AND ENLIVENMENT

Many symptoms of depression, sometimes called the neurovegetative symptoms, are physically manifested in the body: fatigue or energy loss, disruptions of sleep and appetite, weight gain or loss, psychomotor retardation or agitation, and abnormal bodily sensations. It has been suggested (Doerr-Zegers et al., 2017; Rønberg, 2019) that disturbances of one's lived experience of the body are the most fundamental and cross-culturally consistent MDD phenomena. Most often, the embodied experience of a depressed individual is characterized by a sense of heaviness, "deadness," and difficulty in initiating movement. Physically oriented therapies that aim to counteract these qualities through exercise, dance, or intentional movement have shown some efficacy in alleviating depression (Papadopolous & Röhricht, 2014).

Many depressed PAT participants have also indicated that their treatment experiences have alleviated this "deadness" and restored elements of their embodied experience. One qualitative analysis of participant experiences (Watts et al., 2017) found that they had a rich sensory-somatic quality and enabled participants to feel their emotions in their body to a greater extent than usual. Another qualitative analysis of PAT participants' psilocybin experiences (Belser et al., 2017) found that embodiment was a key theme in participant reports. In the authors' experience, PAT participants often leave medicine sessions feeling physically unburdened, as though they have "let go of something" or that something "lifted off" them. They often report that they feel "lighter" and livelier as a result.

These experiences of a renewed, clarified experience of one's body can be developed into sustained improvements in a participant's ability to remain "in their body" and attend to what is occurring in their embodied and emotional experience. In addition to reducing depression in and of itself, this improved interoceptive awareness can be the basis for an increased ability to attend to signals arising in the body that allow for greater emotional self-regulation, sense of grounding and safety, behavioral choice, and self-care. If a participant's experience centers on their relationship to their body, consider working with them during the integration phase to build upon this experience.

Summary: Individuals with MDD often have a de-energized experience of their bodies. A psychedelic medicine experience may leave them with an increased sense of embodiment and enlivenment that, if sustained with ongoing activity, can bring a range of benefits.

Associated EBTs and other clinical approaches: Body-oriented psychological therapies (e.g., sensorimotor psychotherapy, hakomi, somatic experiencing, focusing), dance movement psychotherapies

SOMATIC TRAUMA PROCESSING

It has become canonical to recognize that "the body keeps the score"—our bodies can carry the impact of our emotional experiences and traumas (Van der Kolk, 2014). Many depressed individuals have experienced trauma in their lives, so much so that it has been argued that the diagnostic distinction between depression and trauma should be revisited and a new hybrid trauma–depression condition proposed (Flory & Yehuda, 2022). At the level of the brain, MDD and PTSD show considerable similarities as well. In fact, trauma is a common comorbidity with MDD, as well as other psychiatric indications. So, when working with participants struggling with depression, you should be prepared to respond supportively should their medicine session experience take them in the direction of processing their trauma.

Although ongoing trials using psilocybin to treat PTSD have yet to report their results, psilocybin has long been used to purportedly facilitate trauma work taking place in "underground" contexts. Also, it has recently been suggested (Bird et al., 2021) that its disinhibiting effects on frontal-limbic neural circuits of emotional control are similar to those of MDMA, another psychedelic medicine with established efficacy in allowing traumatic memories to surface and be processed. Like MDMA, classic psychedelics such as psilocybin are generally thought to expand a participant's "window of tolerance" for trauma processing, allowing them to confront trauma-related material with less likelihood of becoming dissociated or disoriented.

In a PAT session, much of this processing may include somatic phenomena, such as trembling, shaking, facial expressions, vocalizing, or other movements, in addition to experiencing and/or discussing episodic memories. A number of somatic therapy modalities have identified these phenomena as forms of working through trauma memories in the body. This idea is based in the increasingly popular notion in trauma work that, when an individual experiences a trauma, the event is "remembered" by the body and the nervous system as a somatic memory in addition to episodic and emotional memories (Van der Kolk, 2014). Somatic therapy approaches to working with trauma take this as their starting point and view the elicitation of these somatic memories as part of resolving trauma.

Psychedelic-induced somatic trauma processing experiences may be relieving for many participants. They may represent a meaningful part of the therapeutic process for participants with trauma histories secondary to depression. Although you are not required to work proactively with these phenomena using any specific skills from a somatic modality, you should be prepared for the possibility that these events may arise and may contribute to therapeutic outcomes. In other words, do not be surprised if the participant begins shaking during a medicine session—instead, support the participant by providing favorable conditions for these phenomena to arise in a way that brings benefit rather than added harm.

Summary: Depressed individuals have often experienced trauma, so trauma and its resolution will likely be a part of some participants' PAT experience. Resolving this trauma may involve expressing it somatically. To do so, you do not need a great deal of expertise in working somatically for this to happen safely, but you should be prepared to respond supportively.

Associated EBTs and other clinical approaches: Somatic experiencing, hakomi, sensorimotor psychotherapy

Affective–Cognitive Mechanisms of Change

> *[I felt] this tremendous rage when I saw the fear, just rage. It was eating me alive. I said, "I won't be eaten alive!" . . . It was rage and then relief when the fear was gone and this overwhelming love and awe.*
> —Edna (Belser et al., 2017; Swift et al., 2017)

INCREASED ACCEPTANCE OF EMOTIONS

Feelings are hard to feel—especially the seemingly intolerable ones. Many individuals struggling with depression have experienced challenging feelings such as guilt, shame, hopelessness, or sadness, often to an overwhelming degree. A common depressive response to such feelings is to dim or deaden one's awareness of them through a kind of automatic, unconscious avoidance. This pulling away from one's emotions is often characterized as feeling withdrawn, numb, and "flattened" as often reported by depressed individuals.

Rather than framing it as "coping with depression," we might begin to think of "depression as coping" or depression as a type of adaptation. In hostile or invalidating home surroundings, participants might have learned to manage unbearable emotions by falling into a depressive state—downregulating both external stimuli (through isolation from people) and internal stimuli (by evading feelings with a flat or blunted emotional response). In some situations, shutting down is actually a way to survive. You may find that for certain participants, the emotional flatness characteristic of their depression may initially have been an adaptive response to a challenging environment but has now become maladaptive as their context has changed. It is motivated by a desire to avoid experiencing seemingly intolerable emotions. A parallel mechanism of avoidance may be at play for comorbid anxiety.

Another way that trauma can overlap with the emotional numbing of MDD is caused by the person never having learned, in early relationships, to attend to, recognize, name, and share emotional experiences with others. Not all alexithymia is avoidance; some is a lack of development of emotional awareness and complexity. For those participants, preparation and integration may require interventions and exercises that cultivate those emotional capacities for the first time.

Psychedelics may provide a temporary invitation to an "approach orientation" to difficult feelings; this may be one of the ways in which PAT elicits positive treatment outcomes (Bogenschutz et al., 2018; Watts et al., 2017; Watts & Luoma,

2020). Participants in PAT clinical trials have often found that they are able to step back from their avoidance and instead approach their emotions with greater acceptance (Wolff et al., 2020). In many cases, participants experience emotional breakthroughs (Roseman et al., 2019) that have been found to predict antidepressant benefit (Murphy et al., 2022).

You will likely find that most participants undergo intense and diverse emotions during their psychedelic experiences (Belser et al., 2017). If they find they are able to tolerate this extended emotional range, participants who have stronger-than-usual emotions may be able to adopt a sustained willingness to engage more with their emotions beyond the end of treatment. In addition to potentially lessening emotional flatness, this may also pave the way for an increased ability to identify, name, and respond adaptively to their emotions.

This expansion of their emotional capacities can bring forth numerous benefits associated with this type of enriched, integrated emotional life, including a sense of empowerment, mastery, resilience, new self-understanding, more confident beliefs about their ability to withstand challenging experiences, and the development of more adaptive forms of coping (Greenberg & Watson, 2006).

Summary: The constricted affect that is characteristic of depression is often due to an avoidant relationship with emotions. By supporting participants' capacity to open themselves to this content in a medicine session, you can help support affective breakthroughs that can be developed into durable posttreatment improvements in their emotional life.

Associated EBTs and other clinical approaches: EFT, ACT, CBT for depression, short-term dynamic psychotherapy

Transforming Emotions and Updating Core Beliefs

As noted above, participants often find that psilocybin gives them an enhanced ability to approach difficult emotions and beliefs about themselves with acceptance and self-compassion. Another potential benefit to doing this in a medicine session is that it allows for experiences that may lead to a durable transformation of these emotions and beliefs. When PAT participants allow themselves to more deeply experience a potent maladaptive emotion (e.g., shame) and the beliefs about themselves that accompany it (e.g., "I am unlovable."), they often find that a more adaptive emotional experience (e.g., self-forgiveness) arises, either on its own or with help from you, and that this comes with a new self-understanding that updates the maladaptive belief. Using the terminology of EFT, the participant can be seen as contacting their "primary adaptive emotions" or "core affect," leading to a type of corrective emotional experience that is directly relevant to their depressed self-concept (Greenberg & Watson, 2006).

Note that this mechanism may be linked to the Mindfulness domain mechanism of a more flexible identity, which focuses on the mindful aspect of developing distance from distressing self-beliefs, whereas this mechanism in the Affective–Cognitive domain is more focused on feeling and transforming core affects.

Summary: Participants who allow themselves to have a heightened experience of a maladaptive emotion may thereby "transform" this emotion and the associated beliefs about themselves into less depressogenic ones.

Associated EBTs and other clinical approaches: EFT, ACT, CBT for depression, short-term dynamic psychotherapy

Relational Mechanisms of Change

> *There was a bit of feeling of conflict, of misalignment. But that kind of dissipated because as soon as I started a sort of blissful connection that included them very much, I really enjoyed their presence for most of that day. . . . I was just really enjoying having them around. I was finding them just charming and funny and enjoyable to be around and I wanted more engagement with them. I wanted nothing more than to just chat and have more connection. I guess my feeling was connecting with people.*
>
> —Dan (Belser et al., 2017; Swift et al., 2017)

RELATIONAL REPATTERNING

In a medicine session, the relational dynamics between therapists and participants in PAT are altered and amplified in many unique ways. Many of these alterations reflect two central elements: a greater likelihood that aspects of the participant's past relational dynamics (i.e., "core scripts") will be played out in the therapeutic relationship and an acutely increased sensitivity to the therapist's responses that may increase the capacity for both healing and harm. In a sense, a PAT medicine session (and, to some extent, the rest of treatment) can be seen as a unique opportunity to make updates to the participant's core scripts for engaging with others.

For example, consider a participant who was neglected as a child. When they notice a small lapse in your ability to be fully present, they may respond toward you with expressions of emotions they felt or repressed in response to their earlier neglect. They may also respond with compensatory strategies they developed: rage, dejection, charming or seductive behaviors, desperation, cloying bids for attention, and so on. A skillful therapist response may call the participant's attention to the pattern, contextualize it, and respond in a way that gives them an opportunity to start moving toward more realistic expectations of others and the quality of care and presence they can provide.

Similar repatterning could occur in response to relational patterns that developed from a range of early life experiences: sexual abuse, experiences of abandonment, narcissistic parents, families that struggled with substance misuse, and so on. Any such pattern may be related to the core beliefs and emotions most commonly found in depression, such as worthlessness, perfectionism, unlovability, or the contingency of love and support. It is particularly common for PAT participants to have strong experiences of shame, and positive relational encounter with a therapist in these moments may offer a potent corrective experience.

Common factor interventions, such as providing empathy, respect, acceptance, genuineness, reassurance, trust, corrective emotional experiences, encouragement to face fears, and working through conflict, can all be catalyzed under the effects of a psychedelic medicine. PAT's heightened potential for relational repatterning offers a unique opportunity to use the therapeutic relationship in the service of treating depression.

Summary: PAT treatment may plasticize a participant's maladaptive rubrics for relating to others, allowing them to be updated in a way that has a therapeutic impact on their depression.

Associated EBTs and other clinical approaches: Relational psychodynamic approaches, interpersonal therapy, EFT, transference-focused therapy

INCREASED INTERPERSONAL CONNECTEDNESS

A key element of depression is social isolation, both actual and felt. This isolation may be based in (and reinforced by) an inability to enjoy social contact, a sense that there is something wrong or unacceptable about oneself (i.e., shame), or a belief that one deserves to be alone. It may also be based on the belief that, if one were to express their emotions (e.g., anger) in the presence of another person, they would risk losing their care and positive regard. Others may have developed a sense of defeat and demoralization around social relationships that leads them to feel that they cannot form relationships or that they are not worth the effort and energy it takes to sustain them. Finally, some depressed individuals may have no difficulty in forming and maintaining relationships with others, though they still feel disconnected.

PAT treatment may reduce a participant's isolation in several ways. For one, if they express emotions such as grief or anger more openly than usual during a medicine session and you respond with care, attentiveness, empathy, and nonjudgmental acceptance, this may upend their beliefs about the safety, value, or possibility of connecting deeply with others and increase their ability to do so in the future with other people. Experiences such as this can help the participant work through any feelings of shame or demoralization that are at the core of their unfulfilling social life. While this mechanism is present in most traditional therapies, its impact on the participant may be amplified in PAT due to the altered relational dynamics present (e.g., heightened sensitivity, transferences).

Even if a participant does not have such an experience with you, a medicine session may give rise to shifts in social cognition that, if built upon during integration sessions, could lead to improvements in their ability to connect with others. These include enduring postsession feelings of social connectedness and emotional empathy, which have been endorsed by PAT participants from previous studies (Carhart-Harris et al., 2018b; Pokorny et al., 2017). By themselves, they are just feelings. But working with them during integration sessions can help the participant become more secure in them and use them as the basis for an improved social life and/or increased openness to support from others.

Summary: A psychedelic medicine session may leave a participant feeling more able to connect with others in a more fulfilling way. You can help them develop this into the basis for reducing depressive isolation, demoralization, and disconnection.

Associated EBTs and other clinical approaches: Interpersonal therapy, motivational interviewing, compassion-focused therapy

Keeping Momentum Mechanisms of Change

Rather than having the [psychedelic-assisted] psychotherapy and then sending them home with a journal and some happy thoughts, what we really ought to be saying is that the therapeutic window is actually open for weeks, if not months, after the acute psychedelic effects have worn off. We need to treat that period of time as precious and have a lot of therapeutic activity during that window rather than just sending them off and letting them be on their own.

—Gül Dölen, MD, PhD, Associate Professor of Neuroscience,
Johns Hopkins University

BUILDING MOTIVATION FOR BENEFICIAL NEW HABITS AND OTHER LIFE CHANGES

Healing is not complete at the end of treatment. In fact, for some participants, the end of treatment may even be the most demanding phase. If psychedelic therapy opens up a critical learning window, it is a window for you to encourage the participant to give up old habits and begin making new habits. It is a time to learn how to make life changes. However, if a participant returns to a way of living that is underresourced, avoidant, or isolated, it is more likely that they will remain at or relapse to their baseline level of depression. In our experience, participants who benefit most in the long-term from treatment are the ones who take advantage of the acute postsession shifts in their experience to create a life that sustains them. This takes both motivation to change and a sustained commitment to doing so.

Thankfully, this crucial juncture for change is often matched by the strong feelings of motivation, clarity, possibility of change, self-efficacy, and commitment to pro-therapeutic changes that arise in PAT (Nielson et al., 2018). In addition, participants may emerge from treatment with an invigorating new set of values or a renewed sense of the values they previously held deeply. All of this, if elaborated on during integration, could form the basis for committed action (Watts & Luoma, 2020). If a participant experiences this type of increase in intrinsic motivation or (re)connection with motivating values, you can work with them to translate this value-driven motivation into the creation of new habits, new skills, and changes to their lived contexts.

Summary: Antidepressive outcomes from PAT may be transient if the participant is not supported in bringing their life into alignment with them. Help participants discover their motivation to make pro-therapeutic life changes and then help to plan and specifically enact them, especially by supporting participants to cultivate and maintain new habits of thinking, feeling, and acting in the world.

Associated EBTs and other clinical approaches: Motivational interviewing, CBT for depression, ACT, compassion-focused therapy

OTHER POTENTIALLY BENEFICIAL PARTICIPANT EXPERIENCES

> *Basically, it seemed like everything that had occurred to me since the day I was born, 'til that very moment, made sense. And not just sense, like . . . not in a rational way, but in . . . there seems like a more cosmic reason, whether it's the good or the bad . . . And then just rolling back all the experiences of my life. Whether it's a sprained ankle, or a delicious meal, or my marriage, or the children, or the clothes I've bought all my life, every meal I've eaten.*
> —Caleb (Belser et al., 2017; Swift et al., 2017)

This section briefly describes several other common treatment experiences that PAT participants have described as supportive to them in their struggles with depression. Although they do not present a clear mechanism of change that overlaps with any of the EBTs we surveyed, they are drawn from existing qualitative data and our own experiences as PAT practitioners and supervisors.

Increased motivation for activities. Many participants emerge from their medicine session with an increased sense of motivation to engage in activities, be they recreational or work-related. They often experience this as a lifting of their amotivation and/or anhedonia. This type of outcome could also be framed as an inroad into behavioral activation.

Autobiographical review. During a medicine session, participants often vividly reexperience moments from their past. Often, there is a shift in the meaning of these experiences, such as a renewal or deepening of the moment's original meaning or the attribution of a new meaning. They may also review a relationship, past or present, and reevaluate its meaning in a similar way.

Feelings of profound gratitude. Some participants connect with a deeply felt sense of gratitude. They are often grateful for their life and all that comprises it, particularly relationships. Others may feel gratitude for the opportunity to be alive in and of itself. Some may feel a paradoxical gratitude for their depression or other adverse life conditions, which have served as learning experiences for them in spite of their difficulty.

Feelings of hope and optimism. The cloud of hopelessness that often accompanies depression can lift for some participants. They have reported that this feeling sometimes persists posttreatment, allowing them to feel less worry, apprehension, or fatalism about the future.

Increased resilience. Some PAT participants have reported that they leave treatment feeling a greater capacity to contend with negative social feedback and the general stresses of life. The reasons they give for this often center on feeling more strongly grounded in a less critical sense of self. This feeling of resilience has been described by at least one participant as a "lightness of being."

Increased sense of acceptance. Some participants experience an increased capacity for acceptance, not just of their emotions, but of the world around them. They come to deeply embody the phrase "That's just the way it is." in a manner that is less about hopelessness and more about resilience and equanimity.

Simultaneous presence of opposites. During a medicine session, many participants report being able to hold two or more experiences that are ordinarily thought to be at odds with each other. Someone may be surprised at their ability to feel joy at the same time as more depressive affects. They often find that this experience allows them to continue to feel more positive affects posttreatment even when their depression is present.

Catharsis. As noted in the previous section, PAT participants often leave medicine sessions feeling physically unburdened and "lighter," often as the result of having expressed powerful emotions, particularly grief. In addition to the opportunities that this presents in terms of their ongoing relationship to their embodied experience, some participants feel that this "letting go" is beneficial in and of itself. Often, they report that the grief they relieved themselves of pertained to lost years and missed opportunities due to their depression.

Letting go of things that don't serve them. Another kind of unburdening may occur in PAT medicine sessions, in which a participant recognizes a long-held self-protective strategy that no longer serves them and makes the decision to let it go. This is often done with a sense of compassion and perhaps even gratitude for the strategy (or defense or protector or maladaptive pattern), as the participant is now able to recognize that it was a sensible response to past adversity, though it has since become overapplied in inappropriate situations.

Shifts in priorities. Another common outcome of PAT medicine sessions is feeling like certain neglected aspects of one's life deserve higher priority. For example, a participant may develop the sense that they need to better prioritize quality time with loved ones.

Experiences of cultural trauma and/or grief. In their medicine sessions, some PAT participants have had deeply felt experiences that pertain to traumatic events suffered by a cultural group to which they belong. For example, a Black American participant may experience immense grief or outrage about the enslavement of their ancestors (Williams et al., 2021). These experiences of cultural traumas may or may not include a sense of connection to the participant's personal struggles. They sometimes come with the sense that their own suffering is "not just theirs," sensing that they are embodying emotions and embodied states with roots that go beyond their personal history. They may feel that their expression of grief about this event benefits some combination of them, their ancestors, and the others with whom they carry this trauma.

Greater openness to new experience. PAT can also increase openness to experience, which is one of the "big five" personality traits and is characterized by a willingness to explore new ideas and experiences. This expanded openness can facilitate a more profound enjoyment of, and curiosity about, a diverse range of life events, possibly combatting anhedonia and providing motivation for behavioral activation. Greater openness may be experienced as liberating to people who have been depressed and living a narrow set of life experiences.

Resourcing. Some PAT medicine sessions are profoundly pleasurable or relaxing, and this can hold great benefit for a participant. This type of experience may provide them with an experience of deep rest and feelings of being psychologically resourced that are normally inaccessible to them. If integrated, a participant could use these experiences to sustain them in the daily struggles of living with depression or further therapeutic work at another time. Refrain from redirecting the participant toward a more challenging place of struggle from a belief that that is where the "real work" of PAT takes place.

A NOTE ON NEUROBIOLOGICAL MECHANISMS

The discourse in the field around how psychedelic medicines exert their therapeutic effects has been largely focused on a set of proposed neurobiological mechanisms. They include a range of competing hypotheses about how classic psychedelic compounds may lead to reductions in psychiatric symptoms. Many of them have made their way into the public imagination about psychedelics by way of the popular media. It is likely your participants will have come across them in some form prior to beginning treatment with you. We offer a brief summary of some of the most popular of these hypotheses here so that you can discuss them with some degree of familiarity with any participant who wishes to do so.

- **Entropic brain hypothesis:** It is thought that under the influence of psychedelics, the organization of brain networks becomes less rigid, as different regions of the brain that do not usually communicate directly start to do so (Carhart-Harris, 2018; Carhart-Harris et al., 2014). This may explain psychedelic phenomena such as synesthesia, in which one set of sensory stimuli (e.g., colors) can be experienced by a different sensory modality than usual (e.g., taste, hearing). One popular theory has posited that this disruption of the usual patterns of brain connectivity might be beneficial for people with rigid thought patterns, as in some depressive presentations. This theory is most often associated with the popular, yet questionable, idea of "resetting" one's brain.

  One of the findings that often gets discussed in relation to this hypothesis is that some studies (but not all) have found a decrease in coherent activity throughout the default mode network (DMN) of the brain. The DMN is a set of brain regions that are known to communicate with each other during resting state activities, such as daydreaming, self-referential thinking, rumination, or even the background process of maintaining one's sense of self. It has been argued that, when the DMN goes offline during psychedelic administration, it may allow for the arising of new patterns of thought and self-beliefs that could have antidepressant effects.

- **REBUS model:** This hypothesis (Carhart-Harris & Friston, 2019) builds off of the entropic brain hypothesis and integrates many of its key findings. The acronym stands for "**r**elaxed **b**eliefs **u**nder **p**sychedelics."

The theory suggests that the disruption of the brain's habitual activity results in a lessening of the "top-down" influence of the participant's preexisting learned beliefs on present experience. When this occurs, there is more opportunity for a "bottom-up" reconsideration of one's beliefs about oneself and the world, which could open the door for antidepressant benefit.

- **The claustro-cortical circuit (CCC) model:** This newer model (Doss et al., 2022) has not yet gained much traction in popular media, but its evidentiary basis in neuroimaging research has been growing. It posits that many of the most clinically relevant effects of psychedelics (including nonserotonergic, nonclassical psychedelics, such as ketamine) may derive from their ability to disrupt neural circuits between the prefrontal cortex and the claustrum, a brain region involved in cognitive control. The disruption of this cognitive control may be what opens the door for the kind of sensory disruptions and changes in executive functioning elicited by psychedelics.

- **Neuroplasticity hypothesis:** In some studies—particularly those done in animals—psychedelic administration has been associated with increases in cortical and subcortical levels of a chemical called brain-derived neurotrophic factors (BDNFs). BDNF is associated with new learning and neuroplasticity, which is the brain's ability to modify or "rewire" the connections between neurons. From this finding, some have suggested that this is a mechanism through which psychedelics can promote new learning. In essence, PAT can open a "neuroplastic window" in which participants are able to rewrite maladaptive patterns of brain activity and behavior. Some who feel strongly that this is the main mechanism by which psychedelics exert their therapeutic effects have suggested that it may be possible to obtain similar benefits from drugs that induce comparable neuroplasticity in the absence of any subjective effects—drugs that have tentatively been labeled "psychoplastogens."

- **Anti-inflammatory hypothesis:** Psychedelics have been found to be powerful anti-inflammatory agents that suppress key inflammatory molecules in the brain. Since inflammation has been linked to a variety of psychiatric conditions, including depression, it has been posited that the anti-inflammatory action of psychedelics might help to alleviate depression by reducing underlying inflammation, perhaps even without the psychedelic effects.

- **Serotonin 2A receptor downregulation hypothesis:** Psilocybin and other classic psychedelics exert their effects, in part, by activating the serotonin 2A (or 5-HT2a) receptor in the brain. In doing so, the number of these receptors available on neurons decreases in a process known as downregulation. This receptor is associated with mood disorders, so the thought is that changes in its quantity may be related to antidepressant benefits.

A full review of these theories, including the many critiques that have been made of them, is beyond the scope of this book and our expertise as authors (for review, see van Elk & Yaden, 2022). We hope to convey that, while these hypotheses have made great strides toward detailing how psychedelics impact the brain during PAT treatment, none of them explain all of the available data and, as such, do not provide a full picture of how therapeutic benefits arise.

Some of these theories have captured the imagination of laypeople and psychotherapists alike. We suggest caution in overweighting the clinical relevance of any brain-based hypothesis of PAT in your work with participants. An overemphasis on proposed *neurobiological mechanisms* in psychedelic research explains participant experiences reductively, offers limited predictive power with little real-life clinical benefit, relies excessively on metaphors that undervalue the importance of active participant participation in the process (e.g., the "reset" metaphor), overlooks social determinants and neglects the role of cultural and contextual factors, de-emphasizes the importance of nondrug therapeutic elements, and sidelines personal growth and transformation.

As clinicians, we can more helpfully look to possible psychological mechanisms of change to help guide our work. Such an approach fosters an integrated understanding of the person, offers strong explanatory power for prediction and decision-making, acknowledges the pivotal role of the therapeutic relationship and alliance, recognizes the significance of personal narratives and subjective experiences, values the transformative power of insight and personal growth, highlights the impact of societal and cultural factors on mental health, emphasizes the potential of psychotherapy as a powerful tool for integration and healing, and maintains the critical focus on the individual's unique trajectory of self-discovery and transformation.

We hope that you'll find the proposed mechanisms of change in this chapter helpful in how you think about working with participants in psychedelic therapy.

> *They would never in a million years convince me that that wasn't real, wasn't true, that was like "oh, something just got activated in part of my brain"...*
> *Yes, you're right. Your experience of God does take place in your brain. So does your experience of your child, your spouse, your coworkers. Yes, things in your brain are activated. It doesn't mean God doesn't exist because there are certain parts of your brain that give you access to it. It's a very reductionist argument.*
> —Baptist Minister (Swift et al., 2023)

OUTSIDE THERAPIES USED IN THIS MANUAL

This section provides a brief introduction to the EBTs and other therapies that most directly influenced the EMBARK approach to MDD. Their contributions can be found throughout the domain-specific mechanisms of change and in the example techniques and interventions provided in the sample session agendas provided later.

Emotion-focused therapy (EFT). This is an experiential psychotherapy approach that treats depression by evoking depression-relevant emotions and transforming them. It does so through validation from an empathic therapist, helping the participant learn to identify and regulate these emotions and bringing them in contact with more adaptive emotions (Greenberg & Watson, 2006). Primary emotions, such as grief or shame, that underlie a secondary, more superficial affective state, such as hopelessness, are evoked. The role of primary emotions in depression can then be better understood and addressed with corrective emotional experience, shifts in one's beliefs about oneself, and new emotional responses. Therapist language and interventions from EFT are often used in EMBARK to support therapists working in the Affective–Cognitive domain, as the treatment goals of EFT largely mirror those in the A domain. EFT is considered an established EBT for the treatment of MDD (APA, 2006), though it has yet to be explicitly incorporated into a PAT clinical trial.

Rumination-focused cognitive-behavioral therapy for depression (RFCBT). RFCBT (Watkins, 2016) is a relatively new adaptation of established CBT approaches that is tailored to specifically target rumination by giving one more control over its automatic occurrence. It differs from traditional CBT for depression in that it focuses less on the content of thoughts and more on addressing the (ruminative) processes of thinking. Its methods consist of functional analysis tools, experiential exercises, and behavioral experiments. Some of these tools, as well as RFCBT's conceptualization of rumination, influenced the development of the suggested mechanisms and integration goals found in the Mindfulness domain. RFCBT has been found to be efficacious in the treatment of MDD (Hvenegaard et al., 2020).

Mindfulness-based cognitive therapy (MBCT). Like RFCBT, MBCT is designed to give one more control over the mind's ruminative thought processes. It does so by increasing one's ability to recognize, understand, and employ disengagement skills to step out of automatic mental processes as they arise. MBCT has so far been found to work best in individuals who are currently in remission, in contrast to RFCBT, which has been found to work best with those who are currently depressed (Watkins, 2016). Like RFCBT, MBCT has been important in the development of treatment goals and therapist interventions within the Mindfulness domain.

Motivational interviewing (MI). This approach (Miller & Rolnick, 2013) focuses on eliciting and building upon a participant's intrinsic motivation to make positive behavior changes in their life. It emphasizes a collaborative approach that identifies, highlights, and builds upon participant statements that are suggestive of movement toward a willingness to change. The Keeping Momentum domain of the EMBARK approach to depression integrates MI's focus on moving participants from a "preparatory" stage to a "mobilizing" stage to the enactment of change through motivated actions. At several points in the manual, the language of MI is used to delineate therapist aims in this domain. Bogenschutz and colleagues (2015; 2018) wove an expanded approach called motivational enhancement and taking action (META; Bogenschutz & Forcehimes, 2017) into their model of PAT treatment for alcohol dependence and found that this combined treatment approach was effective in reducing problematic drinking behaviors.

Spiritual evocation. This method (Miller, 2004; alternatively called *spiritual guidance* by Miller and colleagues, 2008) is an MI-based approach to building a participant's intrinsic motivation to develop their spiritual life. It uses the same interventions and conceptual frameworks as other MI approaches, but specifically geared toward spiritual self-development. Treatment goals in EMBARK's Existential–Spiritual domain borrow its nondirective, collaborative approach to supporting a participant's development of pro-therapeutic spiritual practices. Although MI approaches are well established in the research literature, the only known study on spiritual guidance (Miller et al., 2008) investigated its impact on problem drinking behavior and found that it had no discernible impact. Its status as an EBT is thus questionable. However, the manual written for this approach by Miller (2004) provides potentially helpful guidelines and exemplary language for supporting participants' engagement with any existential or spiritual phenomena that arise in their medicine sessions.

Acceptance and commitment therapy (ACT). This is a third-wave cognitive-behavioral modality that integrates elements of mindfulness, existential thought, and experiential therapies. It emphasizes the cultivation of psychological flexibility by way of six core processes, represented by the "hexaflex" model. The accept, connect, embody (ACE) model of PAT (Watts, 2021; Watts & Luoma, 2020) and the Yale approach to PAT for MDD (Guss et al., 2020) both drew heavily from ACT. The treatment goals that EMBARK adopted for its Affective–Cognitive domain drew influence from several ACT components, including acceptance (of challenging affects) and contact with the present moment. There is also a resonance between the goals of the Mindfulness domain and the ACT processes of cognitive defusion and self-as-context, which both refer to the ability to decrease identification with one's thoughts and feelings. ACT also emphasizes the importance of articulating and committing to one's values as a basis for action as part of its approach to depression, which is a priority that was incorporated into EMBARK's Keeping Momentum domain.

The hakomi method of mindfulness-centered somatic psychotherapy. This is an experiential psychotherapy created in 1979 that has continued to develop in the decades since outside the walls of academic psychology. In its approach, therapists use a set of interventions that invite the participant to attend to their evolving somatic experience (i.e., sensations and feelings) as an entrée into their core beliefs and other psychological material. It also provides therapists with interventions that they can use to help participants attend to their embodied experience that can support the unfolding of an embodied psychotherapeutic process. Many of the example interventions offered throughout this book—particularly those in the Body-Aware domain, for which few EBTs exist, drew inspiration from hakomi. This method was included as one of the therapeutic approaches suggested for therapists in the MAPS MDMA-PTSD manual (Mithoefer et al., 2017).

Compassion-focused therapy. This is a relatively novel (Gilbert, 2009) psychotherapy framework that is intended to address transdiagnostic mental health concerns such as shame and excessive self-criticism. Like ACT, it blends cognitive-behavioral approaches with elements of mindfulness and Buddhist thought. Its approach to therapy aims to increase a participant's sense of safety and self-compassion so that they can better adopt a stance of acceptance toward elements of their internal experience that are felt to be threatening or shameful. Although more evidence is needed before compassion-focused therapy can be considered a fully substantiated EBT, several early studies have proven its efficacy in treating mood disorders (Leaviss & Uttley, 2015) and eating disorders (Goss & Allan, 2014). Its general approach and conceptualization of the motives for affect avoidance were influential in the conceptualization of EMBARK's approach to depression in the Mindfulness and Affective–Cognitive domains. Compassion-focused therapy has been put forward as a potential therapeutic frame for PAT (Pots & Chakhssi, 2022).

Internal family systems (IFS). This approach treats the psyche as consisting of multiple "parts" that play specific roles and exist in complex relationships with each other. Healing is thought to unfold when a participant learns to inhabit their core self; from this position, they can then form new, healthier relationships with their defensive or "protective" parts. These protectors shield various aspects of the psyche that carry pain and negative beliefs stemming from past experiences. Each wounded part is then unburdened through a process of uncovering the specific events, emotions, and beliefs present within it, which in turn allows the protector and its associated defensive behaviors to return to a state of health. The IFS language of "parts" is found throughout this book as a helpful frame for working with the pronounced ways in which participants' inner conflicts often manifest in PAT. For example, this book's concept of self-compassion as something "one gives to oneself" is indebted to the IFS concept of a self that can have familial-type relationships of care with wounded parts of its own broader psyche. Also, the IFS core tenet of respect for defenses/protectors aligns with EMBARK's rejection of aggressive therapist interventions. Mithoefer and colleagues (2017) were heavily influenced by IFS in their development and training of MDMA-assisted therapy for the treatment of severe PTSD.

Relational psychoanalysis. This school of clinical thought is home to several approaches to psychodynamic treatment that share an emphasis on the centrality of relationships to real and imagined others in conceptualizing and treating distress. They are often called "two-person psychotherapies" in order to distinguish them from earlier, "one-person" psychoanalytic approaches, denoting the relative importance they ascribe to real relationships (including that between the therapist and participant) in the healing process, more than intrapsychic drives or object relations. Relational psychoanalysis' emphasis on clinical events, such as transference and enactments, in which opportunities for healing arise within the therapist–participant relationship heavily influenced the approach found in this book to working within EMBARK's Relational domain.

Psychedelic potentiation of common factors. The common factors model in psychotherapy posits that different therapy modalities share several critical elements, and these shared elements, rather than the specific techniques unique to each modality, are responsible for the majority of therapeutic change (Cuijpers et al., 2019). Common factors include known drivers of therapeutic outcome, including therapeutic alliance, empathy, goal consensus and collaboration, positive regard and affirmation, mastery, congruence/genuineness, emotional experience, and catharsis. It may be that psychedelic experiences potentiate the common factors to increase their therapeutic potential as mechanisms of beneficial change (Wolff, 2023). For example, a psychedelic could deepen the therapeutic alliance, increase feelings of empathy, create clarity about participant concerns, facilitate goal setting by promoting introspective self-awareness, increase affirming feelings of mutual regard and self-love, bolster mastery and confidence, activate internal resources, promote authenticity, and facilitate access to a wide range of emotions. A recognition of the importance of these common factors is thus woven throughout much of the approach in this book.

4

Considerations Prior to Meeting With a Participant

Before the first preparatory session begins, there are many pieces that should be in place. Many of them involve your own preparation, such as having your credentials, requisite skill sets, personal commitments, and orientation toward certain aspects of the work in order. Other pieces involve assessing the readiness of a potential participant for psychedelic-assisted therapy (PAT). Others involve concrete tasks that need to be carried out, such as creating a playlist and cultivating a welcoming therapy space. The rest involve tending to the relationships that will support the participant as they go through treatment. This chapter will discuss all of the things that should be thought through long before your first PAT participant crosses your threshold.

THERAPEUTIC CREDENTIALS AND SKILLS

[My two therapists] were really good, like really good, like you must go through many years to be able to do what they did . . . . I would not have been able to make anything out of the trips, you know if they do not focus it onto something specific, but they were really good at guiding the discussion and calming me down when I was going nuts . . . . They have been trained to do that . . . they did it in a really good way. The way they talked to me when I was tripping, and the choice of their words— everything counts everything matters when you are in that state..
                                                    —Adam (Belser et al., 2017; Swift et al., 2017)

The question of who is eligible to become a credentialled PAT practitioner is an important question for the field that remains unanswered as of this writing. For those working in a clinical trial, the U.S. Food and Drug Administration (FDA) is currently anticipating a requirement that two practitioners be present during psychedelic medicine sessions. One practitioner, which they call the "lead monitor," must be "a licensed healthcare provider with professional training

EMBARK Psychedelic Therapy for Depression. Bill Brennan and Alex Belser, Oxford University Press.
© Oxford University Press 2024. DOI: 10.1093/9780197762622.003.0005

and clinical experience in psychotherapy" (personal communication, June 14, 2022) and the other practitioner, termed the "assistant monitor" must have "a bachelor's degree and at least one year of clinical experience in a licensed mental health care setting."

The FDA is also permitting video monitoring, which allows an assistant monitor to oversee multiple therapist–participant dyads simultaneously in separate rooms. This parallel monitoring approach, anticipated by Hanscarl Leuner over 50 years ago (Bill Richards, personal communication, 2017), has been piloted successfully at Sunstone Therapies in Maryland. While this approach may optimize staffing resources, further research is warranted to evaluate its effectiveness and ability to reliably ensure participant well-being.

For those using *EMBARK Psychedelic Therapy* to administer PAT in other settings, we recommend similar psychotherapy training to that outlined by the FDA for the lead monitor, as this book was written for professionals with an understanding of the theory and practice of psychotherapy. We recognize that there are a wide range of safe, responsible, and effective ways of using psychedelics to increase well-being. However, the approach in this manual is a psychotherapy that draws on elements of other psychotherapies in order to effect an outcome defined in clinical terms. It is thus likely to work best when paired with prior expertise in psychotherapy, though it may still be of value to those who practice with psychedelics through a different lens.

Which therapeutic orientation would fit best with EMBARK (e.g., cognitive behavioral, psychodynamic, humanistic, integrative)? We designed EMBARK to integrate well with a broad spectrum of approaches. Still, it would benefit practitioners to seek training in the modalities and practices that inspired the treatment goals in this book, discussed in Chapter 3 (e.g., MI, ACT, somatic approaches).

We also encourage training in relational approaches to psychotherapy, such as relational feminist approaches, transference-focused therapy, humanistic therapy, existential therapy, Gestalt therapy, or any relational or interpersonal psychodynamic or psychoanalytic modality. Training and experience in working proactively with the therapist–participant dynamic may be helpful in creating conditions of trust and safety that increase the likelihood of benefit and decrease the risk of relational harm.

Spiritual intelligence. Regarding other competencies, Phelps (2017) has discussed the perspective of several respected figures in the field who have called upon PAT therapists to develop something that she refers to as their "spiritual intelligence." This term refers to a deeply felt, embodied experience of and appreciation for spiritual concepts, such as the inherent mystery at the core of our existence or the underlying orderliness of reality. Phelps and those whom she cites have suggested that therapists who have developed this "embodied knowledge" (p. 466) in themselves through their own spiritual practices may be more capable of supporting participants who experience mystical phenomena in medicine sessions and later seek to integrate them.

However, one's spiritual life is a deeply personal thing. This perspective is provided as information for you to consider. There are no requirements that you take any particular stance on this topic in order to work within the EMBARK approach. Still, you should be prepared to validate a variety of spiritual or transpersonal phenomena participants may experience in PAT sessions without bias.

Toward this end, work with a mentor or more experienced PAT therapist to explore what countertransference may arise for you when faced with a participant's existential–spiritual content prior to beginning a medicine session with a participant. Develop your awareness of your own preconceptions about religion and spirituality. Harm could be done to a participant by responding to any prior belief or any spiritual event that arises during the treatment with value judgment, doctrinal disagreement, misplaced concern for the participant's sanity, or impositions made on the participant's experience based on your own views.

Some PAT therapists have shown signs of a strong desire to offer specific forms of profound spiritual awakening experience to their participants. Develop your awareness of how your own cosmology informs your desire to do PAT work. In particular, you should reflect on your ability to sit with material that you find to be "dark" or sacrilegious without harboring any hidden agenda that the participant "end up" in a different ideological place. For example, a participant whose experience of depression has led them to a sense of abandonment by God should be allowed to bring this belief to treatment for exploration without feeling pressured by you to "correct" it ("God loves you no matter what."). We encourage you to develop an equanimity toward spiritual events that should characterize your stance throughout the entire course of treatment.

SCREENING AND CONTRAINDICATIONS

Appropriately screening participants is a key element of harm reduction in PAT. In addition to conducting a standard biopsychosocial assessment, you should assess for the presence of a range of medical conditions, psychiatric conditions, and contraindications with other medications. The current state of knowledge on factors to screen for is presented here. However, it is important to note that none of what is written here should be taken as medical advice. All medical screening decisions should be made by a qualified medical professional.

Medical conditions. Classic psychedelics are, to a great extent, physiologically nontoxic (Gable, 2004; Nichols, 2004; Schlag et al., 2022). In all clinical trials conducted in the last 20 years, there have been no reported adverse physiological reactions that have endured after the end of the study (Hodge et al., 2022). The most commonly observed acute physiological events in clinical trials of psilocybin include elevated blood pressure, increased heart rate, and transient hypertension (Breeksema et al., 2022). None of these events have required emergency medical intervention, and some have been found to respond well to therapist efforts to address and reduce participant anxiety. Even in uncontrolled recreational contexts, emergency room visits for classic psychedelics rarely result in hospitalization (Leonard et al., 2018; Winstock et al., 2017).

Still, there remain other risk factors that demand careful participant screening:

- *Neurological conditions.* If a participant has a condition such as epilepsy, other seizure disorder, intracranial hypertension, intracranial bleed, aneurysms, or any other medical condition that is associated with a heightened risk of seizures or convulsions, they should not be administered a classic psychedelic, as it may exacerbate these conditions.
- *Cardiac conditions.* If a participant has a cardiac condition that is not stabilized (e.g., uncontrolled hypertension, marked baseline prolongation of QT interval) or a history of arrhythmia, further medical evaluation should be required before PAT treatment.
- *Other unstable condition.* Any participant with another unstable condition (e.g., endocrine, respiratory, gastrointestinal, hepatic, or renal disorder) should be referred for further medical evaluation prior to beginning a course of PAT.

Psychiatric conditions. In addition to these medical conditions, participants should also be screened for a range of psychiatric conditions:

- *Psychotic disorders.* Participants who carry a current or historic diagnosis of any psychotic disorder (e.g., schizophrenia, schizoaffective disorder), as well as those who have an immediate family history of such diagnoses, are considered to be at risk of adverse outcomes (e.g., psychedelic-precipitated psychotic episodes) and have generally been excluded from PAT clinical trials. However, this conventional wisdom has increasingly been challenged by those who feel that PAT may be of benefit to people with these diagnoses if coupled with a greater degree of therapeutic support than what is provided in a clinical trial (Arnovitz et al., 2022; La Torre et al., 2023; Wolf et al., 2022). In fact, the FDA has recently approved a trial that will explore the use of MDMA to treat the negative symptoms of schizophrenia in participants who carry that diagnosis (Hippensteele, 2023). The approach outlined in this book does not encompass the added clinical considerations required for working with such participants; they are outside its scope.
- *Bipolar disorder, mania, or hypomania.* Classic psychedelics may induce a manic episode in participants who have experienced them previously (Morton et al., 2023).
- *Personality disorders and active suicidality.* To date, these have been exclusion criteria in many PAT clinical trials. However, this may reflect an excess of caution observed in clinical trial settings in order to avoid destabilizing participants with presumed vulnerabilities during short-term treatments with limited follow-up care. In support of this practice, one naturalistic study found that psychedelic users with a history of personality disorder diagnoses were disproportionately more likely to experience persisting adverse reactions to psychedelic drugs (Marrocu

et al., 2023). However, there is also some preliminary evidence that individuals who carry these diagnoses of personality disorder can benefit from psychedelic treatment (Müller et al., 2020; Zeifman & Wagner, 2020), though further research is needed to clarify what treatment components should be present to minimize risks. As with psychotic disorders, the approach in this book is based on what has been found to be efficacious in trials which generally have excluded people with these conditions, so working with people with these conditions may require extra clinical considerations that are beyond the scope of this book.

Contraindications. A qualified medical professional should be consulted to assess potential contraindications with prescribed medications the participant is taking or has taken recently prior to the start of treatment. Drugs that present a known, potentially dangerous contraindication with classic psychedelics include:

- *Lithium.* When combined with classic psychedelics or MDMA, lithium may increase the likelihood of seizures.
- *Monoamine oxidase inhibitors (MAOIs).* Several MAOIs have been found to modulate the effects of several classic psychedelics, with some research reporting an attenuation of drug effects (Halman et al., 2023) and other research noting a potentiation or prolongation of effects (Malcom & Thomas, 2022). However, when combined with MDMA or 5-MeO-DMT, MAOIs may contribute to dangerous serotonin syndrome (Malcolm & Thomas, 2022). This category includes St. John's wort and other naturally occurring substances that have MAOI-like effects.
- *Tricyclic antidepressants.* These drugs have been found to potentiate the effects of classic psychedelics (Bonson et al., 1996).
- *Antipsychotic drugs and benzodiazepines.* These have been observed to reduce the intensity of classic psychedelics (Halman et al., 2023; Pokorny et al., 2016).
- *Selective serotonin/norepinephrine reuptake inhibitors (SSRIs/SNRIs) and norepinephrine and dopamine reuptake inhibitors (NDRIs).* Most psychedelic clinical trials have excluded participants on conventional antidepressant medications or required them to discontinue the medication(s). Recently, a number of clinical trials have been initiated for the treatment of depression in which classic psychedelics are administered to people already prescribed conventional antidepressant medication such as an SSRI or SNRI. More research is needed to fully understand how classic psychedelics interact with these drugs. Two studies have found that SSRIs did not interfere with psilocybin's antidepressant effect (Becker et al., 2022; Goodwin et al., 2023), while another found that SSRIs and SNRIs both had a dampening influence on its subjective effects (Gukasyan et al., 2022; Halman et al., 2023). SSRIs have also been known to significantly mitigate the subjective

effects of MDMA, while Wellbutrin (which inhibits the reuptake of norepinephrine and dopamine) does not (Schmid et al., 2015).

- *Psychostimulants.* When combined with MDMA, these drugs may lead to stimulant toxicity.
- *Central nervous system (CNS) depressants* (e.g., alcohol, opioids, benzodiazepines, GHB), when combined with ketamine, may create excessive sedation.
- *Lamotrigine.* When combined with ketamine on the day of a medicine session, lamotrigine has been observed to blunt the ketamine's effects, but sudden discontinuation may result in nausea and headaches.
- *Nonpsychiatric CYP inhibitors.* Drugs that inhibit members of the cytochrome P450 (CYP) enzymes (e.g., ritonavir, cobicistat) may cause serotonin toxicity when combined with MDMA. These and other CYP inhibitors may also lead to an increase in the blood serum concentration of MDMA with the possibility of resultant toxicity to various organs.

Many of these medications may continue to pose a contraindication risk long after they have been discontinued, as they may have induced durable neurological changes, may still be present in the body, or both. Again, a qualified medical professional should be consulted to evaluate medical concerns and medication contraindications.

Trauma. Assessing the participant's trauma history is also essential. Participants who carry significant trauma do not need to be excluded from PAT treatment, but they will likely require a greater degree of support from you, other providers, and loved ones than participants with less trauma. Ask about trauma during screening to ensure that both you and the participant understand this additional need. Assess for historical events that are commonly acknowledged as traumatizing (e.g., abuse, violence) as well as other life stressors (e.g., racism, transphobic rejection, and other forms of discrimination or oppression) that are often overlooked but are impactful traumas that may surface during PAT treatment (Williams et al., 2020).

Another element to assess is the person's ability to stay with their internal experience without becoming dysregulated. PAT medicine sessions typically involve a great deal of time spent focused internally on one's experience of their emotions and embodied sensations. Individuals who find it overly challenging to retain an inward focus, perhaps due to an excess of internal stimuli that recall past traumas, may be more likely struggle during a medicine session and may not receive much treatment benefit. Such individuals may be better served by a referral to a more suitable treatment modality or a more robust PAT treatment design that involves a longer preparation phase focused on developing their capacity to turn inward without experiencing distress or harm.

Other eligibility considerations. Even with all these screening hurdles, we have seen in many clinical trials (and clinical practices) instances when a participant is enrolled into a study who we later realize was not an appropriate candidate for psychedelic treatment. For example, weeks or months into treatment, the participant is in crisis. This is due to different issues that were not picked up in screening: they are underresourced, under undue stressors, functionally impaired, exhibit problematic interpersonal functioning, or present a high risk of serious adverse event. Sometimes, these risks could have been identified in screening. However, after conducting an initial intake, it is common for dedicated psychedelic therapists to feel a powerful inclination to help the prospective participant and facilitate their access to "the medicine," despite signs that the individual might not be a suitable candidate. Many difficult assessments, such as personological issues, are often "deferred" until later in treatment but could be exclusionary.

When determining eligibility, we have implemented an assessment that serves as a final screen: the Other Eligibility Considerations Assessment (OECA). We have found this single-item assessment helpful and useful in our studies. This assessment is to be completed by each clinical team member who has interacted with a potential participant during the screening process. The question requires a simple response of "yes," "no," or "may require additional assessment":

> Does this participant have any current problem that might interfere with participation or require additional assessment? This includes, but is not limited to preliminary evidence of: underlying personological features or character structure that may require additional support beyond the scope of this research, interpersonal functioning or unstable relationships, unclear or shifting self-image, functional impairment, lack of meaningful social support, antisocial behavior, serious current stressors, impulsive or self-destructive behaviors, personality disorder, or high risk of adverse emotional or behavioral reaction.

A unanimous "no" from all assessors is required for the participant to be deemed eligible for enrollment (Belser & Field, 2022).

ENHANCED CONSENT

As you would at the start of any psychotherapeutic treatment, you should share sufficient information with the potential participant so that they can make an informed decision about whether to participate in the treatment. Clearing this hurdle may be more challenging in PAT than it would be in traditional forms of treatment, as many of the experiences participants may have in a medicine session and some of the enduring shifts in their personality functioning that may result could be very difficult for them to understand in advance (Barber & Dike, 2023; Jacobs et al., 2023; Johnson et al., 2008; Smith & Sisti, 2021).

In response to this unique challenge, Smith and Sisti (2021) have argued that, rather than assessing consent during a brief screening conversation, PAT therapists should facilitate an "enhanced consent" process that begins during a screening visit but continues throughout all preparatory sessions leading up to the first medicine session. By prolonging the informed consent process, participants are given a chance to mull over information provided and generate questions, while therapists are given the opportunity to more thoroughly assess whether the participant has a sufficient understanding of what may await them during a medicine session. Note that enhanced consent is different than EMBARK's "double consent" to touch process, described in detail in the section "Considering the Use of Touch" later in this chapter.

We recommend taking an enhanced consent approach and have provided detailed information about what to expect from treatment in the first preparatory agenda in Chapter 5 for disclosure to the participant. However, you should provide information about the potential risks of treatment in the initial screening visit so that the participant has ample time to ask further questions throughout the preparation sessions. The following list of commonly seen psychedelic effects during psilocybin administration (though generalizable to many psychedelic compounds) includes both adverse events and outcomes that, while potentially elements of a beneficial therapeutic process, represent significant risks and transformations of which participants should be made aware:

In-session (transient):

- Nausea
- Physical discomfort
- Transient heart rate and blood pressure increases
- Headaches
- Auditory, visual, somatic, gustatory, and olfactory hallucinations or synesthesia
- Mood elevation
- Time distortion
- Feelings of connectedness
- Loosening of associations
- Mystical experiences
- Ego dissolution
- Anxiety, agitation, or restlessness
- Confusion
- Emotional distress
- Intense experiences of fear (of dying, of going crazy, of therapist)
- Paranoia
- Disturbing imagery arising with eyes closed
- Resurgent memories, which may or may not be factually accurate

Postsession (persistent):

- Derealization and depersonalization
- Ontological shock (i.e., disturbances to one's sense of what is real)
- Psychiatric destabilization, including suicidality and worsened depression
- Enduring personality shifts, such as increased openness, extroversion, spirituality, connectedness to nature

- Shifts in identity (i.e., one's sense of who they are)
- Hallucinogen persisting perceptual disorder (HPPD) or other visual disturbances that may last years after a medicine session

Note that most adverse events observed in clinical trials resolve themselves by the end of treatment and that the more severe outcomes on this list are rare. However, it is of great ethical importance to inform the participant of the possibility that they may occur and to thoroughly discuss any concerns they may have. Strive to ensure that they understand what each of these terms means and that their consent is well informed and noncoerced.

PREEMPTIVELY ATTENDING TO PARTICIPANT STABILITY

The participant may feel strongly that a psilocybin experience is their only and last hope; thus the participant may idealize the study and feel desperate to participate.

—Jeffrey Guss, MD, Robert Krause,
DNP APRN-BC, & Jordan Sloshower, MD, MSc (2020, p. 10)

PAT treatment is a very intensive form of treatment that may occasionally have a destabilizing impact on psychological functioning in the days or weeks after a medicine session, even when proper screening procedures are in place (Breeksema et al., 2022). This acute destabilization may be due to a number of factors that arise in treatment, including (but not limited to):

- Emergent psychological content (e.g., core beliefs, emotions) of which the participant was not previously aware
- Reconnecting with elements of a past traumatic event in a way that does not feel resolved by the end of treatment
- A sense of having recovered "repressed memories" of a previously unacknowledged abuse history, which may or may not be historically accurate
- Shifts in the participant's identity or values
- Disruptions to the participant's close relationships if the other party feels at odds with any new insights or shifts that arose for the participant
- An urgent, strongly felt need to make significant changes in one's life
- Experiences of friction between the participant's new outlook and the contexts (e.g., workplace, homelife, surrounding culture) to which they must now return
- Disappointment that PAT treatment did not have the hoped for transformative therapeutic effects
- The "therapeutic bends": a period of disequilibrium when a participant has antidepressant effects that are more rapid than gradual. The therapeutic bends are a metaphor for the effects that can occur when a

participant ascends rapidly from great depths (e.g., continuing to rely on old coping styles, distress and grief due to the loss of a habituated identity) (Katzman, 2018)

- Feelings of strong attachment to the therapist that contribute to a feeling of abandonment at the end of treatment, which if not well managed, can cause harm and contribute to psychiatric deterioration

The instructions on how to conduct sessions throughout the rest of this book contain specific in-session actions you can take to minimize the possibility that these phenomena will destabilize a participant. In addition, there are some general considerations to keep in mind before and during the course of treatment:

- *Ensure that a participant is relatively stable before treatment.* PAT should not be treated as a form of crisis intervention. A participant should have adequate stability in their life during treatment, including social support and economic stability. If someone is in the middle of a stressful custody battle or is on the brink of getting evicted, PAT treatment should be postponed.
- *Prepare them for the potential of disappointment.* During the screening and preparation sessions, solicit the participant's hopes and fantasies about what treatment will bring. If they seem unrealistic, be sure to spend ample time unpacking them and tempering them. If they are participating in PAT as part of a randomized controlled trial, prepare them well for the possibility of receiving placebo in order to avoid placebo disappointment, in which hopes may be dashed and depressive symptoms may worsen. Consider using a crossover design or open-label extension in the trial to ameliorate this problem.
- *Request additional written consent to connect with the participant's therapist or prescriber(s).* If a participant is seen by other mental health providers (e.g., psychotherapists, psychiatrists), discuss with the participant the potential value in you being in touch with them in order to provide well-informed, coordinated care with reciprocal information sharing. This may also serve to ensure that you are on the same page as the other providers to avoid the possibility of the participant engaging in triangulation between you and them. Triangulation can lead to miscommunications, inconsistent treatment plans, erosion of trust, validation of maladaptive behaviors such as avoidance or splitting, and increased stress for the participant and providers. As with informed consent, be sure to explore this request with the participant.
- *Ensure that the participant has adequate, informed social support.* Posttreatment destabilization can be significantly worse for those who do not have friends, family, or other loved ones to support them. If a potential PAT participant appears to have nonexistent or low social support, consider working with them to develop some as a precondition to treatment. If they do have support people, help them understand

the basics of PAT and what they might see and need to support in the participant over the course of treatment, especially on the days immediately after medicine sessions, during which the participant is likely to be more emotionally sensitive and vulnerable. Talk with the participant to codetermine whether it would be better to do this through conversations with their loved ones and/or by providing them with psychoeducational materials.

- *Be ready to ensure ongoing care.* In preparation for the possibility that something arises for a participant that requires specialized support at the end of treatment, it would be good to develop your list of trusted providers to whom you could make a referral. This list could include psychedelic-knowledgeable psychiatrists, neurologists, somatically oriented psychotherapists, and so on.
- *Be knowledgeable about peer support.* PAT participants often find it helpful to connect with others who have undergone PAT treatment. Several peer-support organizations have arisen to help participants connect with other participants. Take some time to familiarize yourself with these networks so that you are ready to refer any interested participants toward the end of their treatment.
- *Provide clear information about how to contact a participant advocate.* Informing participants about how to report any concerns they had about the treatment is not only an ethical imperative. They may also feel a greater sense of safety entering into treatment with the knowledge that they have the support of an oversight body.

DEVELOPING THE TREATMENT SCHEDULE

As noted in Chapter 1, the number of medicine sessions (and nonmedicine sessions) is variable depending on the needs of your participant. As of this writing, there is no agreed upon sense of how many medicine sessions are required to attain treatment efficacy, with research groups using anywhere between one and three administrations in their clinical trials.

If you are working in a nonresearch setting, consider determining the number of sessions collaboratively with the participant based on their specific needs. For instance, some participants may need additional preparation sessions to develop a sufficient therapeutic alliance with you, while others may have an unsettling medicine session experience that would benefit from additional integration sessions. It may make sense to collaboratively modify the treatment schedule during the treatment in response to any needs that you or the participant become aware of. You may want to discuss the possibility of such a modification during your first meeting with the participant, including a discussion of how this would impact the cost of treatment.

One of the clinical trials for which this book was originally written included two medicine sessions with a treatment design that looked like the following:

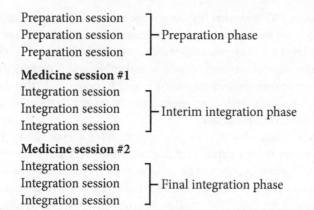

Preparation session ⎫
Preparation session ⎬ — Preparation phase
Preparation session ⎭

Medicine session #1
Integration session ⎫
Integration session ⎬ — Interim integration phase
Integration session ⎭

Medicine session #2
Integration session ⎫
Integration session ⎬ — Final integration phase
Integration session ⎭

However, a shorter treatment design with only one medicine session may be sufficient for your purposes. If so, your treatment design may look like this:

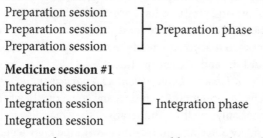

Preparation session ⎫
Preparation session ⎬ — Preparation phase
Preparation session ⎭

Medicine session #1
Integration session ⎫
Integration session ⎬ — Integration phase
Integration session ⎭

In any treatment design, we recommend having at least three preparation sessions prior to the first medicine session. This allows sufficient time for the development of therapeutic rapport and adequate participant screening. At least one of those sessions should be an in-person session, with the rest being either in-person or virtual, so that the day of the medicine session is not the first time you and the participant are in the same room. The deep sense of safety and trust required by PAT is best established through in-person contact, as it allows for familiarization with each other's non-verbal communication and presence. The process of relationship building also requires sufficient time to unfold, both in sessions and between sessions. We advise against compressing the preparation phase; allow adequate time and space for rapport to build.

Since this book was originally written for a two–medicine session design, its later chapters reflect that fact. They distinguish between an "interim" integration phase and a "final" integration phase, which occur after the first and second medicine sessions, respectively. In a treatment design with a single medicine session, treat the subsequent integration phase as a final integration phase. However, if your treatment design includes multiple medicine sessions, treat the integration phase after each session, except for the last one, as an interim integration phase. All other information is applicable to a treatment design with any number of medicine sessions.

DECIDING ON A DOSE

Generally, for a participant's first medicine session, you are advised to provide a dose of the psychedelic medicine you are using that is within the established clinical range for that drug, taking into account all known considerations around specific participant characteristics. If these data are not available, are partial, or leave flexibility for clinical judgment, consider some of the following questions when determining what dose might be right for a participant's first medicine session:

- Have they taken a psychedelic before? Did they know and do they remember what dose they took? How difficult/manageable was that experience for them? How nervous are they about the possibility of repeating a similar experience?
- How much ego strength does this participant have, by your assessment? How resilient do you think they will be if faced with an upswell of challenging personal material?
- How able is the participant to turn toward their internal experience for a significant length of time? Do they experience any distress when they do so?
- How knowledgeable do they seem about the potential effects of the drug? During the preparation phase, how well did they seem to comprehend the intensity of the alterations in consciousness that may occur?

While much is still unknown about optimal dosing practices or the specific participant characteristics that predict adverse reactions to high doses, Aday and colleagues (2021) have presented a helpful review of what is known. They reviewed 14 studies and found that baseline traits of absorption, openness, acceptance, and surrender predicted fewer adverse effects and more mystical effects, while baseline traits of preoccupation, apprehension, and confusion predicted more adverse and fewer mystical effects. Consider the extent to which these traits are present in the participant with whom you are working when deciding upon an initial dose. A participant who exhibits preoccupation or apprehension may be better suited to beginning with a lower dose than a participant who exhibits a capacity for openness or surrender.

Also consider your own orientation toward dose. Do you have a sense that higher doses are inherently more therapeutic? Do you have a predisposition toward wanting to bring about rapid results and transformations in your participants? Do you feel an affinity toward a conceptualization of PAT that sees it as something aggressive that "breaks open the head" or "blows past defenses?" If so, note that there have been observed ceiling effects with psychedelic medicine doses, where higher doses have been found to bring no added therapeutic benefit and more adverse effects (Aday et al., 2021). Consider that trauma-informed care entails respecting participant defenses rather than breaking them down forcefully. Efficacious, transformative PAT does not require an aggressive approach.

For dose selection in subsequent medicine sessions, use the participant's experience of the first medicine session as a basis for determination. Invite the participant to collaborate in this process by sharing their preference for greater or lesser intensity of experience. Of course, all parties should remain aware that many factors other than dose can affect the intensity of the experience and that there is no way to reliably predict that their next experience will definitely be more or less intense.

MUSIC FOR MEDICINE SESSIONS

When I started, not just hearing, but playing the music, my entire body was a musical instrument for every sound, which was coming through my head, and it viscerated from top to bottom . . . I know what a grand piano feels like when it is played.

—Tom (Belser et al., 2017; Swift et al., 2017)

Music is a foundational element of a psychedelic medicine session. The use of music is a consistent feature across all PAT clinical trials and within a wide range of indigenous contexts for the use of psychedelic medicines (de Rios & Katz, 1975). Music has been called the "hidden therapist" of psychedelic-assisted psychotherapy (PAP) (Kaelen et al., 2018) and is thought to play a variety of roles in a medicine session, from stoking a participant's emotional experience to providing them with a crucial kind of guidance and structure as their mind loosens and opens up (de Rios & Katz, 1975). Aspects of a participant's relationship to the music that is played for them in the session, such as the extent to which they like, accept, and resonate with the music, have been found to correlate positively with therapeutic outcomes (Kaelen et al., 2018).

However, playing music in a medicine session is not without its risks. Some clinical trial participants have reported that they felt that the music was "misguiding" them and contributing to their feelings of resistance to the effects of the medicine (Kaelen et al., 2018). This may reflect a poor fit between the music playlist provided by facilitators and the participant's experience. Alternatively, it may signal that the music evoked a challenging emotion that the participant felt guarded against, and perhaps they could have been guided to engage with the music more productively. There remains a lot to understand about the role of music in PAT. We have heard from some PAT practitioners that they just "skip the song," whereas others generally stick with the preset playlist. We recommend that you err on the side of making the participant comfortable, while also attending to the other possible meanings that may underlie a participant's expressed desire to skip a song including personal and cultural associations that may be unknown to you.

The scant data we have so far on the use of music in PAT medicine sessions has provided us with several important insights. First and foremost, Kaelen and colleagues (2018) have found that participants who experience appreciation, resonance, and openness to the music that is played for them showed the greatest reductions in depression. Selecting music that participants like and actively supporting their development of a positive relationship with it should be a priority. Participants in this study also expressed appreciation for what they perceived as the skillful design of the playlists they heard, with many stating that it was helpful to have "calming" music at the start and more evocative music toward the peak of the medicine effects.

What kind of music is recommended? That is a harder question to answer. One study by Strickland and colleagues (2020) suggested that classical music may be less supportive of therapeutic benefit than overtone-based music. However, Kaelen and colleagues (2018) came up with a more complex answer to this question. Their participants had positive associations to the problematically named category of "ethnic music" (e.g., so-called "Indian," "Spanish," or "African"), music that had a human voice (including both English and non-English lyrics), neo-classical music, music that had a crescendo (i.e., a gradual increase in volume or intensity), or music that was "powerful." The distribution of positive preference across these types of music was evenly distributed and seemingly up to personal preference. Other participants reported negative reactions to several of these styles of music, such as vocal music and piano music. Evidently, there is still more to learn about how to fit a playlist to a specific participant, and further research is currently underway.

During a medicine session, participants should be encouraged to listen to the designated playlist throughout the session, though they have the option of requesting that it be turned off at any point. Give participants the option of using either headphones or ambient speakers and allow them to change their preference at any point in the session. Even if they choose headphones, music should be played at a moderate volume through speakers in the room simultaneously so that you have a sense of how the music may be impacting the participant's experience. This also ensures that, if a participant removes their headphones, they will not incur the jarring experience of suddenly being in a silent room. The volume can be adjusted throughout to allow for easeful conversation.

There is a plethora of playlists available on all major music platforms. Some are created and released by universities and other major players in the field of PAT, while others are shared by individuals. If you choose to use any of these playlists, it is recommended that you listen to them prior to using them to discern if they are appropriate for your intended use. You may also create your own playlists. When developing a new playlist or evaluating an existing one, it is recommended that you hew close to the following guidelines:

1. Therapists who work together in a dyad should collaborate when creating the playlists that will be used with participants.
2. Ensure that playlists are long enough for the anticipated duration of the session, given the psychedelic medicine being used, with an allowance for several participant requests to skip tracks.
3. Consider the arc of the medicine experience when constructing a playlist. Start with relaxing, spacious songs and add more evocative ones when the medicine effects are expected to begin and peak. Some have proposed different types of music for the onset, ascension (build-up), peak (plateau), descension (coming down), and return phases of a multihour medicine session (Kaelen et al., 2018).

4. In addition to the main playlist that will serve as a default during the medicine session, it may be helpful to have several song "buckets," or lists of songs that match a particular emotion, such as "reflection" or "grief" or "joy." If a participant moves toward any of these states, you may consider playing one or more songs from a bucket that better matches where they are in order to deepen their experience.

5. Be mindful about using tracks with vocals, as this more "human" musical presence can introduce a potentially distracting element into the participant's experience. It is recommended that you omit all vocals for the first hour or two of the playlist and then only include vocals that are not prominent, such as simple intonations, and do not contain extensive lyrics, particularly in a language spoken by the participant, as it may take them out of the experience.

6. Avoid overwrought classical compositions or any other kind of highly performative music that demands one's attention and active listening (e.g., prominent soloists, jazz music), as these may distract a participant from their process.

7. Avoid music that is too neutral (e.g., background music, "elevator" music). Even the gentler, more spacious tracks should be ones that encourage engagement with and deepening of whatever psychological material is present.

8. Be mindful about the use of prominent, driving rhythms or beats, as these may provide an excess of structure to moments in which the participant may benefit more from a loosening in their thoughts and feelings, such as when they may be approaching a mystical state of oceanic bliss. Consider saving these in a bucket for moments in which they would be most appropriate.

9. Feel free to incorporate different emotional tones in the music that welcome in the full spectrum of the participant's emotional experience (e.g., dark, mysterious songs) while respecting the sensitivity of their altered state by minimizing selections that may be frightening or disturbing.

10. Avoid frequent tonal shifts between songs in the playlist. It is best to think of the playlist in terms of 15- to 30-minute "blocks" of similar songs, perhaps even songs by the same artist.

11. Minimize the use of very short songs (less than ~5 minutes) in favor of longer songs, as the latter give the participant more of a chance to deepen into a specific moment and work with the content they facilitate.

12. Avoid songs that contain applause or other audience noise.

13. Minimize songs that have abrupt starts or endings, as these can be jarring to the participant. You may consider using a cross-fade feature that creates a several-second overlap between successive songs. These features are available in most major music platforms.

14. Be mindful of cultural considerations when choosing songs:

a. If there is a song that you imagine you would feel uncomfortable playing for a person from a social location that differs from yours, be attentive to reasons why this might be.
b. Avoid using sacred songs without cultural context and permission, as this can be a form of cultural appropriation that should be avoided. Likewise, many White recording artists have appropriated sacred music from both Eastern and Indigenous cultures. Make every effort when including music from any other culture to be sure the artists are members of the culture in which the language and the song originates.
c. Given that music and the appreciation thereof are always deeply informed by culture, consider collaborating with participants from differing social locations in order to tailor your playlist to their specific preferences (Williams et al., 2020). Ideally, this should be done in a way that does not detract from the experience of novelty that should generally accompany the music played in medicine sessions, rather than creating a playlist full of songs with which they are already familiar.

WORKING WITH A COTHERAPIST

Each therapist will bring their unique combination of training and perspectives to their encounters with the participant. This includes their identity as a therapist, personal history with depression (or not), personal experience with psychedelics (or not), and experience treating participants experiencing major depression. Therapists also carry their own experiences, transferences toward the study, feelings about their home institution, transferences between therapists, and transferences between disciplines and the psychedelic community.

—Jeffrey Guss, MD, Robert Krause, DNP APRN-BC, & Jordan Sloshower, MD, MSc (2020, p. 14)

In the majority of clinical trials to date, therapists have worked in therapist dyads (see Chapter 1). This practice is generally thought of as a way of reducing the possibility that relational harm (e.g., therapist sexual abuse) will occur (Harlow, 2013, as cited in Passie, 2018, p. 12), though it has also been framed as a way of enhancing clinical benefit via increased support and more opportunities for transference (Eisner & Cohen, 1958). It can also be seen as a way of bringing complementary sets of expertise into the room.

However, for many therapists, working alongside another therapist in support of a single participant is an unfamiliar experience. It brings with it a range of unique challenges.

Before beginning work with a participant, spend time with your cotherapist. Get to know them and get a sense of how they work as a clinician. Talk through any notable differences in approach that arise in your conversation. Explore how your styles and your personalities may complement each other during treatment. Discuss what fears, anxieties, and points of excitement you have about PAT work or about working in a dyad specifically. You and this person will be expected to retain your therapeutic presence in moments of great intensity during a medicine session. It is imperative to develop as much comfort interacting with one another as you can before the first preparation session.

It may also be helpful to discuss some of the more concrete aspects of how the session will be conducted. Consider mapping out any division of roles that you imagine would be helpful. For example, you may be the therapist who leads the discussion of participant expectations during a preparation session, while your cotherapist conducts the somatic awareness exercise.

Prior to the first medicine session, discuss how the two of you might communicate with each other in the space, such as using a particular kind of eye contact to signal a need for the other to intervene or discussing how you imagine you will communicate during silent moments (e.g., by using a pad). However, when working with an attentive, alert participant during a medicine session, it is advisable to use transparent communication rather than furtive communication so that the participant is not encouraged to feel suspicious or left out of the interpersonal dynamics in the room. For instance, you might clearly state, "I'm going to ask [cotherapist] to go find you some water while we keep talking" rather than asking your cotherapist to do so with whispers, silently mouthed words, or subtle gestures. Transparency can defuse paranoia. For example, some therapists choose to tell the participant early on, "During the medicine session, we might write little notes to one another because we don't want to make noise. We will show these notes to you so you can see them."

During a medicine session, be mindful of the fact that the participant is likely to be very sensitive to the quality of the relationship between you and your cotherapist. They may sense the presence of any amount of discord between the two of you, and this will enter their experience. Attend to your working relationship throughout the session, as well as your own internal experience, which may contain feelings of being excluded, needing to assert yourself, or other challenging experiences. Keep in mind that a harmonious relationship between cotherapists is likely to be most supportive to the participant, and make any internal adjustments of accommodations you can that help you bracket your feelings of discord for the day and return to being a calm and supportive presence.

Both therapists should also enter the treatment with the expectation that the participant will likely gravitate toward one therapist or the other. This could be due to a number of factors and, in most cases, does not need to be corrected, though it may be worth naming and exploring for some participants. Talk to your cotherapist (and perhaps your supervisor) about how each of you thinks you will react, emotionally and behaviorally, if the participant evidences a preference for the other therapist. This is a good way to minimize any resentment that may arise and adversely impact the treatment.

Before meeting for the first integration session, meet briefly with your cotherapist to discuss what curiosities you each have about the participant's experience during the medicine session. Some therapists have found it helpful to set aside separate blocks of time during the first integration session to explore each of their curiosities and questions for the participant (after the participant is given ample time to discuss their own). Otherwise, the session may become confused if both therapists play tug of war, simultaneously trying to turn the discussion toward their own curiosities and resulting in a disjointed session.

The language of this book is geared toward individual work, though its approach is equally applicable to dyad work. If you intend to work with a cotherapist, keep this in mind as you read through the book. As you read about each intervention, recall that you will be conducting it with a cotherapist and spend some time imagining how this will look in practice.

INVOLVING OTHER PROVIDERS

If the participant coming to you for a course of PAT is seeing another mental health provider or other healing professional, they should be aware of this treatment. Some PAT therapists have found it helpful to speak directly with the participant's other providers (with the participant's consent and buy-in). This can be helpful in determining appropriateness of fit for PAT, developing a holistic plan for medication discontinuation and recontinuation (if medically advised and necessary), and ensuring continuity of care. It may also help to avoid unhelpful dynamics of splitting, in which the participant idealizes you (the practitioner who has yet to disappoint them) and devalues their other providers, which could reduce the total amount of support available to them.

Some PAT therapists have also (with the participant's consent and buy-in) invited the participant's weekly psychotherapist into medicine sessions. The weekly therapist will often play a supportive role rather than participating actively in guiding the session, but their presence can be beneficial in several ways. Their presence may provide a greater sense of safety and comfort for the participant. The presence of both therapists can enhance the therapeutic alliance and provide increased validation and support for the participant. In witnessing the material that arises, the weekly therapist may be able to more effectively work with these themes in their weekly sessions. They may also learn about how to support the participant's more vulnerable parts by watching how the PAT therapist does so during moments in which they arise.

The clinical challenges of this collaboration include managing and defining roles (who is the primary therapist, who takes the lead in the joint session), aligning therapeutic approaches, and effectively communicating about participant matters. The participant might feel uneasy with two therapists in one session, potentially impacting the therapeutic relationship and the participant's openness during sessions. There could also be frictions between various understandings of the participant's psychedelic experience, as the weekly therapist might lack specialized training in PAT, and the PAT therapist might lack sufficient back-ground on the participant's history and a well-established therapeutic relationship. Careful coordination, communication, and respect for the participant's comfort and therapeutic process are crucial to overcome these challenges. Although this book does not provide further instruction on how to integrate a participant's weekly therapist into the work, it is worth noting as a practice you may wish to explore.

INVOLVING FAMILY MEMBERS OR LOVED ONES

> *You can't tell people more than they're ready to hear . . . and I want to keep the sanctity of it.*
> —Jewish Renewal Rabbi (Swift et al., 2023)

Participants undergoing PAT treatment do so from a place of embeddedness in their close relationships. Any new behaviors or other changes they are in-spired to make will occur within the context of these relationships. Any need for posttreatment support that arises will be met, to some extent, by these relationships. Long before the participant came to you, their depression was inextricably linked to these relationships, impacting them and being impacted by them in turn. As such, attending to these relationships throughout the whole course of treatment is essential. This is particularly true for participants who come from a cultural background that emphasizes family and other forms of relational embeddedness.

Talking about your psychedelic experience with people can be hard. For all participants, you will need to provide support in how to talk to their loved ones about PAT treatment. This is important for many reasons. Loved ones may be suspicious of psychedelic drugs, even in approved, legal contexts. Loved ones may also have reactions of confusion, disbelief, or condemnation when the partici-pant shares with them any nonordinary content that arose during their medicine session, and this may inspire shame, doubt, or other detrimental feelings in the participant in regard to their treatment experience. Or, even when their loved ones are open and receptive, the participant may simply have difficulty finding the words with which to talk about their experience. Loved ones may react with wariness to any sudden changes they notice in the participant's personality or be-havior, even if positive, and this may discourage the participant from continuing to progress. While a participant retains the right to discuss their experience with loved ones to whatever extent they wish, it is important that you work with all parties to help create the conditions that ensure that the participant does not feel they *have* to refrain from sharing.

You can provide support in a number of ways. For example, you can work with the participant to normalize the fact that their loved ones may have unsupportive reactions and provide them with communication skills or scripts for navigating this. You can provide psychoeducational materials about PAT that you create spe-cifically for family members and make yourself available to address any questions they might have about its content. You can invite their loved ones into early consultation meetings about treatment or dedicated family meetings to give all parties a chance to hear about PAT and react to it in a context of support and psychoeducation. Consider that the need for this type of support may be higher to create safety for families from communities that have been disproportionately impacted by the War on Drugs.

Some participants may wish to have their family members in the room during a medicine session or to invite them to a preparation or integration session. This may be potentially beneficial for many of the same reasons it can be beneficial to invite the participant's weekly therapist, as discussed earlier. Involving family members in psychedelic psychotherapy can provide insights into the participant's behavior and strengthen their support system but can also raise confidentiality concerns and potentially complicated family dynamics. Clinically, therapists must balance the family's and participant's perspectives, establish clear boundaries, manage possible conflicts, and navigate diverse expectations. Despite its challenges, with caution and skillful handling, family involvement can contribute significantly to the therapeutic process. It may also be a culturally attuned practice when working with participants from collectivist or family-centered cultures. Additionally, participants who rely greatly on their caregivers for medical or other reasons may benefit from having them involved in treatment (Peterson et al., 2022).

If you are open to having direct contact with family members, or even inviting them to a session, we encourage you to explore this possibility collaboratively with the participant, imagining together what it will be like to have their loved one present during a range of possible treatment events. If you both agree to invite them in, incorporate them for the entire process rather than inviting them to show up on the day of a medicine session. This book will not provide any further instructions on the specifics of how to work with a family member in the room, as it is a complex topic, but it is noted here as a potentially beneficial addition to the work. Further information on this topic may be found in the evolving literature on conjoint approaches to PAT (Monson et al., 2020; Wagner et al., 2019).

DEVELOPMENT OF THERAPEUTIC PRESENCE: CUSHION

The intensity of the therapeutic experience for the participant is affected by the therapist's capacity to remain calm in the face of highly intense emotion and expressiveness.

—Jeffrey Guss, MD, Robert Krause,
DNP APRN-BC, & Jordan Sloshower, MD, MSc (2020, p. 22)

It can make all the difference to conduct PAT with a presence that conveys safety, calm, relatedness, and authentic positive regard. It could even be said that one's presence is the primary, foundational intervention that one can offer to a participant in PAT. If your presence is somehow at odds with the state of surrender and receptivity required of the participant during a medicine session, it will diminish the treatment in ways that cannot be reversed by any skillful intervention or demonstration of technical know-how.

In EMBARK, you are encouraged to adopt a presence that reflects the following attributes, which can be represented by the acronym "CUSHION" (Figure 4.1):

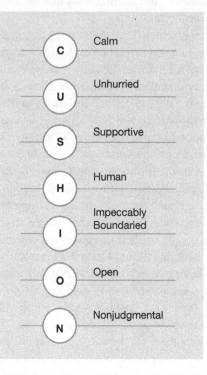

Figure 4.1. CUSHION

Calm. You should model the kind of open receptivity and acceptance that you ask the participant to adopt. This entails remaining nonreactive and unperturbed in the face of any material that arises for the participant. To these same ends, it is also advised that you engage in your own personal therapeutic process to cultivate your own self-acceptance to present as an implicit model for the participant.

Unhurried. A sense of spaciousness and slowness signals to the participant that they can attend more fully to the content of their experience, which will contribute to therapeutic outcomes. You should make the participant feel that you have all the time they need, lest the two of you collude in an avoidance of important content and/or an overly industrious approach to treatment.

Supportive. Your consistent demonstration of support should make participants feel that they can safely surrender to the experience of the medicine. Any distraction you may experience due to outside or personal concerns will likely be evident to the participant in their state of heightened sensitivity, and this may detract from their experience.

Human. You are advised to be mindful of the ways your self-presentation may give an impression of being aloof, distant, "false," or authoritative, as this may evoke distrust in a participant during a medicine session and adversely impact their treatment. PAT participants often experience a dissolution of boundaries and a sensitization to interpersonal dynamics that could lead them to experience any nongenuine action or self-presentation on your part as disruptive.

Impeccably boundaried. Although a "human" presence may entail a different approach to one's professional role than is found in talk therapy, holding firm boundaries is still vitally important—possibly even more so. It is your responsibility to provide this at all times. Remain mindful of the participant's heightened suggestibility and impaired autonomy and minimize the imposition of harmful or unwanted suggestions or interpretations, either implicitly or explicitly. These impositions may occur if you are too authoritative (i.e., being a "guru") or too loose (i.e., being a friend). Clear, firm boundaries not only prevent ethical transgressions; they may also contribute to therapeutic outcomes in and of themselves for a participant who was not afforded such boundaries earlier in life.

Openhearted. In a medicine session, participants are likely to benefit from a therapist who expresses genuine positive regard for them, particularly during moments of challenging affect. This is a basic element of the healing that may occur in the Relational domain. Ideally, your presence will exude a faith in the participant's process and their ability to bring themselves toward healing. An openhearted presence is also one that resists pathologizing the participant's symptoms and defenses, instead choosing to see them as strategies that were once supportive but have outlived their usefulness.

Nonjudgmental. To best support the participant's ability to welcome all material that arises in the medicine session, you should refrain from judging the rightness, value, or moral quality of all material that comes up. This phase of the treatment works best when a noncorrective approach is adopted and you maintain a faith in the "rightness" of what the participant is experiencing, even if it seems dark, regressive, or counter-therapeutic on its surface.

Developing your CUSHION presence does not need to follow any universal formula. There is no personal development practice that fits everyone. There are likely to be as many ways to do this as there are people doing it. For readers of this book who wish to take their first steps in this direction, we offer a few practices that may be supportive: Sit with the words that make up the CUSHION acronym. Watch Manuela Mischke-Reeds' video on therapeutic presence in the Body-Aware module, accessible online via the EMBARK Open Access platform. Consider engaging in some of the personal care practices laid out in Appendix A. Schedule a conversation on the topic with someone whose presence has touched you the way that you hope to touch others. Enroll in a training that offers experience in attending to someone in a nonordinary state and listen openly to their feedback. Or bring this idea of therapeutic presence to your personal therapist, clinical supervisor, or peer consultation group.

For many, this acceptance of the invitation may feel like crossing a line from "career path" to something more significant and deeply personal. If that is true for you, we encourage you to welcome that feeling. The rewards to be reaped by pursuing presence as a path will likely benefit, not just your work with PAT participants, but your personal well-being. This could mark the start of a beautiful connection between your vocation and your own personal path, one that can lead you to a deeper presence to the things in your life that nourish you most.

DEVELOPMENT OF THERAPEUTIC PRESENCE: FRAZZLE

Pursuing a career in therapy is not for the faint of heart; it can be a high-stress endeavor teetering on the brink of burnout. We have often seen psychedelic therapists dash into sessions, coming directly from a grueling day at the hospital, or even dedicating their Saturday to a medicine session after an already packed week at the clinic. We have seen that baseline traits of preoccupation, apprehension, and confusion predict more adverse events and fewer mystical effects in participants (Aday et al., 2021). How about these traits in the therapist?

While we strive to cultivate a therapeutic presence exemplified by CUSHION, it may also be useful to spotlight and prevent the typical pitfalls that threaten the integrity of PAT. To this effect, we introduce the counter-acronym FRAZZLE, a cautionary assembly of therapist characteristics that could jeopardize the therapeutic process (Figure 4.2). You should strive to avoid FRAZZLE:

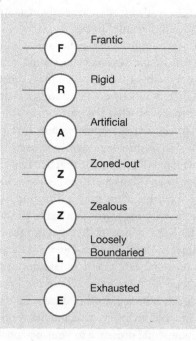

F — Frantic
R — Rigid
A — Artificial
Z — Zoned-out
Z — Zealous
L — Loosely Boundaried
E — Exhausted

Figure 4.2. FRAZZLE

<u>Frantic</u>. Therapists who are reactive and perturbed, unable to maintain a calm demeanor in the face of administrative hiccups or challenging material that arises for the participant.

Rigid. Therapists who are inflexible in their orientation, conceptualization, or techniques, failing to adapt to the individual needs of the participant. This can harm the therapeutic alliance and make the participant feel pressured or disempowered in session.

Artificial. Therapists who lack authenticity or genuineness in interactions with the client or hide behind "shrinky" artifices. Try to "be real" with participants.

Zoned-out. Therapists who are not fully present during sessions, checking text messages or daydreaming during multihour sessions or displaying a lack of attention or focus, which can make the participant feel unheard and unsupported.

Zealous. Therapists who become overbearing, performatively charismatic, or falsely authoritative. Overzealousness or a seeming inauthentic enthusiasm can make it difficult for a participant to feel trust and get comfortable.

Loosely boundaried. While it is important to establish a human connection during PAT, maintaining necessary boundaries is crucial. A loose approach can lead to blurred boundaries, dual relationships, and ethical transgressions. Also strive to avoid looseness in your clinical thinking, your case conceptualization, your selection of interventions, and your maintenance of an appropriate frame (times, durations, cancellation policies, fees, etc.). Avoid just "wingin' it" as a general therapeutic approach.

Exhausted. Therapists who are too tired or fatigued to provide effective therapy. Avoid overburdening your schedule by trying to fit psychedelic therapy sessions into your evenings or weekends alongside your standard practice without allowing ample time for personal rejuvenation and recovery.

FRAZZLE serves as a reminder of potential pitfalls for psychedelic practitioners. While therapist "self-care" in the form of yoga and massages is often touted as a necessary set of practices to avoid therapeutic dysregulation, we remind you that FRAZZLE is in the system. There are systemic reasons why therapists are frantic, exhausted, and zoned-out or why they revert to overly scripted behaviors. Remember, the first step to avoiding a FRAZZLE-like presence is to be aware of it, then to gently encourage yourself to pause, breathe, connect, recharge, and express. Lather, rinse, repeat.

COMMITMENT TO PERSONAL THERAPEUTIC WORK

Do your work. [laughs] Do your own work, do your own work. I think that's how you can help your clients the most. The more we go into different territories and more work with grief, with shame, whatever, with anger, rage, with sexuality, with Eros, the more work we've done on ourselves, the more we'll be able to support our clients through those spaces, the more we'll be able to actually be accountable, to be aware of our shadows.

—Psychedelic guide (Brennan et al., 2021)

Because PAT makes unique demands on therapists (Taylor, 2017), we strongly suggest that you be actively engaged in your own ongoing process of personal healing and development. This may take the form of personal therapy or a range of other healing practices. This suggestion is in line with perspectives held by experts (Phelps, 2017) and experienced PAT practitioners (Brennan et al., 2021), who posit that a practitioner's commitment to their own healing, growth, and development will improve their ability to serve participants in a variety of ways. For example, this commitment may bring you a greater sense of self-acceptance and an inner settledness, both of which will help you provide the kind of CUSHION presence that best serves the people with whom you work.

Additionally, engaging in your own work may help you to develop a capacity for self-awareness that augments your ability to notice when you are entering into a problematic dynamic or engaging in a harmful form of intervention with a participant. Self-awareness and self-knowledge can serve as important first lines of defense against ethical boundary transgressions. Also, by attending to your own woundedness and unmet psychological needs in your own personal healing practice, these part of you will be less likely to "take the wheel" during a session with a participant and lead to you making poor clinical choices or even doing harm. As noted in Chapter 2, the need to protect against these possibilities is even higher in PAT than it is in traditional therapy due to the greater intensity of relational dynamics (e.g., transferences, enactments) in the former. So, even if your personal material does not normally disrupt your ability to remain ethically grounded in your traditional therapy practice, you may find that the dynamic terrain of psychedelic work requires further personal work from you.

This commitment may feel at odds with what is required of you in other contemporary clinical settings. This type of focus on the personal qualities of the therapist has become an increasingly spurned aspect of professional development despite the demonstrated relevance of these qualities to professional competencies (Bennett-Levy, 2019). Fewer and fewer psychologists-in-training have chosen to undergo their own personal therapy as part of their training, with most feeling that they do not need it (particularly those who endorse a cognitive-behavioral orientation) and others worrying about its emotional stress, disapproving judgments from their training programs, or simply not being able to find space for it within the time demands of graduate school (Schwartzman & Muir, 2019).

A focus on personal development may be challenging in other ways as well, particularly to those with less clinical experience or "impostor syndrome." It can feel unsettling for them to consciously link their personal woundedness to their professional ability to work with participants. Any sense of themselves as still-developing practitioners may start to feel like an admission of their privately held sense of personal inadequacy. This can be understandably painful.

However, there are also contemporary precedents for this focus on personal development, including psychoanalytic approaches to training, in which aspiring analysts must first undergo analysis themselves to minimize problematic countertransference toward participants (Nierenberg, 1972). Also, many indigenous approaches to sacred plant medicine apprenticeships include a years-long process of developing the person of the healer. We encourage you to see your personal development in a similar light as these traditions and to hold it as an important part of what you offer to participants.

COMMITMENT TO RECEIVING SUPPORT

I think the process, actually long before transgressions, is to have a place where people can really openly and safely talk about the edges that they're running . . . . I think places where peer consultation comes with a sharp lens, you know, so that it's not just brushing each other.
—Psychedelic guide (Brennan et al., 2021)

It is highly recommended that all PAT providers participate in regular meetings with a clinical supervisor and/or a peer supervision group. In addition to continually developing your PAT skills, these meetings provide a space for examining the ways in which your personal material (i.e., reactions, emotions, needs) may be showing up in your work with participants. PAT is thought (Anderson, 2020b; Phelps, 2017; Taylor, 2017) to elicit counter-transferential reactions from therapists more readily than traditional talk-based therapies. This makes it essential to regularly discuss how your unacknowledged personal material is entering into the treatment, even if you are a highly experienced provider. We encourage you to find a supervisor who does not hold professional power over you so that you may approach supervision with an openness to being vulnerable and exploring the deeply personal dimensions of your work with participants.

Additionally, we encourage you to seek out or create a peer consultation group for yourself and your colleagues. These meetings can provide a different kind of support and feedback on one's work. Some PAT practitioners have felt that their tight-knit communities of practice have provided them with a compassionate context of accountability and a sense of shared commitment to doing the work well. Of course, as in any group or community, there is the potential for groupthink and other forms of shadow, so be sure to devote enough time to intentionally naming and exploring the relational dynamics present in the group.

CULTURAL CONSIDERATIONS

The potential impact of various cultural factors on the treatment should be taken into account before the first session. As various experts have pointed out (Michaels et al., 2018; Morales et al., 2022; Thrul & Garcia-Romeu, 2021; Williams et al., 2020), the clinical protocols used in most PAT trials today have been developed on the basis of clinical experience and research evidence drawn from work with homogenous participant populations consisting of White, Western individuals. The approach laid out in this book is no exception, as it is based largely on the same pool of research. As such, it is essential that you consider the social location of the participant you will serve and what shifts you need to make to elements of your approach to accommodate their needs and preferences. The intent of doing so should be to help the participant experience a maximum of safety, comfort, and confidence in accessing the treatment.

The following nonexhaustive list of suggestions by experts on cultural competence in PAT (Smith et al., 2022; Williams et al., 2020, 2021) may provide a helpful starting point:

- Allow more time for establishing safety for people from social groups that have experienced historical and/or contemporary oppressive treatment from medical providers (e.g., Black Americans, LGBTQIA+ people). This may mean providing additional preparation sessions, conducting a longer assessment of symptoms to give them more time to open up, and so on.
- People from communities that have been impacted by the disproportionate criminalization of drug use of the racist War on Drugs and/or high rates of substance misuse may have more concerns, fears, and questions about ingesting mind-altering substances. Devote as much time as needed to responding to them before moving into treatment.
- People from marginalized groups often arrived at treatment having had less lifetime access to mental health treatment, which may mean that they have less familiarity with mental health language. Avoid the use of jargon and provide as much psychoeducation as the participant needs to ensure that they are able to communicate their symptoms, questions, and treatment goals to their satisfaction.
- Seek education and consultation on the culture-specific ways in which depression may be experienced, expressed, and coped with by the participant (Chapman et al., 2014).
- Ensure that the art in the room and the music used in medicine sessions are representative, culturally attuned, and free from any exoticization or fetishization of nondominant cultures.
- When assessing for the presence of trauma, explicitly invite participants to consider that their experiences of oppression (e.g., racism, transphobia, homophobia) may have been traumatizing or had important impacts, as they otherwise may not recognize them as such. For support in assessing racial trauma, consider using the UConn Racial/Ethnic Stress & Trauma Survey.

To best serve participants from social locations that differ from yours, you are strongly encouraged to also be continually engaged in your own process of developing your capacity for cultural humility. To do so, NiCole T. Buchanan (2021), an EMBARK faculty member, advises that PAT practitioners must continually work to "better understand [their] privileged identities, how they complicate [one's] ability to work effectively with others, and that experiences are dependent on the matrices of identities one holds (race, gender, sexuality) and their particular historical and contemporary context" (p. 143).

PERSONAL PSYCHEDELIC EXPERIENCES

Some significant authors and institutions recommend a minimum of five controlled self-experiences for the education of therapists using [PAT], ideally with the (different) substances which will be used by the specific therapist . . . . It is our opinion that direct experience with psychedelic therapy is valuable in training to become a [PAT] therapist and furthers the safety of treatments.

—Recommendations for a model training curriculum for PAT by leading psychedelic researchers (Passie et al., 2023)

It has been suggested that personal experiences with the nonordinary states of consciousness brought about by psychedelics may contribute to PAT therapists' ability to support participants by giving them an enhanced understanding of what their participants may undergo in a psychedelic medicine session (Nielson, 2021). To put it plainly, How can you help facilitate a nonordinary state of consciousness if you, yourself, have never experienced one?

It has also been suggested that doing so may also give therapists a firsthand sense of the vulnerability and suggestibility engendered by psychedelic medicines in a way that could help them minimize relational harm to participants (Brennan et al., 2021). Accordingly, a survey of 32 therapists working on a phase II clinical trial of psilocybin for MDD found that 88% had personal experience with at least one serotonergic psychedelic, with 81% having used psilocybin (Aday et al., 2023).

Participants may also prefer a therapist who has personal experience with psychedelics. An online survey of 800 people with depressive symptoms found that they ranked personal experience with psilocybin as the most important characteristics they would want in a psychedelic therapist (Earleywine et al., 2022). Similarly, a thematic analysis of online discussions about harm reduction among people who used psychedelics in nonclinical contexts found that approximately 80% felt that it was important that the people supporting them had had their own psychedelic experiences (Engel et al., 2022).

As such, some research groups have attempted to provide their facilitators with opportunities to experience the effects of the drugs they will administer. The Multidisciplinary Association for Psychedelic Studies (MAPS), an organization funding and administering clinical trials assessing the efficacy of MDMA in the treatment of PTSD, obtained FDA permission to conduct a "healthy volunteer" trial that allowed study therapists to undergo a medicine session as a participant (MAPS, 2021). However, providing experiential training with psychedelics has proven challenging for other research groups due to the high costs of doing so, various legal factors, stigma around drug use, and this practice's affront to the institutional logic of psychiatry, which does not value or require personal experience with medications administered to participants (Nielson & Guss, 2018).

In research settings, this practice has also come under scrutiny for potentially introducing a source of bias in that therapists who take a psychedelic medicine for the first time as preparation for working on a clinical trial may develop an inflated sense of the drug's capacity to heal, which could have implications for research blinding and objectivity in the presentation of results (Anderson et al., 2020b). Also, one study found that investigator self-disclosures about personal experience with psychedelic drugs degrades perceptions of their integrity as a researcher held by psychedelic-naïve observers (Forstmann & Sagioglou, 2021).

Dr. Charles Grob, a physician and pioneering psychedelic researcher at Harbor–UCLA Medical Center, points out the bind. In public talks, when he is asked if he has ever tried psychedelics, he says, "I'm damned if I have, and I'm damned if I haven't. If I have, then my perspective would be discounted due to my own personal bias, and if I haven't, it would be discounted because I would not truly understand the full range of experience the drug can induce" (Chapkis & Webb, 2008, p. 1).

EXPERIENTIAL TRAINING

Given this set of important considerations, training in the EMBARK approach has not required personal experience with psychedelics. However, prior to becoming a certified EMBARK facilitator as required to participate in a Cybin clinical trial, therapists have been required to undergo at least one session that involves them being the participant who experiences a nonordinary state of consciousness. This can be done in a variety of modalities, including PAT, as well as various alterative techniques, such as holotropic breathwork, which, despite some important differences, can elicit equally profound states of consciousness with comparable utility for educating therapists about what it is like to be in the role of participant.

We consider experiential training a necessary part of preparing therapists to work with participants in an altered state of consciousness. The unique sensitivity, lability, vulnerability, and extremity of affect that they experience can only be understood experientially, and such understanding is important for maintaining an appropriate and ethical therapeutic approach.

For practitioners who elect to experience psychedelic medicines for themselves, we advise that this be done in a context of adequate support. This entails not just the level of medical and psychological care appropriate for each specific practitioner but also sufficient peer and/or supervisory support to ensure that personal experiences inform clinical practice in a responsible way by protecting against the risks of ego inflation, guruism, or other reactions that may adversely impact one's clinical judgment.

PREPARING THE SPACE

I have wonderful feelings about this room.
                                   —Augusta (Belser et al., 2017; Swift et al., 2017)

As noted earlier, participants are particularly sensitive to external factors during a medicine session. This includes the physical details of the space in which the session is taking place. You should prepare the space before the participant arrives so that they enter a space that is free from commotion. The space should signal to them that they are being cared for in a thoughtful and thorough way.

Ideally, the manner in which the space is prepared should also communicate to the participant that they are entering a space that is designed to support them in an experience that is distinct from the everyday.

Specific items that should be present in the space include:

- Tissues
- Music system with headphones
- Eye mask
- No noticeable smells (e.g., cleaning materials), as participant will be very sensitive
- Climate adjustment control readily available
- Space in the room that allows for the participant to stand up
- Writing materials for you to take notes
- Clean emesis basin, not prominently displayed
- Medicine, with dosage already measured out
- Optional items:
  - A weighted blanket
  - Art and/or writing materials for participant (for later in the session)

The space should have a bathroom that is easily accessed from the treatment area. The lighting should be soft in all areas that a participant may experience during the drug effects, including the bathroom. We have found that it is helpful to cover the mirrors in the bathroom so that the participant does not get caught up in and possibly disturbed by their distorted reflection.

CONSIDERING THE USE OF TOUCH

[My therapists] couldn't have been better. It was as though they were as guided as I was and at times—when the emotion was becoming really intense, two or three times, they reached out and put their hands on me. One put their hand on my shoulder, another held my hand, and it was at the precise moment when I needed that contact. They could not have been better prepared, or done a better job, or shown greater care for me. It was incredible, it really was.

—Mike (Belser et al., 2017; Swift et al., 2017)

One distinguishing practice within PAT that has generated a lot of heated conversation is the use of touch-based interventions. These interventions are most often light forms of touch, such as handholding or an arm around the shoulder.

Influential voices in the field have insisted upon its importance, while others have questioned this assertion. The question of its necessity remains unsettled as of this writing. Ultimately, it remains up to you and the participant to decide if and how much touch will be incorporated into treatment. This section will provide some background and suggestions for how to make this determination. See also the instructions on how to navigate touch with a participant throughout the chapter on medicine sessions (Chapter 6).

Historical and Current Perspectives

During the early wave of PAT research, therapist–participant touch was commonplace. It was a popular ground for innovation, with several well-known researchers creating their own practices around it. Betty Eisner (1967), known for pioneering male–female therapist dyads with Sidney Cohen, advocated for the use of "supportive touch," stating that "during moments of fear and anxiety it was found extremely helpful to the participant to have some sort of physical contact" (p. 544). She also suggested a type of "restraining touch", stating that "the participant . . . seemed to request and at the same time enjoy struggling against the firm physical restraint of the male and female therapists. Afterward, the participant pronounced it one of the most 'freeing' experiences of his life" (p. 544). Joyce Martin (1964) suggested a third type of touch akin to a kind of "reparenting," in which the unmet infantile needs of regressed participants were satisfied with maternal actions, such as caressing, rocking, and sometimes even bottle-feeding. Reactions were polarized at the time, but this notion of providing corrective experiences laid the theoretical foundations for much of the touch used in later PAT settings.

Some voices that remain influential in the field in the current wave of research have also advocated for touch—primarily supportive touch. Stan Grof stated in his seminal *LSD Psychotherapy* that "the importance of physical contact in LSD psychotherapy is unquestionable" (1980). Bill Richards, a widely respected PAT researcher whose work has spanned both waves of research, has written that "the therapist's hand on a shoulder or arm, or the therapist holding the volunteer's hand at appropriate times may provide critical interpersonal grounding and affirm safety." Michael Mithoefer, who pioneered the modern research of MDMA in the treatment of PTSD, included the following passage in his treatment manual:

> Mindful use of touch can be an important catalyst to healing during both the MDMA assisted sessions and the follow up therapy . . . Withholding nurturing touch when it is indicated can be counter therapeutic and, especially in therapy involving non ordinary states of consciousness, may even be perceived by the participant as abuse by neglect. (Mithoefer, et al., 2017, p. 15)

Current Controversies

However, this historically widespread perspective on the value of touch in PAT has been called into question recently by accounts of harmful touch and sexual boundary transgressions by PAT practitioners in the underground and in clinical trials (McNamee et al., 2023; Goldhill, 2020). These instances of in-session touch that was either inherently sexual or may have contributed to a therapist–participant dynamic in which sexual abuse later occurred have sparked an important, far-reaching conversation in the field about how to better prevent this type of relational harm. This has led some to call into question the necessity of touch altogether, noting that that there remains a lack of empirical data or consensus around the efficacy and safety of therapist–participant touch (Devenot et al., 2022b). These voices have argued that, until touch-based interventions can be administered more safely, a precautionary approach that minimizes touch is warranted.

The field of PAT has only just begun to reckon with the potential for this type of abuse and relational harm. It has started to interrogate historical perspectives in light of more recent advances concerning trauma-informed care and the asymmetrical power dynamics involved in psychotherapy. The value of welcoming the voices of clinical trial participants into these conversations has begun to be appreciated. Some organizations have created basic guidelines for administering touch-based interventions (MAPS, 2019). Still, this reconsideration of the place of touch in PAT is ongoing, and most clinical trials to date have allowed therapists to use it with little standardization of how and when this occurs.

Why Touch?

Despite the lack of PAT-specific research on the subject, we have some nonpsychedelic research to draw from to develop our understanding of how touch may help. The rationales most commonly put forth by therapists for the use of touch include that it offers encouragement, a sense of acceptance, a sense of being supported, implicit permission to express affect, soothing, grounding, and missing developmental experiences of care (Durana, 1998; Goodman & Teicher, 1988; Mintz, 1969). When participants were asked how they have been impacted positively by therapist–participant touch, they report that it often helps them do the following in therapy (Alagna et al., 1979; Horton et al., 1995; Pattison, 1973; Stockwell & Dye, 1980):

- Engage in deeper self-exploration
- Have more positive feelings about the therapy
- Experience a sense of trust and openness
- Feel a greater sense of safety and containment
- Feel more bonded to their therapist

- Feel more reassurance
- Experience more acceptance
- Feel a greater degree of connection to external reality and the world
- Glimpse a new mode of relating
- Feel less alone
- Get in touch with bodily sensations
- Experience higher self-esteem
- Experience "breakthroughs" in therapy

Some of the therapists interviewed in these nonpsychedelic studies noted that supportive touch may confer the greatest degree of benefit to participants who are in a regressed state in which core emotions and beliefs relevant to their unmet developmental needs are activated. As noted earlier, these states are frequently elicited by psychedelic medicines, suggesting that the purported benefits of touch-based interventions may be particularly accessible in psychedelic therapy.

Some research has also focused on the question of how to determine when therapist–participant touch is appropriate. When researchers examined what factors entered into therapists' thinking about this question, they found that their theoretical orientation, understanding of the participant's personality features, and consideration of therapist–participant dynamics were the most common considerations (Goodman & Teicher, 1988; Holroyd & Brodsky, 1977; Hunter & Struve, 1997; Lamb & Catanzaro, 1998; Smith et al., 1998). When participants were asked what made therapist–participant touch feel okay for them, they noted features such as clarity of its purpose, a sense of control, congruence with the content under discussion, and a sense that it was for their benefit rather than that of the therapist (Gelb, 1982; Horton et al., 1995). Notably, none of this decades-old research considered the impact of the participant's social location or trauma history on their experience of touch in therapy.

Why Not Touch?

Other research has highlighted the ways therapist–participant touch can be harmful (Alyn, 1988; Bacorn & Dixon, 1984; Durana, 1998; Holub & Lee, 1990; Jourard & Rubin, 1968; Kertay & Reviere, 1993). These reasons include:

- Serving as a means through which the therapist's unmet need (e.g., for affection, validation, closeness, sexual contact, professional potency, intimacy) enter into the therapeutic relationship
- Sending confusing signals to the participant that disrupt the therapy, such as leading them to believe their therapist wants to have sex with them
- Exploiting power differentials in the room insofar as the therapist likely feels more comfortable initiating touch than the participant

- Serving as an entrée to sexual contact, though some research has suggested that this is most often not the case (Holroyd & Brodsky, 1980)
- Retraumatizing the participant by recalling past instances of abuse that involved touch
- Disrupting the imaginal play of the therapy space with the inherent concrete reality of touch
- Distracting the participant from their therapeutic process
- Signaling that they need to calm down, which could be received as invalidating of their emotional experience
- Encouraging feelings of dependency on the therapist as a source of stability or grounding
- Encouraging them to accept support from another person to the detriment of drawing upon their own intrinsic ability to support themselves

Many of these risks may also be exacerbated by the addition of a psychedelic medicine to the treatment. Recall from the Chapter 2 section on ethically rigorous care that when a participant takes a psychedelic, it can lead to increased suggestibility, impaired autonomy and ability to consent, and amplification of therapist–participant dynamics. When touch-based interventions are used in the presence of these phenomena, the meaning they hold for the participant may be different than it would be under normal circumstances. For instance, if a participant is experiencing elements of a past instance of sexual abuse, and their therapist places a supportive hand on their shoulder, this may contribute to feelings of unsafety and could lead to harm.

Touch in EMBARK

> If you're going to use touch, get supervision and or ongoing consultation around it. Having more eyes on the situation is better than having just you. And anytime . . . you feel like, "Oh, I should just make an exception for this client" or "Oh, maybe this is what they really need," you should question yourself and why you're doing that and get consultation. If it's anything that you wouldn't feel comfortable talking about with a colleague, talk about it with a colleague [laughs] . . . . If you are going to loosen up your boundaries in any way, shape, or form, don't just do it in isolation. Get consultation around it.
>
> —Psychedelic guide (Brennan et al., 2021)

As should be apparent, there is still a great deal that the field needs to learn about the place of touch in psychedelic therapy. The approach laid out in *EMBARK Psychedelic Therapy* takes a precautionary approach that limits the types of touch used, attends vigilantly to consent practices, and encourages therapists to prioritize nontouch interventions. These consent practices, both in preparation and during the medicine session itself, are described in the next section.

In the EMBARK approach, only supportive touch is recommended. Within this approach, we advise against the use of touch that restrains or contains (e.g., placing the weight of the therapist on top of the participant and inviting them to struggle to escape) or involves more intensive touch (e.g., full-body spooning). The following list of forms of touch is recommended as an upper limit for practitioners with no prior experience offering therapeutic touch:

- Handholding
- Placing a hand on the participant's arm or foot
- Placing an arm gently around the participant's shoulder
- Allowing the participant to place their arm around your shoulder
- Allowing the participant to place their head on your shoulder
- Hugs, when requested by the participant, in the standing position

Consent to touch is reciprocal—you are advised to honor your own comfort levels around touch and not feel as though you need to push beyond them. Even if asked, you do not need to hug your participant. Refrain from adopting an automated or cookie-cutter approach to touch. No one is served by you forcing yourself out of your comfort zone when it comes to touch.

Consider each participant's unique background and needs and attend to the constantly shifting therapist–participant dynamics present within a psychedelic medicine session. Finally, whenever possible, make decisions about touch in communication with others: your cotherapist, your supervisor, and your peer consultation group.

Double Consent for Touch

If any forms of supportive touch will be available to the participant during the medicine session, it is essential to assess their consent for the specific forms of touch that may be used. EMBARK employs a "double consent" protocol in which the participant's consent for touch is assessed twice: during preparation (when the participant has not taken a psychedelic medicine) and again during the medicine session. This two-stage protocol is important because the altered state that the participant will enter during the medicine may disrupt their capacity to give proper consent. In addition, by giving them a sense of what forms of touch may be used prior to the day of the medicine session, you give the participant time to consider further what is or is not comfortable for them. This gives them a chance to rescind their consent and thus further contributes to the validity of their consent. This double consent protocol is becoming standard practice in the field of PAT (e.g., MAPS, 2019).

Assessing Consent During Preparation

During the preparation phase, engage the participant in a conversation about their levels of comfort and consent around the forms of touch that will be available:

1. Tell the participant that some participants, but not all, have found it helpful to have the option of requesting basic supportive touch during a medicine session.
2. Ensure that they know this is optional and that they can decide not to receive any touch at this or any other point in treatment.
3. Emphasize that you will reassess consent during the medicine session before touch is offered. Today's consent conversation is giving them an opportunity to say if there are any forms of touch that they know for certain would not be okay at any time. If they say they are open to something today, they will still maintain the opportunity to turn it down during the medicine session. Note that they can also ask for touch to end at any time, and this request will be honored.
4. Discuss each specific form of touch, assess the participant's level of comfort with each one, and assess their consent.
5. Encourage the participant to honestly express their level of comfort about touch. If they are ambivalent, do not try to convince them to consent.
6. If you are working with a cotherapist, give the participant the opportunity to provide different levels of consent for each of you.
7. Tell the participant that they may actively request these mutually agreed upon forms of touch during the medicine session, but you will also use your discretion to determine whether or not it would be safe and supportive in that moment.
8. Note that there is a remote chance that an emergency will arise that requires you to use touch to protect them from physical harm (e.g., they begin to fall when walking to the bathroom) or if they become nonresponsive, regardless of consent agreements, but this is very unlikely.
9. Encourage the participant to keep thinking about and feeling into any affirmative responses they gave and empower them to let you know the next time you meet if anything has shifted for them.

Assessing Consent During the Medicine Session

If you feel that a supportive touch intervention would be helpful to a participant's process during a medicine session (see Chapter 5 for scenarios in which it may), assess for consent again. The following practices compose the second half of the double consent process.

First, check in with yourself in the moment to identify your motivations for providing touch before offering it. For some PAT therapists, an urge to touch a participant is often born of either a compassionate, yet misguided desire to take a challenging experience away from a participant, a lack of trust in the participant's process, or a desire to be skillful by "making something happen." Your impulse may also reflect a desire to have one or more of your own needs met, such as for closeness, physical contact, or intimacy. You should only offer touch if it is primarily motivated by sound clinical discernment as to what would benefit the participant. When considering touch, you should first ask whether nontouch interventions may provide equivalent support while providing the added benefits of bolstering the participant's autonomy and minimizing the potential for feelings of dependence to arise.

Assess for the participant's consent before initiating:

1. Ask whether the participant would appreciate touch, using simple but clear language ("Would you like my hand?" or "Here is my hand if you'd like").
2. Shortly after the touch begins, check in about the participant's sense of its rightness ("Is this good?"). Make any adjustments they ask you to make.
3. Remain attentive to the participant's nonverbal responses to the touch, as these may also indicate discomfort and a need to adjust.
4. Recognize the potentially strong impact that sudden cessation may have. When possible, solicit consent before doing so ("I'm going to take my hand back, okay?").

General Considerations Around Consent

Be attentive to the many complexities of consent. If the participant is a survivor of sexual abuse, use additional caution when assessing the participant's openness to touch, as they may have developed a belief that they must consent from past experiences of having their boundaries disrespected. Take added care to ensure that they feel that they can refuse all touch, during preparation and medicine sessions. If working with a cotherapist, be sure to ask them whether they would feel more or less comfortable receiving touch from either therapist, particularly if the therapist's gender identity is similar to that of the perpetrator of the participant's abuse.

Be aware that power dynamics present in the therapeutic relationship (e.g., therapist–participant, researcher–subject, male–female, White–Black, well–unwell) can complicate a participant's "yes." You should check in with yourself, the participant, your cotherapist, and your supervisor to ensure that potentially coercive dynamics have been integrated into your understanding of affirmative consent given by a participant. If you or anyone else feels that such a dynamic is present, give the participant more time and space to check in with their response, perhaps between sessions. Help them feel that they are fully welcome to say "no," perhaps by explicitly discussing the feelings of coercion that might be present for them.

Also, be sensitive to cultural differences in comfort levels around discussing the body or having another person attend to one's body. For some participants, even providing information to you about what is happening in their body (e.g., "I feel a tingling in my hands") and having you attend to it through vision and/or touch may be uncomfortably intimate or even inappropriate given their culture's attitudes toward embodiment. Additionally, cultural differences around touch may mean that even basic supportive touch (e.g., a hand on the shoulder) could become a confusing or intrusive experience. Neglecting these differences may disrupt the therapeutic alliance, diminish treatment benefits, and even do harm to the participant. You should attend to these factors by proactively noticing any unspoken discomfort the participant may be experiencing and explicitly inviting them to note any cultural attitudes toward touch you may be unaware of.

5

Preparation Sessions

I think that's probably the value of having the sessions before [the medicine session] . . . because it's not like it's a couple of strangers watching you—it's a couple of people that I had already opened up to, that already knew me and who I was, and that I felt comfortable with. So that was OK. It was nice, it was nice. I was so protected—my goodness—I couldn't have been more protected. It couldn't have been done better.

—Erin (Belser et al., 2017; Swift et al., 2017)

The preparation phase of PAT marks the start of treatment. It is an opportunity to create a therapeutic container of safety and a strong therapeutic alliance that will guide the rest of the treatment toward positive outcomes. In this book, we are outlining a preparation phase that consists of three 90-minute nondrug sessions. This is where the groundwork is laid for the participant to potentially receive benefit in any of the six EMBARK domains.

You will not yet know which of the domains will become the most salient for this participant, so during preparation all parties should remain open-minded about what will happen during the medicine session. The approach here is more generalist than in subsequent phases. You will provide psychoeducation, develop skills, respond to participant questions or concerns, and work to develop an alliance characterized by deep trust and support.

Your overall approach during this phase should be one of empathic listening, unrushed education, and consistently demonstrated respect for the participant's autonomy and capacity to, with your gentle guidance, bring themselves to healing.

Embark Psychedelic Therapy for Depression. Bill Brennan and Alex Belser, Oxford University Press.
© Oxford University Press 2024. DOI: 10.1093/9780197762622.003.0006

PREPARATION: AIMS

Aim to accomplish the following during this phase:

- Build a rapport characterized by trust, connectedness, and empowerment
- Learn about the participant's experience of depression
- Continue to assess participant suitability and informed consent for treatment
- Explain elements of the treatment
- Explore consent for supportive touch
- Develop the intentions that the participant will bring to the medicine session
- Identify and build upon participant skills that may be supportive during the medicine session:
  - Emotional self-regulation
  - Attending inwardly to feelings and somatic sensations
  - Meeting all that arises with open receptivity

Much of what happens during preparation sessions may feel like the initial sessions of a course of traditional therapy: getting to know each other, building a therapeutic alliance, learning about what brings them to treatment, explaining to them how treatment will look, assessing capacity and consent, and so on. However, it can be helpful to remember that there are four PAT-specific treatment elements that you should be sure to work on with the participant prior to a medicine session, which are summarized here but discussed further throughout the chapter:

1. Inner-focused awareness. Above all, a participant should be prepared to enter their medicine session with the ability to tune into their thoughts, emotions, and sensations with clarity and receptiveness. This is the primary participant capacity that will lead to benefits arising during the medicine session. You will guide the participant through a somatic awareness practice that help them develop this ability (see agenda #2 in this chapter), as well as regularly practicing it throughout the preparation sessions by noticing what is present in their present experience.

2. Adopting an approach of open receptivity to what arises. Encouraging the participant to notice and consider engaging more openly than usual with their emotional experience (i.e., turning toward feelings rather than away) will likely open the door for greater potential benefit. As such, you will work with them to increase their ability to approach and embrace their emotions, including both challenging ones and stronger-than-usual positive ones. When doing so, be sure to support their autonomy by emphasizing that they will still retain the ability to decide how they engage with the emotions and other psychological material they encounter.

3. Emotional self-regulation. In the event that a participant becomes destabilized by the intensity of their internal experience during a medicine session, it is important that they have a go-to way of regulating their emotional state should they need to do so. In the preparation sessions, you will help them develop at least one self-regulation practice for use if needed. This skill should generally be worked on before the other three on this list as a way to support the participant in other preparation practices that invite them to turn inward (e.g., somatic awareness practices).

4. Intentions. What would be beneficial for the participant to explore during the medicine session? Having an answer to this question by the end of preparation can lend structure and forward momentum to the participant's experience of the psychedelic medicine. You will work with them to clarify and connect with their intentions as part of preparation.

THE PSYCHEDELIC PREPAREDNESS SCALE

McAlpine and colleagues (2023) developed a scale for assessing a participant's readiness to benefit from the use of a psychedelic medicine. When they administered this scale to 46 people who were about to attend a 5- to 7-day psilocybin retreat, they found that high scores predicted self-reported benefits. The scale assessed the following 10 aspects of preparation (with example items for each):

1. *Psychoeducation.* "I have learned about the effects of the substances through conversations with other people."
2. *Intention setting.* "I have a clear intention for the psychedelic experience."
3. *Expectation management.* "I know that my experience will be somewhat unpredictable."
4. *Psychological mindedness.* "I am going into the experience willing to learn more about the meaning behind my thoughts."
5. *Emotional readiness.* "I feel ready for the psychedelic experience."
6. *Willingness to surrender.* "I am ready to experience whatever 'comes up' during the psychedelic experience."
7. *Psychophysical robustness.* "I feel as though my mind and body will be 'strong enough' for the upcoming experience."
8. *Safety/security.* "I feel a trusting, positive experience with the people who will be around me during the psychedelic experience."
9. *Prepared for change.* "I feel ready to accept some big changes that might occur in myself as the result of the psychedelic experience."
10. *Preparatory practices.* "I have dedicated time to preparing for the psychedelic experience."

These 10 conditions are a starting point for PAT treatment that is likely to support benefit. They are also very congruent with the approach detailed in this section.

PREPARATION: WORKING WITHIN THE EMBARK CLINICAL DOMAINS

This section provides a general sense of how to prepare a participant to potentially receive benefit in each of the six EMBARK clinical domains. Remember that the significance of each domain in a particular participant's treatment remains to be seen. You are preparing them to potentially go down any path that arises for them by ensuring that they have the skills and supportive conditions they will need to do so.

Existential–Spiritual: Preparation

> *I was prepared for the dark. I was prepared for being alone. I was prepared for the death experience. So I was not afraid. Had I not had those conversations with [the study team] and then found myself lying in a grave with dirt coming in on top of me, I don't see myself going "oh, death is beautiful," which is what I did.*
>
> —Methodist Minister (Swift et al., 2023)

GOAL FOR PREPARATION: CREATE THE CONDITIONS FOR EXPERIENCES OF EXISTENTIAL AND SPIRITUAL CONTENT TO ARISE

Psychedelic medicines have been used for centuries as a way of engaging with spiritual and existential dimensions of human existence, and these dimensions have shown up in the experiences of many PAT trial participants. Your work to prepare the participant to potentially receive benefit in this domain should focus on building space within the treatment for the possible arising of experiences the participant deems sacred. To do so, you should simply name that this might occur and explore their openness to it.

There is no need to go into great detail about the specifics of any one type of spiritual or mystical experience, be it from a specific culture or a specific study. If the participant expresses curiosity, it is okay to give a brief overview of some of the content that could arise (see Chapter 3). When you do, be sure to describe it in a way that is not voyeuristic or exaggerated, which may be tempting given the fantastic quality of these experiences. Also, ensure that they do not develop a rigid expectation of attaining a specific kind of experience (e.g., ego death). If the participant is ambivalent toward the possibility that their medicine experience might contain such content, this is fine. There is no need to convince them of anything. The goal of this framing is to simply "open a door" for the participant so that, during their medicine session, they know they have the option to walk through it.

If a participant mentions an existential theme (e.g., death, mortality, meaning/ meaninglessness, cosmic justice/injustice) or a spiritual question (e.g., the existence or nonexistence of a higher power), collaboratively assess if and how this theme is relevant to their depression and whether it would be useful for them to set an intention of exploring this theme during the medicine session. If a participant specifically mentions religion, spirituality, and/or spiritual practices as a valuable resource for coping with their symptoms, either presently or potentially, it is appropriate for you to affirm this and to collaboratively determine if it would be helpful to set an intention of exploring it further as a resource during the medicine session.

When discussing a participant's religious, spiritual, or existential "big picture" beliefs, keep an ear open for those that might indicate the presence of trauma. For example, a belief that the world is a fallen, dangerous place or that it's not safe to trust anyone but God might indicate trauma. If such a belief arises and you are concerned that it might be a reactive belief that does not serve the participant well, devote some time to collaboratively assessing with the participant whether they feel it would be helpful to develop an intention of exploring this belief during the medicine session. Avoid becoming argumentative or directive or attempting to "take away" the participant's belief. The goal is not to transform these beliefs in the preparation sessions; it is to bring a curiosity about them to the medicine session.

Mindfulness: Preparation

Learning to be, just be.
—Charismatic Episcopalian Reverend (Swift et al., 2023)

GOAL FOR PREPARATION: HELP THE PARTICIPANT LEARN HOW TO ATTEND TO THEIR INTERNAL EXPERIENCE AND TO SOOTHE THEMSELVES IF NEEDED

Preparation in the M domain focuses on helping the participant enter the medicine session with as much capacity to attend to their inner experience as they can muster. Benefits in this domain will arise most readily if they are able to approach any material that arises with openness, acceptance, and compassion. Your role in supporting this ability is twofold: (a) guiding them through specific practices that develop this capacity (see agenda #2 in this chapter for an example of an embodied awareness practice) and (b) encouraging them to slow down and attend to their inner experience at many points throughout the preparation sessions.

This slowing down should suffuse your time with the participant during the preparation sessions. Notice when they may be overlooking an aspect of their experience that is present, invite them to pause and guide them toward their internal experience. For example, if they are speaking about how their relationship with their partner has been adversely impacted by their depression and they look downward with a slightly pained expression on their face, ask them to pause and attend to what is coming up for them. You may make observations about what you see to attend to what is there (e.g., "It looks like there might be some sadness there."). Normalizing this kind of moment of self-attentiveness now will make it easier to encourage the same during a medicine session.

This kind of mindful moment can also present an opportunity for the participant to practice their ability to look at their feelings with equanimity and self-compassion. If they notice sadness but appear motivated to turn away from it, see if they would feel comfortable simply noticing that it is there. Empower them to set the terms for their relationship with it, finding a sustainable place between denying its presence and allowing it to engulf them. You can use the language of "parts," "self-states," or parallel concepts to help participants recognize that they can experience themselves as distinct from specific feelings or states that arise. If they are open to it, they can engage in compassionate conversation with these parts now and later, during the medicine session. For example, a participant experiencing fear or anxiety about the medicine session during preparation can be encouraged to validate and be curious about their fearful part.

In general, any invitation to the participant to turn inward should be conducted in a trauma-informed way that recognizes the stressful, dysregulating experiences that this might elicit. Specific instructions on how to conduct specific awareness practices in a trauma-informed way are provided in agenda #2 in this chapter. Similar caution should be applied to any spontaneous moments of mindfulness you invite the participant into.

Body-Aware: Preparation

I can't begin to describe it to you other than to say it's sensory based on all my senses—could be all the colors, what I get to hear, what I get to touch, what I get to smell . . . it informs my vision, but it wasn't something that was calculated up here, it's something that literally went through my body.
—Caleb (Belser et al., 2017; Swift et al., 2017)

Goal for Preparation: Develop the Participant's Ability to Tune in to the Wisdom of the Body

Similar to the Mindfulness domain, the primary aim of preparation in the B domain is to help develop the participant's capacity to attend to their *embodied* experience during the medicine session. You can help them to understand the importance of tuning into their body and to gain a basic sense of how to do so; this will lay the groundwork for benefits that may spontaneously arise in the medicine session.

As in the M domain, you can support the participant in developing this skill through specific practices (see agendas in this chapter) and continual attentiveness to the participant's embodied experience during preparation sessions. This continual attention can be integrated with the moments of slowing down mentioned earlier in the M domain section. You can remark on moments in which the participant spontaneously attends to their embodied experience. You could also make use of any statements they make about how their depression or an emotion shows up in their body (e.g., "There's a hollowness in my chest."). Use these moments as an opportunity to appreciate their ability to notice these phenomena in their body and to recognize their relevance to psychological material. You may also choose to encourage the participant to attend to their body when you notice that they may not be aware of something meaningful to their therapeutic process that is happening there (e.g., when their posture changes).

Many participants will not initially understand why somatic awareness is important to treatment. It may be helpful to provide psychoeducation on why it is. The participant should arrive at their medicine session with a clear sense of the value of following the body's sensations, rather than pathologizing or ignoring them, even if they still struggle to do so.

Affective–Cognitive: Preparation

These emotions that I had not dealt with . . . a deep sadness and a loss of that childhood thing. I know now why I wouldn't want to have dealt with that. Because it was overwhelming.
—Brenda (Belser et al., 2017; Swift et al., 2017)

GOAL FOR PREPARATION: INVITE THE PARTICIPANT TO
REMAIN OPEN AND RECEPTIVE TO THEIR EMOTIONS
AND SELF-BELIEFS

Preparation in the A domain is the time to lay the groundwork that will support the participant in having a full experience of important psychological material that arises, including powerful emotions and beliefs about themselves that may ordinarily be inaccessible or too challenging to open themselves to. One key part of your role in supporting their openness to such experiences is to help them understand the potential value of taking an open and receptive posture toward this material. You can do so by having a discussion with them about this topic (see agendas in this chapter) and by encouraging the spontaneous arising of any emotional experiences during the preparation sessions, deepening them, and framing them as a good example of the kind of open receptivity they may benefit from adopting during their medicine session.

For example, if a participant becomes tearful when discussing their hopes for treatment, ask them if it would be okay to shift attention toward the emotion that's coming up. Begin by asking simple, emotion-focused questions (e.g., "What are you noticing coming up?") or reflections that use the participant's emotional vocabulary (e.g., "It looks like that grief is here right now, isn't it?"). Give them ample time to experience the emotion before gently exploring what is present in it (e.g., "Are there any words that are coming up with the grief?"). If the participant expresses any beliefs associated with their emotions that seem relevant to their depression (e.g., "I really can't imagine myself in a relationship."), collaboratively decide if it would be worth exploring them further during the medicine session.

Gently redirect any attempts by the participant to develop a firm conclusion about how to resolve these feelings (e.g., "I just need to leave the past behind me") toward an open curiosity about the feeling and its origins. You should also refrain from making a concerted effort to confront or modify any maladaptive self-beliefs that arise during the preparation phase. Instead, such beliefs should be framed as a rich area for exploring during the medicine session. Resist the urge to make premature interpretations or to try to organize the meaning of emotional patterns for the participant. The preparation phase should generally focus on naming and deepening rather than analyzing, transforming, correcting, or adjusting.

Cultural and structural dimensions of emotion. Be attentive to cultural differences in how participants relate to their emotional life. These differences may show up in many places, such as their comfort level around expressing or discussing emotions. This may present additional challenges for some participants in remaining openly receptive to their emotions. Allow them to decide within their own cultural self-understanding whether or not a particular way of relating to their emotions would serve them. Explore how they imagine it will be for them if they do have an emotional opening in their medicine session, particularly in the presence of a therapist.

Also, avoid pathologizing or minimizing negative emotions or beliefs that may reflect valid responses to the cultural or structural conditions in which the participant lives. Some feelings of anger, rage, frustration, or sorrow may be caused by persistent outside conditions (e.g., systemic racism, widespread ableism) and would thus be inappropriate to frame as emotions that would benefit from being transformed during psychotherapeutic treatment. Similarly, some beliefs about the world that seem self-defeating (e.g., "Nobody wants to hire me." or "People look down on me.") may point toward real conditions, such as pervasive racist, transphobic, or ableist discrimination.

Coaching the participant to "get to the core" of these feelings in the implicit hope that they will unravel into something more psychological, like a maladaptive belief learned in early life, may be invalidating to the participant. Additionally, encouraging participants to develop their ability to manage these emotions may also send the implicit signal that unjust conditions should be accepted. Consider that seemingly maladaptive beliefs may be a source of empowerment. As a queer, trans participant said, "Looking back on that first experience with psilocybin, I can see now that the freedom I felt came from finally realizing that there was nothing wrong with me. It was not me who was fucked up, but the world that was fucked up." (PatientNB, Belser & Keating, 2023, p. 131).

You should use your clinical judgment and consultation with subject matter experts to learn how to better hold emotions and beliefs that reflect broader contextual conditions appropriately. Consider holding these emotions as something that could be valuable to feel and explore during the medicine session without any implicit hope that they resolve themselves by the end of treatment.

Relational: Preparation

> *They were so exceptional in their care of me through the therapy sessions, and we developed a very close bond. I felt very comfortable with them—I felt I was in very good hands, and I wanted to share the things that were pertinent to our communal intent that we had spoken to.*
>   —Mike (Belser et al., 2017; Swift et al., 2017)

GOAL FOR PREPARATION: BUILD A RELATIONSHIP THAT CONVEYS SAFETY, ACCEPTANCE, AND EMPOWERMENT

Throughout the preparation phase, the most important thing you can do in this domain is to build an appropriate working relationship with the participant. The potential benefits in this domain are contingent upon this type of relational container. Whenever it would be helpful, explore what the participant needs in order to feel connected, safe, accepted, and empowered with you. Communicate to them that they are encouraged to bring up any thoughts, feelings, or concerns they are having about the working relationship that you are building together.

When building the relational container during this phase of treatment, be sure to attend to the following elements:

Expectations of the relationship and relational boundaries. During preparation, it is helpful to remember that, during the medicine session, the participant might feel shifts in their experience of the interpersonal boundaries between you and them. They may feel a deep connection with you and/or find themselves seeking a stronger than usual degree of closeness with you. After this experience passes, they may find it hard or confusing to return to a more boundaried way of relating to you. Preemptively attend to this possibility during this phase by ensuring that both you and the participant are clear about the boundaries, nature, and duration of the relationship. You may even want to discuss the possible arising of feelings of closeness to name them and normalize them.

Cultural differences and social locations. Attend to how any differences between you and the participant in terms of race, culture of origin, gender, class, sexual orientation, ability, or other cultural factors may impact your shared understanding of the therapeutic relationship. Any underexplored cultural differences in meaning ascribed to the relationship may impact the participant's experience of treatment. For instance, participants from some cultures may expect you to be a strongly boundaried professional, while others would prefer you to be more open and personable. Consider adjusting your stance in the relationship to better meet these expectations, provided you remain within the realm of what is comfortable for you and ethically rigorous in terms of maintaining appropriate boundaries.

Ability to request and receive support. Proactively discuss how the participant feels about accepting support and care from others in their life (e.g., romantic partners, coworkers, helping professionals). Invite them to discuss past experiences that have impacted their ability to access support. Let them know that they may perceive a degree of care and support available from you during the medicine session that is unfamiliar or new to them. Ask them what challenges they might have around this, as well as how they would like the two of you to navigate these challenges together. If it would be beneficial to the participant's treatment and they are amenable, consider having them set an intention of allowing themselves to receive care from you and/or exploring any challenges they have in doing so.

Support for their autonomy. Communicate your faith in the participant's ability to bring themselves to healing. Help them feel that the benefits of treatment will come from within them rather than by way of something you "do" to them and that they have everything they need within them for this to happen. This can be communicated through explicit assurances and by implicitly demonstrating it in how you invite them into each part of the treatment process. Additionally, if you sense that the participant is giving you too much of the credit or responsibility for their treatment outcomes, work with them to shift the locus of control back to them. This may involve taking yourself off a pedestal, reminding them that you have only played a supporting role in their healing process, highlighting the strengths and resources they have brought to bear, or helping them distill what was helpful about the support you offered them so that they can find it for themselves outside of their relationship with you.

Consent and collaboration. Instructions on how to explore consent for touch and PAT treatment are both provided in Chapter 4. However, you should adopt a more general stance of continually assessing the participant's consent for other aspects of treatment, such as any awareness practices you use with them during preparation (e.g., "Would it be all right if we tried a awareness practice?"). Give them a sense that they are an active collaborator in their own treatment process and that they can question, modify, or reject most elements of it.

Enactments. Proactively address the possible influence of the participant's history of trauma on their way of interacting and forming relationships. Those who have experienced significant relational trauma will likely experience a variety of challenges in connecting with you, including fear, reluctance, or dependence. It can be helpful to think of these relational patterns as enactments of prior traumatizing relationships. They may include transferential projections of you as being dangerous, abusive, smothering, overbearing, or neglectful. Enactments may also arise during experiences of intense attachment and abandonment at the end of treatment, despite the participant knowing that treatment is time limited. If you notice indications of these dynamics early in the work, gently and carefully address them in the preparation sessions. This may help mitigate or manage their emergence during medicine sessions, in which the participant is more vulnerable and may experience heightened emotions and transferences.

Self-awareness. Keep in mind that much of what happens in the relational field between you and the participant is outside of both parties' habitual awareness.

For this reason, it is important for you to engage in practices that support you in growing your awareness of your own personal psychological material and how it may show up in session.

Keeping Momentum: Preparation

I really want to enjoy every minute. I want to enjoy being alive and I knew that before the study but afterwards I became able to do it much more often. I have found ways to make that happen.

—Edna (Belser et al., 2017; Swift et al., 2017)

GOAL FOR PREPARATION: BEGIN INSTILLING THE IMPORTANCE OF MAKING POSTTREATMENT CHANGES

The main preparatory aim in this domain is to ensure that the participant understands that there are essentially two parts to PAT treatment: what happens during the treatment itself and the work of carrying it forward after treatment ends. Let them know that sustaining benefits requires them to allow their medicine session experiences to inspire changes in their life. This will include the cultivation of new habits in several areas of their life to replace old, maladaptive ones, as well as taking action to change the circumstances around them that have anchored them in their depression.

Devote time to exploring any preconceptions the participant may have that contradict this framing. For example, they may enter treatment with the notion that the medicine produces the cure in a mechanistic way that requires no behavioral changes, like many other psychiatric medicines. Or they may have read simplified accounts of PAT in the media or in popular science writings that present PAT as something that automatically brings benefits. Help them to understand that the way PAT has its therapeutic effects involves more of a sustained effort to cultivate new habits of thinking, feeling, and relating than any of these notions would suggest.

Importantly, the preparation phase is also the time to begin encouraging the participant to refrain from making any major life changes (e.g., divorce, marriage proposal, quitting a job) in the days or weeks immediately following a medicine session, as their inner decision-making equilibrium may be in flux for some time and regrets may arise later.

PREPARATION SESSION AGENDAS

Having those massive counseling sessions with Seema and Steve were—I've never spent time trying to remember being, my entire life, I've never spent time looking back to try to remember my childhood because I've forgotten so much of it. Not the psilocybin part, but just having all of that leading up to the psilocybin made such a huge difference to me because it helped give me so much understanding as to who I am and why I am the way I am, and a little bit more forgiving to myself.

—Mary (Belser et al., 2017; Swift et al., 2017)

This section contains three suggested agendas for the preparatory aims that should be conducted before a participant's first medicine session. When using them, please consider the following important notes:

- Agendas are meant to be used flexibly. Aims can be conducted out of order or moved from one session to another, in most cases, in response to a specific participant's needs. If your clinical judgment indicates that something else is "in the room," such as a recent event in the participant's life, make contact with it rather than pretending it is not there in service of sticking to the agenda. You can frame this process of slowing down and paying attention as exemplifying the approach the participant should take in their medicine session.
- These agendas are designed for a preparation phase that consists of three sessions. You and your participant may determine, either before beginning treatment or during the preparation phase, that it would be best to schedule additional sessions to allow more space to be devoted to these aims.
- These agendas presume that the participant is new to psychedelic therapy. A returning participant may not need to complete all of these aims with you again, though they may need to review them. As such, fewer preparation sessions may suffice. However, we recommend a minimum of three 90-minute sessions (or session time equivalent) for a first-time PAT participant.
- These agendas also presume that a screening visit has already taken place in accordance with the guidelines laid out in Chapter 4 and the participant has been deemed eligible.
- It is recommended that the italicized language suggestions not be recited to a participant verbatim, in order to avoid coming across as stilted.
- Although you should keep the EMBARK 6 + 4 domains and cornerstones in mind, we discourage you from presenting the entire EMBARK framework to participants. It may be overwhelming and not relevant to their experience. It is fine to describe aspects of EMBARK to the participant, especially as relevant clinical content emerges. Also, when providing psychoeducation to the participant during consent about potential psychedelic experiences, you may find EMBARK's six clinical domains helpful as an internal organizing principle.

Preparation Session 1 Example Agenda (90 minutes)

1. Begin to build rapport and establish trust.
2. Set the agenda for the day's session with the participant.
3. Solicit participant's story of what brings them to treatment.
4. Explore participant's history of psychedelic use and/or preconceptions about use.
5. Provide education about the medicine experience.
6. Discuss the course of treatment.
7. Explore existing self-regulation skills and/or develop new ones.
8. Introduce intention-setting.
9. Begin discussing outside support.

1. Begin to build rapport and establish trust

Building the relational container for the work starts in the first encounter between you and the participant. Begin the process with a presence marked by genuineness, calm, relatedness, attentiveness, authentic positive regard, and empowerment (see "Development of Therapeutic Presence" in Chapter 4). Specific interventions that may facilitate such rapport-building include questions showing genuine interest about aspects of the treatment so far, such as the recruitment and screening process or the participant's interactions with other staff. Be spacious and generous with the amount of time devoted to this part of the agenda. Signal to the participant that this treatment rewards slowing down and being attentive to what is present. At some point early in the session, review the expectations around confidentiality and documentation that were covered during the screening visit to explicitly bring these agreements into your relationship with the participant.

2. Set the agenda for the day's session with the participant

Outline the agenda for the participant with language such as:

> We'll start the session today by hearing a bit about your hopes for this therapy process, your depression, and what the path that has led up to this treatment has been like. After that, we'll ask a set of questions about you, your background, and how life has been for you recently. Then, we'll give you a sense of what to expect from the medicine session, and we'll go over any questions you have at the moment about that. We'll also talk a bit about how these preparation sessions will go and what the rest of our work together will be like. Then, we'll practice one of the skills that can be helpful to bring into a medicine session, called "self-regulation." Finally, at the end of today, we'll go over some of the logistics that you can start to think about. How does that sound? Do you have anything you'd like to add to the agenda?

3. Solicit participant's story of what brings them to treatment

Allow the participant to begin by telling the story of what they're hoping to get from the treatment and their struggles with their depression (and other) symptoms and suffering in a largely uninterrupted way. This will set a collaborative, yet focused frame for the treatment and provide a rich source of clinical information for you. Prompt them with a request such as *"We'd like to hear about how it has been for you to live with depression and also about your hopes for this therapy."*

Attend to the participant's story in a way that is congruent with your clinical orientation and empathic listening skills. Be sure to note several pieces of information:

- Any material that pertains to EMBARK's six clinical domains or care cornerstones.
- The participant's motivations, expectations, and hopes for treatment, including a sense as to what acute life conditions may have most inspired them to come in.
- A lived sense of how the participant experiences their depression: the specific symptoms that they struggle with, how they experience those symptoms, what triggers them (if known), the specific ways these symptoms disrupt their lives, and so on.
- Coping mechanisms and other resources or strengths that the participant has found supportive.
- Any information about the function of their depressive symptoms. For example, a participant's restricted affect or ruminative thought processes may serve to keep trauma-relevant emotions at bay. The participant may either disclose this explicitly or show it in a way that requires your interpretation.
- Indications that the participant has experienced any traumatic events (particularly traumas that have relational aspects, such as child abuse or sexual assault) and/or trauma-related symptoms.
- Structural and cultural conditions that may have impacted the participant's experience of depression (e.g., difficulty finding employment, experiences of racism, participant's sense of the messages about depression they receive from the surrounding culture).
- Any history of other treatment modalities (e.g., talk therapy, SSRIs) and how the participant experienced them.
- If the participant has undergone PAT before, how they experienced it, and how they are carrying that experience into their treatment with you.

Express gratitude for their willingness to share their story, particularly any parts of it that seemed to require additional courage to speak about. While it is important to allow for this telling to unfold in a way that feels spacious, be sure to limit its duration to ensure that other aims can be completed. Remember that a course of therapy in this form is a time-limited treatment, so this is not a comprehensive psychological history that may take many sessions to complete.

In her presentation on the Culturally Competent care cornerstone (available online via the EMBARK Open Access portal), Dr. NiCole T. Buchanan mentioned the DSM-V Cultural Formulation Interview (CFI) as a potentially helpful tool for assessing a participant's experience of their challenges in a culturally attuned way (APA, 2013). If you find that its structure would help you ensure that you attend to cultural and structural elements as you get to know a participant, feel free to use it, either in full or in part.

4. Explore participant's history of psychedelic use and/or preconceptions about use

The participant may have used psychedelic substances prior to treatment. It is worth exploring this use insofar as it might influence their expectations of treatment. If they have prior experience, ask whether it was challenging or well tolerated and whether it occurred in a healing context (e.g., in an Indigenous ceremony or with the support of an "underground" psychedelic guide). Ask them what, if anything, they found beneficial or challenging. Validate their experience but also ensure that they understand that every medicine session may be entirely different than the last and that it is best to temper any expectations based on prior psychedelic use.

For some participants who have not previously used psychedelics, there may be concern about the use of a potent mind-altering medicine. Check to see if this is the case. If so, seek to understand these concerns. If the participant is concerned about stories they have heard from people who have used psychedelics recreationally, explore with them whether these concerning outcomes would still be likely to arise in a more structured treatment setting, as many of them would likely not.

Finally, be sure to modulate the participant's expectations about how effective the treatment will be for them. Psychedelic therapy has been the subject of a lot of glowing popular media coverage in recent years. If participants have read any of these articles, they may enter treatment with an unrealistic sense of its ability to cure their depression. It is important to address these beliefs at the outset of treatment to minimize posttreatment feelings of disappointment that may trigger a relapse of depressive symptoms. Assure them that the data on PAT have been promising so far but that it is not a "magic bullet" and any durable benefits will require the participant to be engaged in the work rather than be a passive recipient.

Participants from social groups that have received disproportionate consequences for substance use due to the racist biases of the War on Drugs may respond differently to this conversation than those from dominant social groups. They might find this discussion of their own history of substance use challenging and may require more time to build trust with you before feeling safe enough to engage in it. They may also benefit from more time spent on this conversation (or revisiting it in future preparation sessions) due to greater levels of fear or concern about using mind-altering substances. Circle back around to this topic as many times as the participant needs in order to feel their concerns are addressed.

5. Provide education about the medicine experience

Convey a broad, general sense of what might arise in the medicine session. Providing this sense in the first preparation session helps the participant begin the gradual process of settling into a state of readiness and acceptance that will serve them well in the medicine session. At a minimum, be sure to cover the following key boldface points.

Common Experiences With the Medicine

- The medicine affects everyone differently, but you will likely **experience strong shifts** in your perceptions, sensations, thoughts, feelings, and sense of what is real. I am sharing all of this with you so that you have some sense of what to expect, you feel more comfortable knowing that these effects are likely normal experiences of the medicine, and you can feel prepared.
- **Visual changes:** With your eyes closed, you might see vivid images, shapes, or patterns. You might also see entire scenes play out. You might see entities, like religious figures or strange beings. What many people have found most helpful when they encounter such things is to welcome it all with open arms. I might remind you to do that if need be.
- With your eyes open, the room and the people in it might look very different. Things might change their appearance as you look at them. This can be distracting, so I might invite you to put your eye mask back on so that you can focus on what's going on inside you. **Focusing inside tends to help the medicine work best.**
- Thoughts: Your **thinking may also change.** You may have new thoughts, insights, or feelings of understanding. You might feel like you understand things in a deeper or more "sacred" way. You may also feel like you are somewhere else in time or space. Sometimes, your thoughts might seem strange to you, like "Why am I thinking that?" It is best to let yourself go with the flow of these thoughts and ideas, rather than judging them. It is usually helpful to trust that the arising of these thoughts is part of the therapeutic process. See if you can accept their presence and be curious about what you can receive from them.
- Body perception: Your **sense of your body might also change.** It might feel very hot, very cold, very tight, or very relaxed. No matter what you're feeling in your body, know that I will be monitoring you to help keep you safe from harm. These body sensations are a normal part of the therapy, and the best thing to do with them is to, again, embrace them.
- Overall, during the medicine session, you may take on some very different perspectives on things. These **new perspectives** can sometimes inspire positive changes in your life. Having these new perspectives will not solve everything overnight. But, if you open yourself up to new perspectives, they can create openings and opportunities you can build upon over the coming weeks and months.
- You may also feel a **profound sense of connection.** This could be with important people in your life, with me, here in the room, with people you've never met, and maybe even with plants, nature itself, or all of reality.

- Your main role in the medicine session can be summed up in two words: **openly receive.** The therapy works best when you remain open to whatever thoughts, feelings, or sensations come your way instead of judging them or rejecting them. Allowing them all to flow and unfold— no matter how challenging or strange they may be—is the goal. If you do this, your mind and body will usually know where to take you so that you can have positive treatment outcomes. The best thing you can do is let them do so.

Difficult Experiences

- There may be moments in which you feel **very uncomfortable,** nauseous, scared, anxious, or **very emotional.** Your thoughts might race more quickly than you can understand them. You might see or think frightening things. Even though these experiences might be intense, these are normal potential experiences of the medicine.
- If you experience any difficult thoughts, feelings, or sensations, first see how it is to **remain open** and turn toward them rather than to turn away or reject them. It may seem strange, but this will help them to pass or transform more quickly. It's more likely to be helpful and healing. Try to approach them with **openness and curiosity** about what they might be trying to tell you.
- Some say that these difficult moments may represent some of the hard things you've experienced in your life "moving through you." **Letting them run their course** can turn into a way of letting go of a lot of the "stuff" you've been carrying.
- However, if your experience ever comes to feel like "too much," there are **techniques that you will be more than welcome to use to support yourself.** We'll be reviewing those in the next two preparation sessions.
- If you need **support from me,** you can always feel free to ask. I can offer reassurance or advise you to try something different. If it feels okay to you, I might offer some **basic physical support,** like handholding, to help you feel grounded. We'll discuss touch in the next session and talk about how you feel about that.
- Importantly, some people who take this medicine feel **nothing at all.** It is possible that you may not feel strong effects. This may be relieving or it may be frustrating. If this happens, I'll invite you to keep doing what you're doing, which is staying open to whatever comes up and paying attention to how you're feeling. This kind of experience may still be valuable. If it disappoints your expectations, we will certainly have time to talk about that afterward.

Roles of the Participant and Therapists

- In the next two preparation sessions, we'll get to know each other a bit more, hear more about your experience of depression, and do some practices that will help you prepare for the medicine session.
- The medicine session will be different. On that day, what will happen is you'll come in, I'll check in about how you're doing, we'll do a brief

awareness practice, and then you will lie down on a bed, put on an eye pillow and headphones (unless you'd prefer not to), and you'll spend the rest of the session listening to music and **focusing on your inner experience.** You won't need to do anything else. All you'll be asked to do is **turn your attention inward and be present toward whatever arises in your mind and body.**

- Of course, you should **feel free to feel, express, and say anything** that comes up in you to whatever extent feels right to you. You can do whatever comes naturally to you. I will take on the responsibility of **making sure that no harm comes to you or me, that nothing inappropriate happens, and that the therapy space is not damaged.** If anything you do goes outside of these bounds, I will work gently with you to redirect you.
- There may be times when it feels like it makes sense for you to sit up or move, but the **default will be lying down.** You can ask to change things about the room, like the temperature.
- I will spend some time talking with you before you take the medicine that day, but once you start feeling the effects, **I will remain mostly quiet** and not interfere with your experience of the medicine. I may check in briefly every so often to see how you're doing, but the session will be primarily you focusing inside and being openly receptive to your emotions, thoughts, or anything that else that comes up in your inner experience.
- You might want to talk about something you are seeing or thinking, and I will certainly talk with you if that's what you really want and need. But it is generally best to **stay in your own experience as much as possible** and tell me later. But you are always welcome to reach out to me for support if you feel you need it.
- When the session is winding down, you can share a bit about what you experienced with me. I'll bring you some light snacks.
- In the **integration sessions** that follow, I can hear in more detail about what came up for you, and we'll discuss how you hope to take it forward.
- The session is expected to last [insert info about timeframe of medicine being used]. You will be **required to stay** until we both feel that it is safe for you to go home. **Does this all sound okay to you?**

Practical Preparation (at This Point in Time)
- There are some things to do to prepare in the week or so leading up to your medicine session. People often find it helpful to think of the session as a multiday experience with a "runway" leading up to the experience and another that gives you time to land afterward.
- Before the medicine session, **leave lots of space in your schedule** in the days leading up to and the days after the session. Try not to work too much or go to big social events. If possible, minimize contact with stressful or difficult people and relationships. If you are a parent or

caregiver and have access to support, consider using it during this time. You should try to enter into a **slowed down and self-reflective state** during the days before the session. Make time to do relaxing things in the days before, like going for walks in nature. If you have a spiritual practice, like prayer or meditation, spend time doing this. Perhaps try some journaling. **Prepare to be off your phone and not contactable** for almost an entire day during the medicine session.

- Also, **take care of your body** during the days before. Try not to eat any heavy foods that are hard to digest, like dairy, red meat, or processed foods. Avoid alcohol consumption and other intoxicants during these days. All of this will serve you well in the medicine session. Also avoid using cannabis or medicines we haven't discussed. If you begin using a new medicine in response to any symptoms you are having, please let me know ASAP.

- Notice if any **thoughts or feelings are calling for your attention** in the days before. Sometimes, when people know they are going to have a medicine session, their mind starts to prepare by bringing things up for their attention. Sometimes, people have powerful or significant dreams. If this happens for you, note these things and bring them to sessions.

- After the medicine session, see if your schedule would allow you to **take a day or more off from work.** If you can't, at least make sure that your day is not too heavily scheduled. If you are a caretaker and have access to support, you may consider using it in the days after your medicine session. You will want to give yourself ample time to stay in touch with the thoughts, feelings, imagery, and bodily experiences that came up in the session. Many people find that the therapeutic process supported by the medicine is still unfolding in the day or two after the session. Consider continuing the changes to diet and substance intake that you made during the preparation to help support this unfolding.

- We will talk about more "day of" logistics as the session grows closer, but for now, plan on making these openings in your schedule and making these changes to your diet.

- Aftercare: Also, you will need a **support person to pick you up** after the session, as you should not drive a vehicle for 24 hours after taking the medicine. It would be good to arrange that person now, as I will need to speak to them before the session to make sure they are able to support you.

- It would be good to **be thoughtful about how to communicate with the other people in your life about your treatment,** both before and after the medicine session. It is natural to be at least somewhat excited or nervous and to want to share this with others in your life. They may also ask you questions about your experience, even though it might be hard for them to understand the process. If you need support in figuring out how to talk to people about the treatment, I would be happy to help.

The authors acknowledge that this language draws inspiration from that of Guss and colleagues (2020), who in turn drew inspiration from that of Bogenschutz and Forcehimes (2017).

6. Discuss the course of treatment

Provide the participant with a sense of what to expect from the structure of sessions going forward. If they do not already have one, give them a clear timeline of when the sessions will occur. Give them a sense of the purpose of preparation and integration sessions, as well as their quantity and timing. This may be a good time to explain that the preparation sessions will include, in addition to getting to know each other and building trust, a focus on developing several key skills: self-regulation, open receptivity, and focusing on their inner experience of their feelings and their body.

7. Explore existing self-regulation skills and develop new ones

Explain to the participant that it can be helpful in medicine sessions to have one or a few ways of resourcing themselves if they begin to get dysregulated. You can frame these as "self-regulation skills," "internal resources," or anything similar that feels like a more accessible term for you and the participant. These skills include any practices that help the participant do any of the following: titrate the amount of challenging material they are working with, ground or soothe themselves, or access their internal resources (e.g., resilience, strength, self-compassion).

Ask the participant if they currently have any techniques that they use when they feel agitated or stressed out. If they have been in therapy before, ask if they have ever learned anything like that with a previous therapist. It may jog their memory if you provide them with a list of examples.

If they are able to name a skill they already use, invite them to practice it with you in this session so that both of you will have a sense of how you can deploy it in case it is needed during the medicine session. It may be helpful to support them in deepening and expanding their go-to skill through further practice with you or an invitation to practice on their own between sessions.

If they are unable to name any existing skills, use this time to help them cultivate a relationship with a new one. Any self-regulation practice that can be employed in a moment of distress is acceptable. Provide them with a "menu" of the different types of techniques (listed below) and ask them if they have a sense of which might be the easiest for them to work with. If they do not express a preference, suggest they try a breathing practice. Types of practices may include:

- Breathing techniques
- Self-touch or self-hug techniques
- Touching fabrics
- Grounding stretches or postures
- Visualization
- Sensory refocusing practices

- Tapping
- Rocking

Remember that the practice you choose with the participant is one that should be accessible and easy to use in moments of dysregulation or emotional distress. Practices that involve a lot of verbality (e.g., distracting oneself by listing objects in the room of a specific color) may be less effective than simpler ones that prioritize the body.

Note that these practices are intended to alleviate only experiences of distress that threaten to derail their medicine session and not all experiences of challenging emotions. It may be helpful to frame this skill as something to keep in their back pocket just in case, though they will likely not have to use it.

Here is an example of a breath-based practice that can be used:

STOMACH BREATHING EXERCISE

Take a moment to let your body settle into a comfortable, relaxed posture. Feel your feet flat on the floor. Let your spine feel supported in an upright position without having to be too rigid. Keep an attentive yet relaxed posture. Notice any tensions in your shoulders or neck and give them a chance to release if they'd like. Just notice the places where your body comes in contact with the chair. Your back, your seat, the back of your legs. Let yourself feel secure and supported by the chair. You can choose to either close your eyes gently or keep them open.

Whenever you're ready, start by putting one hand, either one, on your stomach and the other on your chest. As you breathe in and out, see if you can feel your stomach moving your hand. Pushing into it as you breathe in, and collapsing as you breathe out. Practice this for a few more breaths. Just noticing, with your hand, each breath going in and each breath going out.

Next, we'll do this with deeper breaths. As you breathe in, really let yourself feel the breath going in through your nose, down through your throat and chest, and into your stomach. See how much you can expand your stomach into your hand. When you breathe out, see how much you can exhale, without using your hand to push. With each breath, notice the air going in and going out.

Do this for a few more breaths. Fill up your stomach and your hand with each breath in, and flatten out with each exhale. Notice the whole path that each breath takes: nose, throat, chest, stomach, into your hand. It's okay if you get distracted. Gently bring yourself back to noticing your breath as many times as you need.

As the exercise winds down, you can let yourself start to breathe normally again. No need to take big breaths anymore. Just let your breath do what it wants, little by little. If your eyes are closed, feel free to keep them closed as long as you'd like.

Gently, at your own pace, let your awareness start to come back to the room around you. As you come back, notice whatever you can about how you feel.

8. Introduce intention-setting

Toward the end of the session, invite the participant to begin thinking about their intentions for treatment. Begin by defining intentions as questions or curiosities pertaining to their depression that the participant can use to focus their upcoming medicine session. Some examples include:

- "I want to better understand why I think so poorly of myself."
- "I'd like to know more about this sunken feeling in my chest I have felt for years."
- "I want to look at why it is so hard for me to maintain healthy relationships."

For a participant's first medicine session, they may also reflect a wish to successfully engage with basic elements of the treatment:

- "I would like to let myself experience my emotions more than I usually do."
- "I want to see how it is to feel open and emotional with the therapist around and maybe see if I can accept their care."
- "I want to be more in my body and less in my head."

Intentions are not specific changes that the participant wants to make to their life or specific problems they want to solve. The following examples are *not* suitable intentions, as they are specific life changes or specific problems. Work with the participant to look to the motivation behind these statements to formulate intentions:

- *"I want to spend more quality time with my partner."* ➔ "I would like to look at why I struggle to connect with my partner."
- *"I want my parents to start respecting my choices."* ➔ "I want to look at the pain I feel about my relationship with my parents."
- *"I have to stop getting caught up in these negative thought patterns."* ➔ "I would like to see where these negative thoughts come from and why they take me over."

VALUES AS INTENTIONS

Dr. Sarah Bateup (personal communication, 2022) has invited participants to focus on a specific personal value they hold as important, such as dependability, faith, or self-acceptance, as a form of intention-setting. Over the course of treatment, their intention is to grow their ability to embody and act from this value.

The participant does not need to come with a fully formed intention by the next session. They should be asked to simply begin thinking about where they would like to learn more about themselves and/or seek support in shifting something. One intention is ideal, though having two or three related ones is acceptable. Intentions should be relevant to the participant's depression. Ensure that the participant understands that the content of their medicine session is ultimately not something under their control and that their intentions are merely requests that should be held lightly.

Note that some participants may set an intention that reflects a desire to adapt to harmful circumstances (e.g., an abusive relationship, exploitative working conditions). If you notice this during the preparation phase, evaluate whether such adaptation is advisable or if it might be more beneficial for them to focus on altering these circumstances. Explore with them whether they would be willing to broaden their intention around this particular issue to leave room for shifts in their context. For example, if they wish to ask the medicine for help in "finding peace" with their problematic spouse, gently offer alternative approaches to the same concern that are more likely to increase their sense of their capacity to respond with more agency and understanding ("I want to better understand what I need in relationships.").

CHANGE TALK IN MOTIVATIONAL INTERVIEWING

In *Motivational Interviewing* (Miller & Rolnick, 2013), therapists are advised to listen for their participants' "change talk," or statements that reveal a consideration of, motivation for, or commitment to change. The acronym DARN CATS comprises seven types of change talk that may be helpful to listen for in PAT preparation sessions, as they may reflect an area to explore as a basis for an intention that resonates with a participant's intrinsic motivation for change.

Desire/longing	"I really want to be healthier."
Ability	"I know I can do this all differently."
Reason	"If I don't fix this now, I might fall apart."
Need	"I can't keep doing this to my body."
Commitment	"When I leave, I'm doing it differently."
Activation	"I can feel my will to live coming back."
Taking Steps	"I'm going to start therapy again."

9. Begin discussing outside support

Before undergoing PAT treatment, it is essential to make sure that the participant has sufficient support in place, for both during and after treatment. This may include family, close friends, other providers, and/or having a list of as-needed professional referrals. Collaboratively explore with the participant how much support they will need, what might get in the way of obtaining it, and how you can work with them to troubleshoot any issues before proceeding to a medicine session. Also, let the participant know that they should begin making plans with a reliable person who can pick them up after the medicine session.

As mentioned earlier, this may also be a good time to talk to the participant about how to communicate with their loved ones about their treatment experience (see Chapter 4 for further discussion). Let them know that it is their choice how much to share, but that you are there to help them try to troubleshoot any challenges that may be in the way of them communicating as they would like. For example, you could work with them on how they will communicate or how they will navigate unwanted reactions.

End the session on an encouraging note. For instance, you may let the participant know that they are doing something meaningful or convey your feeling that they are taking good steps to work on their depression.

Preparation Session 2 Example Agenda (90 minutes)

1. Set the agenda for the day's session with the participant.
2. Check in about intentions.
3. Help the participant understand the importance of welcoming challenging material.
4. Introduce and practice a somatic awareness exercise and suggest practicing it at home.
5. Discuss logistics and at-home preparation.

1. Set the agenda for the day's session with the participant
Briefly discuss the expected content of the session, using language such as:

> *In today's session, we'll start by talking about your intentions for treatment that we started discussing last time. We'll spend some time going over them and developing them together so that they can set the frame for the rest of the process. After that, we'll go over two more important things that you can bring into your medicine session. The first one we'll cover is the importance of going toward your feelings instead of away from them during that session. After that, we'll go through an awareness practice that could help you develop your ability to turn inward and pay attention to your body, which is what you'll mostly be doing during the medicine session. After that, we'll wrap up with some logistics. How does that sound? Is there anything you'd like to add to our agenda?"*

2. Check in about intentions
Begin by asking the participant how they have been since the last session. Ask them if any questions or concerns have arisen since the previous session and respond to them. Use your clinical judgment to determine which anxieties you should work to resolve (e.g., safety concerns, concerns about the therapeutic alliance) and which should be normalized (e.g., nervousness about the potential intensity of the medicine effects).

Ask the participant if they were able to come up with any ideas for intentions since the last session and use these as starting points. Your role in this process is to:

- *Link the participant's intentions to their struggles with depression.* Participants may bring in ideas for intentions that do not clearly relate to their depression. Ensure that there is a meaningful connection. Note that some seemingly unrelated intentions may actually have an intuitive connection to the participant's depression that they should be helped to articulate.
- *Guide a deeper exploration of the experiences, feelings, and beliefs informing the intentions.* An intention should not feel like an uninspiring item on a to-do list. It should feel alive for the participant. Work with them to feel their intentions more, both in session and through continued reflection on them between sessions.

- *Gradually develop one (or a few) intentions to bring into the medicine session.* By the time the preparation phase has concluded, the participant's intentions should be in a clear enough format that concise reminders can be given to the participant during their experience with the medicine, if need be.
- *Coach the participant on how to hold their intentions.* Remind the participant that intentions are important but should be held loosely when entering the medicine session. They serve as guiding suggestions, not rigid expectations.

3. Help the participant understand the importance of welcoming challenging material

Let the participant know that the next part of the session is meant to give them a sense of how to work with the feelings and thoughts that come up during the medicine session. If helpful, psychoeducational materials from your modality of choice may be used, as long as they speak to the following six points:

1. When challenging thoughts and emotions come up, we often do not want to face them because of how overwhelming they can be.
2. When we continuously avoid our feelings by "shutting down," "checking out," or using alcohol or other drugs to avoid them, they can have ongoing negative effects on our life (e.g., depression, anxiety, addiction, sleep problems).
3. In psychedelic medicine sessions, people often find that they have a greater capacity than usual to face these thoughts and emotions without getting overwhelmed.
4. During the medicine session, you are invited to try to be open and curious about them, as this may reduce the negative effects they have in the long run.
5. It can be helpful to try to engage compassionately with these experiences and with yourself as you approach them.
6. These feelings and beliefs usually have causes in our life experiences, and it can be productive to be curious and compassionate toward these as well.

The notion of remaining open to challenging experiences should be framed as a noncompulsory process that does not undermine participant autonomy. Resist the temptation to use "tough" or overly provocative language when describing it (e.g., "No pain, no gain."). Ensure that the participant feels empowered in the knowledge that their autonomy and intuitive sense of how to respond to a feeling will always be honored and that the encouragement to remain open and receptive should not be taken as a mandate to push past their better judgment. Assure them that their self-protective strategies and parts will be welcomed as a valued, important voices in determining a stance toward whatever material comes up.

To point 5 from the list above, helping participants to understand the value of bringing compassion to any phenomenon that arises—challenging emotions, self-critical beliefs, upsetting memories, feelings of "stuckness" or inability to change—is a crucial part of preparation. Suggested metaphors for highlighting this approach include:

- Welcoming everyone to the table
- Befriending the monster in the closet
- Being gentle and kind with yourself no matter what comes up
- Relating to yourself as you would to a friend who's having a difficult experience

To make these points, feel free to draw from any instances of compassionate self-understanding that have already arisen in treatment. You are also welcome to bring in any materials or exercises that would aid in applying these principles to the participant's lived experience of depression.

Be attentive and responsive to the possibility that self-compassion may feel inaccessible, uncomfortable, or overwhelming for your participant (Gilbert et al., 2011). For many, this kind of positive emotion can come with associations to past aversive experiences, such abuse and neglect. They may worry about becoming dependent on self-compassion, fear that they will become weak as a result of it, or see it as a form of letting their guard down that will invite negative consequences. Do not pressure participants who struggle with self-compassion to push past these difficulties to adopt it. Instead, consider inviting them to set an intention of exploring this difficulty during the medicine session.

4. Introduce and practice somatic awareness

Explain to the participant that being able to attend deeply and consistently to what is coming up in their embodied experience during a medicine session will likely help them move toward therapeutic outcomes. Invite them to join you in practicing a somatic awareness exercise that will help them develop their ability to do so.

If helpful, begin by discussing some of the embodied experiences that may arise during a medicine session (see Chapter 2 for examples). Give the participant time to share their reactions, concerns, or questions about them. Now and throughout treatment, adopt a stance of normalizing any non–physically threatening embodied experiences so that the participant will be less likely to interpret them as events that require medical intervention. It may be helpful to direct the participant toward data demonstrating the relative safety of psilocybin. Encourage the participant to relax into the fact that you (and the team physician, if one is present) will pay strict attention to their physical well-being at all times.

In addition to helping them feel that most common somatic events are safe, help them understand how they can be valuable. The specific way you discuss this is up to you, as long as it is accessible to the participant. Encourage the participant to welcome any bodily sensations that arise and to remain openly receptive to them. Discussing all of this with them may help them relax into the understanding that they may trust in the healing wisdom of their body during the medicine session. The value of cultivating inward awareness in the medicine session should be the main focus of this discussion. Save any exploration of the potential value of this kind of awareness in everyday life for the integration sessions. The use of metaphors to convey material is encouraged. Next, guide them through a practice that helps them strengthen their ability to turn their attention inward in this way. Exercises from a range of modalities are welcome, as long as they focus on inviting the participant to remain attentive and receptive toward sensations in their body and any associated feelings or reactions that arise. Care should be taken to keep the participant "in their body" and passively observing, rather than intellectualizing or trying to make sense of their experience.

The way the exercise is taught and practiced should meet the participant "where they're at" by providing space for the validation and processing of whatever challenges arise for them. For example, an attempt in which the participant's thoughts were racing and distracting them should be framed as valuable learning insofar as they were able to turn inward and notice these distracted qualities, which required mindfulness.

Some participants may associate awareness or mindfulness practices with the religious traditions from which they most often derive, such as Buddhism or Hinduism. If they are members of another religious group, such as Christian or Jewish traditions, they may feel that engaging in awareness practices puts them at odds with their own faith. If such discomfort arises, be respectful of it and devote ample time to discussing it. Ask the participant if their faith provides any practices that teach them to attend to their inner experience. If so, invite them to bring that practice into the preparation work. Alternatively, the participant may be relieved by the knowledge that the type of inward awareness practiced in this treatment is a form that is free from any elements of a specific faith (e.g., devotion to a deity, recitation of mantras in a specific language). Consider sharing with them that nonreligious mindfulness and awareness practices have been studied by secular science and have been found to provide benefits that are independent of any religious tradition. In all of these discussions, be respectful of discomfort and avoid rushing past participant concerns.

As with any awareness or mindfulness practice used in treatment, ensure that your approach is trauma-informed. Participants should never be encouraged to sustain an inward focus if it generates distress, dissociation, or dysregulation. Let the participant know that, while the exercise might be difficult, it is not meant to elicit strong discomfort, panic, or fear. It is most important that they feel safe at all times. Tell them that, if they feel frightened by anything that arises during the exercise, they are encouraged to tell you, and that the exercise can be stopped. Invite any questions or concerns they may have before jumping in. Let them know that they are welcome to keep their eyes open from the outset, open them at any point during the exercise, or stand up if they feel activated. Feel free to explain these considerations to them using common metaphors such as "pumping the brakes."

Some participants may become dissociated during an awareness practice without recognizing that they are doing so. In addition to empowering them to give voice to any distress, you should remain attentive throughout the exercise for signs that trauma is arising, such as overly loose or rigid muscle tone, shifts in breathing, sweating, emotional lability, or increased paleness of the skin. If your selected practice is too activating for the participant, use an alternative exercise that uses a form of attention that is more comfortable and accessible for them (e.g., focusing on a sensory experience, a guided imagery practice that gently involves the body).

Any selected exercise should invite the participant to cultivate a receptive state. Exercises that involve visualization or chanting are discouraged, as they may not teach the same state of surrender and receptivity to what is naturally present, which is the stance that would benefit them most in a medicine session.

Feel free to use the following example or a comparable practice of your own:

BODY-FOCUSED AWARENESS PRACTICE

Take a moment to let your body settle into a comfortable, relaxed posture. Feel your feet flat on the floor. Let your spine feel supported in an upright position without having to be too rigid. Keep an attentive, yet relaxed posture. Notice the places where your body comes in contact with the chair. Your back, the seat, the back of the legs. Let yourself feel secure and supported by the chair.

You can choose to either close your eyes gently throughout this meditation, or you can let them stay open and rest on a spot on the floor in front of you if you'd prefer, keeping your gaze soft and still. Remember that you can always choose to open your eyes later if anything too stressful comes up for you.

Let's begin by turning the attention inward, focusing on the sensations present in the body. Take a moment to notice how your body feels right now. Scan from the top of your head to the tips of the toes, gently observing any areas of tension, discomfort, or ease. We're not looking to change or correct anything. Simply noticing and giving your attention over to whatever is there.

If you come across any tension or discomfort, try to approach it with curiosity, like a gentle investigator exploring the landscape of the body. Notice the qualities of these sensations—are they tight, heavy, tingly, or achy?

As you continue to breathe, direct your attention to any areas that are calling for your awareness. Allow the breath to be a soothing companion, gently guiding you toward these sensations.

Now, imagine you can have a conversation with these sensations. If they could speak, what would they say to you? Listen attentively without judgment or trying to change anything.

If you notice your mind wandering, kindly acknowledge the thoughts and gently bring your focus back to the sensations in the body.

As you maintain this gentle awareness, see if you can welcome and hold the sensations with compassion. Embrace whatever arises with an open heart, knowing that it's okay to feel whatever you feel.

As we come to the end of this practice, take a moment to express gratitude to yourself for dedicating this time to connect with your body and its sensations.

Gently, at your own pace, let your awareness start to come back to the room around you. You can keep your eyes closed (if they're closed) as you slowly come back to your chair, the room, the other people in it, maybe make small movements with your hands or feet if you'd like. As you start to slowly open your eyes and come back, see if you can take with you this quality of noticing that you used. Let it come back to you now and then throughout the rest of your day.

Once the exercise is complete, briefly discuss the participant's experience and normalize any common difficulties they had (e.g., distractions, self-judgment). Leave them with a sense that whatever success they had was adequate and representative of an increase in their capacity. Recommend that the participant practice this exercise at home on their own unless it would feel too risky for them to do in an unsupported setting.

If the participant found it distressing to "go inside," you should take this into consideration when assessing their readiness for a psychedelic medicine session, which typically favors some degree of turning inward. It may be that this participant needs additional preparation sessions that focus on resourcing them further. If their distress is sufficiently severe, it could also indicate that they are not a suitable candidate for psychedelic work at this time and would be better served by a thoughtful referral to another modality of care.

5. Discuss logistics and at-home preparation

As the session comes to a close, check in with the participant about their arrangement for a support person who will pick them up from the medicine session. Respond to any questions, concerns, or needs for troubleshooting.

Now that the medicine session is approaching, you should also review week-of dietary and other restrictions with the participant. Frame this conversation with them collaboratively, as diet is a personal concern that will carry different meanings for each participant. First, ensure that the participant is abstaining from any contraindicated medications for the psychedelic you are using. Also, advise them to eat in a way that puts minimal strain on their digestive system for at least 4 days before the medicine session. For many participants, this means avoiding heavier foods, such as meat and dairy, as well as spicy foods and any other food that is contraindicated for the specific psychedelic drug being used. Participants may also be well served by avoiding the use of any other mind-altering substances (including alcohol) for at least 3 days prior to the medicine session, or as long as they can. Some participants also find it helpful to taper down their caffeine intake as much as they can, as caffeine use or withdrawal on the day of the medicine session may impact it adversely. You may even want to frame other consumptive activities—watching TV or movies, reading the news or social media, and so on—as something to be mindful about and suggest that they limit violent or disturbing content during their preparation, as anything that is in recent memory may be taken into their medicine session (Garel et al., 2023).

In nonmedical psychedelic healing contexts, it is sometimes advised to abstain from sexual activity for at least 3 days prior to dosing, which is a restriction you may explore with the participant. All of these restrictions are often also applied to the 3+ days after the medicine session to allow the participant's body to ease back into normalcy. Work with the participant to develop a specific plan that suits their needs.

Invite the participant to continue practicing the somatic awareness exercise at home several times before the next session. Invite them to write down any difficulties or questions that arise when they do so that can be discussed next time. Encourage them to practice from a relaxed place of self-compassion as much as they can, rather than an intensely driven or self-punishing place.

Additionally, if the participant's intentions are still unformulated, encourage them to spend more time feeling into them before the next session.

Preparation Session 3 Example Agenda (90 minutes)

1. Set the agenda for the day's session with the participant.
2. Check in about intentions and at-home practice.
3. Revisit somatic awareness and/or self-regulation practices (if helpful)
4. Invite a relational check-in.
5. Assess consent for touch-based interventions.
6. Discuss logistics and at-home preparation.

1. Set the agenda for the day's session with the participant

Briefly discuss the expected content of the session, using language such as:

> *In today's session, we'll start by checking in about the intentions that we worked on last time to see how they've been sitting with you. Then we'll check in about how the practice exercise you did on your own* [if they did so] *was for you. After we do, we're going to build off of that one and work on another kind of awareness exercise together today* [if you feel it would be helpful and accessible for them]. *After that, we'll check in about how it's been for you to be working with me so far. Finally, we'll spend some time talking about the kinds of physical support you'd prefer to have or not have, and we can talk about anything else you'd like before we go into the medicine session together. Then, we'll talk logistics again and wrap up. How does this sound? Is there anything you'd like to add?"*

2. Check in about intentions and at-home practice

As in the previous session, ask the participant how they have been since the last meeting. Ask them if any questions or concerns have arisen and respond to them. It may be helpful to let the participant know that it is often said that the session truly begins a few days before the medicine is taken, so the appearance of anxieties or other unexpected emotions may be an expected part of the process. Encourage them to begin the practice of welcoming these feelings or at least trying to let them be present.

Ask the participant how they are currently feeling about their intentions and whether they have shifted or evolved at all since the last session. By the end of the preparation phase, the participant should have a clear depression-relevant intention (or two) that will frame their medicine session.

Ask the participant how any at-home practices (self-regulation, somatic awareness) have been going. Frame any difficulties as part of the process and respond compassionately to any self-judgment that arose.

3. Revisit somatic awareness and/or self-regulation practices (if helpful)

If you or the participant feel that it would be beneficial to revisit any of the skills that they are bringing into the medicine session, devote some time to doing so. Even if they are mostly confident about their grasp of these skills, err on the side of practicing them together in this session to deepen them and refresh them prior to the medicine session. This practice will be particularly important if this session is the first in-person meeting, as using these skills together in the treatment space will give all parties a more robust sense of how to call upon them during the medicine session.

4. Invite a relational check-in

It's important to have an explicit metacommunication with the participant about how it is going before a medicine session. In the final preparation session, leave ample room for a check-in about any concerns that either you or the participant may have about your relationship. This may include therapist–participant dynamics that have yet to be explicitly brought into shared awareness, participant misgivings about you that have not been adequately attended to, participant concerns about differences in your respective social locations and your competence in navigating this difference, or any other unexpressed feelings the participant may have toward you, such as attraction or aversion. If left unaddressed, these relational factors may later disrupt the relational container in a way that impacts the participant's ability to feel safe enough to adopt the receptive, open approach that is asked of them, which may lead to diminished therapeutic outcomes.

Encourage the participant to give voice to any relational dynamics they feel need to be discussed. If you feel that you have become aware of any such dynamic, and the participant does not mention it, use your clinical judgment to determine whether offering it to the participant for discussion is in their best interest. Be mindful of the ways therapist–participant power imbalances that derive from inequalities in the surrounding culture may influence the participant's willingness to mention how these imbalances affect them. For example, a dyad of straight therapists working with a queer participant should consider being more proactive in empowering the participant to acknowledge that this dynamic is worthy of discussion and speak to how it affects them.

Example language to use in this check-in may include:

> Before we go into the medicine session together in a few days, it would be helpful if we could spend some time hearing from you about how it has been to be working together with me. Take a moment to check in with yourself and see if there is anything about me or the working relationship we've built together that feels like it needs to be talked about. I really encourage you to be as open as you can. I've found that the more of this kind of thing that we can name and talk through, the more productive of an experience you'll have in the medicine session. Maybe there's something you want to ask about me or something you want to ask from me. Maybe I did something that made you uncomfortable or upset. Anything like that, I'd be very open to working it out with you so it doesn't interfere with your medicine session.

5. Assess consent for touch-based interventions

If you intend to offer touch to the participant, it is very important to begin the process of assessing their consent for any forms of touch that may be used. Do so in accordance with the double consent procedure described in the "Touch in EMBARK" section of Chapter 4.

6. Discuss logistics and at-home preparation

Check once more to ensure that the participant has arranged a support person to pick them up after the medicine session. Remind them of the minimum number of hours they will be required to stay on site. Let them know they can eat a very light breakfast (avoiding dairy, meat, or spicy foods) as soon as they wake up on the day of the medicine session and that all other dietary needs throughout the day will be provided for by you. Inform the participant what to bring to the medicine session, such as the following:

- Comfortable, loose-fitting clothing
- Clothing layers to accommodate subjective fluctuations in temperature
- Photos of important loved ones or oneself, if desired
- Meaningful objects to have in the space, if desired
- A totem to hold throughout the process that can later symbolize it, if desired
- A journal for taking notes toward the end of the session

Explore the participant's openness to beginning the dosing portion of the medicine session with a brief "opening" as a way to mark the movement from an ordinary moment into a nonordinary moment. If they are comfortable with the idea, invite them to decide what form it will take, perhaps drawing from their spiritual or religious practices. Allow them to take more time to think about it between now and the medicine session if they would like. If they ask for suggestions, consider offering them the following:

1. Reading a poem
2. Lighting a candle
3. Sharing a moment of silence
4. Singing a song
5. Building an altar of meaningful items
6. Performing a knot-tying ritual
7. Having an exchange of supportive, heartfelt words between you and them

Invite the participant to continue practicing any somatic awareness or self-regulation exercises that were a part of preparation in the days leading up to the medicine session. Remind them to practice from a relaxed place with as much self-compassion as they are able to access.

Remind the participant to continue to abstain from any contraindicated medications and to observe the dietary restrictions to which they agreed. Encourage them to not overhydrate themselves on the morning of the medicine session to avoid frequent trips to the bathroom. Encourage them to limit stressful activities and allocate extra time for reflection in the days leading up to and following the medicine session. Wish them a restful and reflective time between now and the day of the medicine session, assure them of your faith in their ability to bring themselves where they need to go during the medicine session, and bid farewell to them in a way that communicates again the promise of compassionate support that will be offered to them that day.

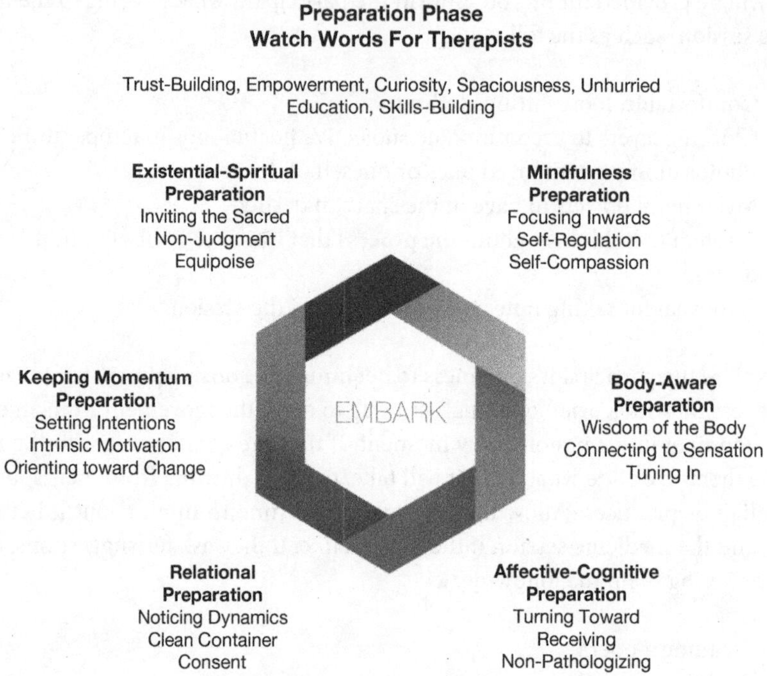

Preparation Phase
Watch Words For Therapists

Trust-Building, Empowerment, Curiosity, Spaciousness, Unhurried
Education, Skills-Building

Existential-Spiritual
Preparation
Inviting the Sacred
Non-Judgment
Equipoise

Mindfulness
Preparation
Focusing Inwards
Self-Regulation
Self-Compassion

Keeping Momentum
Preparation
Setting Intentions
Intrinsic Motivation
Orienting toward Change

EMBARK

Body-Aware
Preparation
Wisdom of the Body
Connecting to Sensation
Tuning In

Relational
Preparation
Noticing Dynamics
Clean Container
Consent

Affective-Cognitive
Preparation
Turning Toward
Receiving
Non-Pathologizing

Figure 5.1. Preparation Phase: Watch Words for Therapists

6

Medicine Sessions

When you're a little kid and the first time you jump off the high board, you know it's like—you know you can swim, and you'll probably be fine, but it's pretty scary. It was more than that though—it was even scarier than that because you're really going. For me it was like I was getting to go into my mind and explore a whole new world that I had not known.
—Brenda (Belser et al., 2017; Swift et al., 2017)

Medicine sessions are the main event of psychedelic therapy. They are the sessions in which the psychedelic medicine is administered. The therapeutic stance to take during these sessions in one of support, responsiveness, and skillful following. For each participant, a unique array of psychic material will arise without any consciously willful attempts on your part or theirs to control or determine it.

This chapter is structured similarly to Chapter 5, though it contains several new sections. Like the last chapter, it begins by detailing the specific therapist aims for the session, followed by general advice for working within each of EMBARK's six clinical domains. The therapist's aims are then woven into an agenda for the first part of the session. The chapter also includes three sections that give specific guidance on how and when to intervene during the medicine effects. It concludes with advice on how to work with a participant who is not experiencing strong medicine effects or believes they received placebo.

In contrast to the preparation sessions, your interventions will be less preset and more responsive in the medicine sessions. This is because, once the psychedelic medicine takes effect, that is when your role shifts from preparing the participant for the whole potential range of experiences that could arise to helping them benefit from the actual experience they are having. You have shown them the trail map, but now they are the one embarking on the journey.

EMBARK Psychedelic Therapy for Depression. Bill Brennan and Alex Belser, Oxford University Press.
© Oxford University Press 2024. DOI: 10.1093/9780197762622.003.0007

In the medicine session, you may also begin to see which of the six EMBARK clinical domains may become emergent for your participant. This transitional moment signals a shift from a neutral but curious stance toward responsive attention to particular domains (e.g., E domain, B domain, R domain). The emergent domain(s) may continue to shift during the time between the medicine and integration sessions. There is no need to do anything with this information just yet, but it is advisable to keep your eyes open for clues as to what directions the path might take during integration.

MEDICINE SESSIONS: AIMS

Generally, your role in medicine sessions is to:

- Prepare the space
- Provide the medicine
- Provide mindful, compassionate attention, even when the participant is focused internally
- Maintain appropriate boundaries
- Ensure participant safety and well-being
- Supportively listen to the participant's first impressions as the medicine wears off
- Ensure that the participant departs from the session safely

Additionally, you might be called upon to provide the following forms of support, if indicated by the situation (which will be explained in greater detail in the agenda that follows):

- Encourage the participant to remain open and receptive to material that arises
- Respond to participant needs or concerns
- Provide relational support and care when appropriate
- Remind the participant of their intentions if they become unfocused
- Take notes of significant statements or themes that arise for the participant
- Provide supportive, consensual touch when appropriate
- Respond appropriately to some challenging events that may impact participant well-being

More so than any specific aim or intervention, the quality of your presence during the medicine session is of the utmost importance. During a medicine session, participants will be exquisitely sensitive to everything about your presence, including your level of anxiety, your facial microexpressions, the tone of your voice, and the quality of your eye contact. Remember to sit on your CUSHION and avoid FRAZZLE.

C	Calm	F	Frantic
U	Unhurried	R	Rigid
S	Supportive	A	Artificial
H	Human	Z	Zoned-out
I	Impeccably boundaried	Z	Zealous
O	Openhearted	L	Loosely boundaried
N	Nonjudgmental	E	Exhausted

Some important reminders on the topic of presence:

- Refrain from engaging in other activities (e.g., reading, looking at your phone) while the participant is focused internally. Stay focused on them in order to remain attuned to what is going on for them.
- If you are working with a cotherapist, the participant will be very sensitive to the dynamic between the two of you. If you notice yourself experiencing any tension or dissonance with your cotherapist, find a way to dissipate or resolve it, or it will likely have an impact on treatment.
- When communicating with your cotherapist in front of a participant, minimize any attempts to communicate anything outside of the participant's awareness (e.g., the use of subtle gestures, facial expressions, whispers, private notes not shared with the participant). The participant is likely to pick up on these and feel curious about them. It is better to communicate transparently.
- Avoid a pathologizing, industrious attitude that views the medicine session as a 5- to 7-hour window for "fixing" something. The participant is better served by a presence that communicates that they are doing everything right and that there is nowhere they are required to go.

Many practitioners find it helpful to cultivate a practice of their own that helps them settle into an appropriate therapeutic presence before a medicine session. This is strongly recommended, as it may improve the participant's treatment experience and make the work more sustainable for you. Examples of these practices are listed in Appendix A.

MEDICINE SESSIONS: WORKING WITHIN THE EMBARK DOMAINS

This section provides a sense of the basic conditions that need to be present for a participant to potentially move toward benefit in each of the six EMBARK clinical domains. Remember that there is no way to guarantee that a particular domain will become important in any given medicine session. Following the general guidance in this section is just a way to make sure that all doors are open for them.

Existential–Spiritual: Medicine Session

> *How do you explain infinity? What do I tell you? What word do you want me to use to explain infinity? Because that is what I am feeling. I am experiencing infinity.*
>
> —Adam (Belser et al., 2017; Swift et al., 2017)

GOAL FOR MEDICINE SESSION: CREATE A SPACE THAT IS RESPECTFUL OF THE SACRED

Your role in supporting healing in this domain during the medicine phase is mostly subtle and supportive. The emphasis should be on creating a physical and relational container that is conducive to the participant's exploration of any existential or spiritual elements that may arise in the medicine session.

Your inner and interpersonal disposition should be open, facilitative, and genuinely respectful of events that the participant experiences as sacred. Many of the phenomena that fall within this category are delicate, so it is crucial that you show respect for them and make efforts to not disturb them. Avoid unnecessary movements or noises as much as possible, as the participant will often be very sensitive to sensory disruptions when they are experiencing existential or spiritual phenomena.

If the participant reaches out for support or other interactions while experiencing such content, remain receptive and humble. Refrain from imposing any interpretations, judgments, or overt redirection, even if the content appears "dark" or counter-therapeutic.

Mindfulness: Medicine Session

> *[During psilocybin] there's just this sweetness of being—sweet, tender quality of being and seeing the world. And I remember saying the second [medicine session], that it takes a week of sesshin practice to sort of reach this sweet spot … you're looking out of these eyes that's like a newborn baby, really . . . And I think that is similar to what happens on a retreat. And this is powerful in that way. You see the world with new eyes.*
>
> —Zen Buddhist priest (Swift et al., 2023)

GOAL FOR MEDICINE SESSION: MODEL AND ENCOURAGE A MINDFUL, SELF-COMPASSIONATE PRESENCE

Many of the treatment mechanisms in the M domain are founded upon the participant's ability to be attentive to their inner states in a curious, accepting, and compassionate way. This type of "observer consciousness" often arises in a profound way on its own during a medicine session. You can best support this process by modeling a similar presence. To develop your ability to do so, you may find it helpful to engage in your own mindfulness practice, either right before the session or on a more regular basis throughout your life as a support for the cultivation of such a presence (see Appendix A).

It may also be helpful to prime this kind of self-attentiveness before the medicine is provided by engaging the participant in a brief reiteration of one of the awareness practices they were taught during the preparation phase. However, it is generally not advisable to suggest to the participant that they engage in any *formal* mindfulness practice while feeling the effects of the medicine, as this kind of focused activity may interfere with their ability to be receptive. If they seem distracted, simply invite them to turn inward using the interventions discussed in later sections of this chapter. It is also important that the participant be engaged with any emotions that arise, so in most cases, both you and the participant should refrain from using any mindfulness practice that minimizes or "bypasses" emotional experience.

Body-Aware: Medicine Session

> *I saw everything that has happened to my body, all the food I have eaten the drugs I have taken, the alcohol, the people I have had sex with, the chemo, the exercise, everything that has ever happened to my body, I took it in at once. Then I made this decision, like, okay, I need a body to go on, so I will choose this body. So, I kind of accepted this body.*
> —Victor (Belser et al., 2017; Swift et al., 2017)

GOAL FOR MEDICINE SESSION: HELP THE PARTICIPANT STAY PRESENT TO THEIR EMBODIED EXPERIENCE

For benefit to arise in the B domain, the participant should be supported in tuning into the wisdom of their body. The main role that you will likely play in this process is to gently encourage them to attend to their embodied experience when they show evidence of not doing so. This inattention may show up as excessive talkativeness, tonic muscle rigidity, restriction of breath, or other idiosyncratic signs (see later sections of this chapter for specific guidance). These behaviors may serve a self-protective or defensive function that operates outside of the participant's awareness. When you notice any of these signs, gently guide the participant back toward listening to their embodied experience so that somatic processes of healing are given an opportunity to unfold.

Affective–Cognitive: Medicine Session

> *I felt a kind of joy and sorrow all at once. It probably looked more like sorrow, but sorrow has never been so beautiful . . . I just felt indescribably sad, grateful, and joyful—all at once.*
> —Caleb (Belser et al., 2017; Swift et al., 2017)

GOAL FOR MEDICINE SESSION: SUPPORT THE PARTICIPANT IN WELCOMING AND EXPLORING EMOTIONS THAT ARISE

In the A domain, benefits are most likely to come from the participant experiencing their emotions, or at least engaging with any challenges that arise when they attempt to do so. To best support this, you can:

- Remind them to attend to what is present in their emotional or embodied experience if they become distracted
- Reflect on any emotions that are present but perhaps not being attended to
- Reassure them with encouragement and support if they have difficulty
- Resource them if they become dysregulated

Specific interventions for providing these forms of support can be found in later sections of this chapter. Also, as in other EMBARK domains, your therapeutic presence could be a key facilitator of beneficial experiences. Your embodied presence is a major part of how you can communicate your confidence in the participant's ability to have emotional openings, which may be just what they need in order to go to the places they need to go inside themselves.

Relational: Medicine Session

> *I was flying through space with the spirit guide, and I encountered three people who are dead who were very close to me. My dad's dad, my mom's mom, and my best friend in college who died. And they all gave me reassuring messages in space. From my friend Tim, "I'm sorry for everything that has happened. I just wanted you to know I love you, man." My grandfather gave me a hug, and my grandmother kissed me on the cheek. That was powerful.*
>
> —Victor (Belser et al., 2017; Swift et al., 2017)

GOAL FOR MEDICINE SESSION: PROVIDE A CONTAINER OF ETHICAL, COMPASSIONATE CARE THAT COULD SUPPORT RELATIONAL REPATTERNING

To support benefit in the R domain, provide an empowering relational container that can welcome and hold a range of interactions that might be beneficial to the participant. Maintain a CUSHION presence that signals your willingness to provide an abundance of care without any pressure on the participant to accept it or respond to it in a specific way. This presence should be maintained even in sessions where the participant remains mostly internally focused.

In general, your default approach to a participant who engages interpersonally should be to limit your interactions with them to the forms of support described in the "Basic Interventions" section of this chapter, which gently guide them back to their internal experience. However, you should also use your clinical judgment to decide whether a more sustained interaction may provide an opportunity for benefit.

Remember the altered therapist–participant dynamics that are likely to be present during a medicine session. The following two dynamics are common:

Enactments. As mentioned in Chapter 2, enactments are generally thought to be coconstructed in a relationship between the participant and the therapist. In enactments, the therapeutic relationship may become a staging ground for the unconscious playing out of both your and the participant's prior relational patterns. For example, participants may become more likely to engage you in a way that reflects unmet developmental needs (e.g., love, validation, and appropriate boundary-setting from caregivers) or past relationships of abuse, often in the unconscious hope of obtaining a better outcome from you (e.g., setting more appropriate boundaries). Enactments require a self-reflexive process of developing your own awareness to work through them skillfully with the participant, often requiring clinical supervision or peer consultation.

In traditional therapy, enactments are often dynamics that arise in the therapeutic relationship over time. Psychedelic therapy may accelerate this process. Enactments often show up in sudden and pronounced ways over a course of treatment—particularly in a medicine session—that are important for you to recognize and respond to skillfully. Although an enactment can be a confusing, unsettling experience for all parties involved, as the therapist, it is always up to you to work with awareness and respond to the underlying dynamics to minimize relational harm.

Potential indicators of an enactment include:

- *Strong transferences:* The participant may treat you like a significant person from their past. For example, they might bristle at the basic rules you set for the session or vie for your attention in childlike ways. They may display an unusually high degree of emotional intensity toward you.
- *Strong counter-transferences:* You might notice yourself having a disproportionate emotional response toward the participant, such as feeling unusually angry, "stuck," charmed, fatigued, or bored by them. You may feel as though you are being pulled into a certain role.
- *Problematic interpersonal patterns:* You may notice that the participant has begun to be consistently late for sessions with no compelling reason, or they may have started bringing you gifts on a regular basis. You may also notice yourself making exceptions to your typical practices, for example, around cancellation policies or communication boundaries.
- *Shifts in the therapeutic field:* Sometimes a therapist can sense an enactment as a hard-to-name disruption in the therapeutic alliance or another unsettling or unexpected change in the therapeutic field.
- *Shifts in the participant's verbal or nonverbal communication:* In a medicine session, you may notice a pronounced shift in how the

participant is interacting with you, such as a different posture, different facial expressions, or a different tone in their voice. These may indicate that the two of you have entered into a dynamic that echoes one from their past.

Enactments are generally thought to be an inevitable part of therapy. As one of our teachers has said, "It's not whether you get into them, it's how you get out." It is not simply a binary issue of a therapist responding "appropriately" or "inappropriately," but rather how the process can be identified, worked through, and exited skillfully and ethically.

For instance, a participant who suffered early childhood sexual abuse from a male caregiver may act in certain ways with a male therapist (e.g., flattering the therapist, attempts to form a special relationship with him, offering favors, trying to make the therapist feel special or needed, seeking to make contact with the therapist in the hallway, teasing flirtatiously or making provocative overtures, etc.). These behaviors may emerge in a way that is outside of awareness for both the therapist and the participant. For example, the therapist may not be aware of how gratifying it feels to be flattered or to feel needed by the participant, that is, how their own counter-transferential material is involved in cogenerating the enactment. It is essential that you remain alert to the possibility of such enactments and to respond to them in a way that provides a healthier resolution to the traumatic interaction being reenacted.

During medicine sessions, a therapeutic response to enactments typically begins with becoming aware of them, which then leads to the compassionate provision of a response that protects the participant from reexperiencing the type of harm they experienced in the past. In the prior example, a therapeutic outcome would more likely result from the male therapist responding with compassion and an assurance that he cares for the participant in a way that does not involve sexual contact. The healthier boundaries he sets provide the protective response, while the compassionate framing avoids the risk of eliciting a new enactment of other early life experiences of rejection, shaming, or abandonment (which may have resulted from a response that relied on a stern recitation of the rules of treatment). During integration, it may even be possible to work with this enactment as a basis for the participant's growth in awareness of themselves in relationships and freedom to choose how they engage with other people. This involves understanding the enactment within the context of the participant's history, linking it to past relationships, and making sense of the roles that both you and the participant have unconsciously adopted.

Regression. This is a general term used to refer to the resurgence of emotions, memories, needs, behaviors, and relational dynamics from an earlier developmental stage in the participant's life. Although this term has not been used much in contemporary clinical trials of PAT, it has historically been considered an important constitutive part of treatment (Abramson, 1966; Eisner, 1967; Grof, 1980; Meckel, 2019) and is frequently evoked in underground psychedelic healing contexts (Brennan et al., 2021). Regression could be distinctly noticeable, such as when a participant begins to act in a childlike way, or it can be subtle and easy to miss, such as when an early life wound gets activated for a participant and they need age-appropriate reassurance.

Remain attentive for any regression, subtle or obvious, that may be occurring and impacting the relational dynamics in the room. Look out for shifts such as shifting or rocking in an uncharacteristic manner, adopting a higher-pitched tone of voice, demonstrating excessive clinging behavior, seeking reassurance, avoiding eye contact, laughing inappropriately, resorting to habits such as thumb-sucking or nail-biting, and speaking in a childlike or babyish manner, as these can all indicate that a regression is occurring. The participant may be unaware of a wish for support or less capable than usual of making it known verbally.

If there is regression, resist making metacommunications that might be appropriate for a non-PAT therapy but are likely to be less effective during a psychedelic medicine session. For example, "I noticed that your voice has become softer and you're avoiding eye contact. Can you tell me more about what you're feeling right now?" Use shorter sentences that require less adult cognition, such as "Are you feeling shy?"

Use your clinical judgment to decide whether it might be helpful to ask if and how they want to engage with you. You can also encourage, validate, and reassure with nonverbal support.

Keeping Momentum: Medicine Session

> I said, "Wow, it's vitally important to get this down as soon as possible," because so much of what happened was so intense and so fleeting that it would drift off into the wind. And to write it down, even if you don't get every step, if you get enough steps so you can travel along them, the other steps then will be reminded.
>
> —Mike (Belser et al., 2017; Swift et al., 2017)

GOAL FOR MEDICINE SESSION: LISTEN FOR AND RECORD STATEMENTS OF MOTIVATION OR INTENTION TO MAKE LIFE CHANGES

The medicine session can be thought of as a powerful time of self-persuasion. It is often a time of burgeoning motivation for posttreatment changes. In most cases, there is not much need for you to intervene in this process, other than to direct the participant back toward a stance of curiosity if you feel they have prematurely resolved their process of exploration in favor of a solution. In general, it is advisable to avoid actively engaging the participant in the process of planning specific changes during the medicine session. Save that for integration.

One helpful thing you can do during the medicine session to support the building of momentum to note any expressions of intent to change to revisit in the subsequent integration sessions. If it would be helpful, revisit the "Change Talk in Motivational Interviewing" text box in the first session agenda found in the chapter on preparation (Chapter 5).

MEDICINE SESSION AGENDA

> *And then um, I remember breathing, feeling my breathing, and then kinda feeling that I was coming up against a membrane of some sort. Then at some point, I came through to it, and that was just like amazing, I was in some sort of like what I call a great plane of consciousness is what it really felt like. It was beautiful, it was very comforting, and I felt like I could reach out to anybody and connect with them. So names of family and friends kind of came to mind, and I also started to, I think that's when I also started really feeling grateful, and kept going "thank you thank you thank you" in my head, and I also started feeling like I was surrendering into something.*
>
> —Chrissy (Belser et al., 2017; Swift et al., 2017)

This section contains an agenda for the first portion of this session, prior to the administration of the medicine. For guidance on how to intervene once the medicine takes effect, see the subsequent sections of this chapter.

Plan approximately 4–8 hours for the medicine session, depending on the drug used and individual participant factors.

Agenda

1. Help the participant get comfortable in the space.
2. Provide the agenda for the day.
3. Open the space.
4. Check in about intentions and agreement to stay for the duration.
5. Invite a brief somatic awareness exercise.
6. Provide the medicine.
7. Support participant's experience.
8. Check out with a short debrief and provide food.
9. Attend to any persisting distress, dysregulation, or dissociation.
10. Remind the participant of next steps and ensure safe departure.

1. Help the participant get comfortable in the space
It is best to have the physical setting in order before the participant shows up so that they arrive in a space that is free from commotion; this signals that they are

being cared for in a thoughtful and thorough way. Specific suggestions for the physical setting are provided in the "Preparing the Space" section of Chapter 4.

The participant is likely to arrive with some nervousness. Greet them in a warm and attentive fashion that lets them know that they are entering a space in which they can feel at home and cared for. It is also helpful to greet them in a way that is consistent with any established understandings about their needs or boundaries around touch. Be mindful that some participants may experience, for example, hugging or other forms of touch as unsettling, despite your intention to use touch to signal warmth and welcoming.

Provide them with clear and gentle guidance from the moment they arrive, such as letting them know where to place their belongings. If you held the preparation sessions elsewhere, orient them to the space. Encourage them to explore on their own a bit if they feel called to do so in order to help them feel comfortable and grounded. If it would increase their sense of safety, invite them to notice where the exits are. Once they are somewhat settled, ask if there is anything about the space that they would like to change (e.g., temperature, art placement).

2. Provide the agenda for the day

Orient the participant by giving them a clear sense of what to expect for the day. Specific language may include the following (with adjustments for the specific medicine):

> *"Before we begin, I just want to give you a sense of how the day will unfold. Right now, you can take some time to settle into the space at your own pace. Whenever you're ready, we'll open the session together. If you would like to bring in anything from your own religious or spiritual practice, like a prayer, you can feel free to do so then. Next, we'll spend a little time checking in about your intentions, just to bring them into the session today. Then, I'll guide you in a brief awareness exercise like we did in the preparation sessions so that you can start moving into that inward focus we've talked about. After that, you'll take the medicine and wait for it to take effect, which usually takes between 30 to 60 minutes. Once it does, you will have your experience with the medicine for a few hours. When it's over, we'll talk for a bit, and then you'll get picked up by your [partner/spouse/family member]."*

Before moving on, ask if they have any questions about the agenda.

3. Open the space

At this point, open the space with whatever opening practice or ritual the participant decided would feel helpful and appropriate since your discussion about this during the preparation phase (e.g., reading a poem, a knot-tying ritual). Ask them how they would like you to participate, if at all. If they would like to skip this opening, allow them to. If they feel that an opening is important but are unsure of what to do, you can suggest that they bring their intentions for the session into their heart; then invite them to speak them out loud or hold them silently for a moment.

4. Check in about intentions and agreement to stay for the duration

Before the participant takes the medicine, it is useful to bring the intentions they developed for the session during the preparation phase back into their awareness. This check-in should be brief—1 to 5 minutes. Its goals are to remind the participant of what they hope to explore in the session and to reawaken their sense of its importance. Attend to the potential presence of any rigid expectations and remind the participant that it is best to hold their intentions lightly. If possible, try to make contact with any emotions that seem present around the intentions and encourage their expression. Begin with language such as *"Let's take a moment to check in about the intentions that you've set for today. Do you recall what it is that you would like to focus on today?"*

Conclude with language like: *"Great. Keeping these intentions at the back of your mind will help guide your session today. At some point, I might remind you of them."*

It is important to make an explicit agreement with the participant to stay for the duration of their experience. You might say,

> *"Feel free to feel, express, and say anything that arises in you to whatever extent feels right to you. I will help you make sure that your actions and expression stay within safe bounds, like not hurting yourself or me, holding safe boundaries between us, or damaging the space. If any of your behaviors go outside of these bounds, I will work gently with you to change course. It's also important to make two agreements: (a) We all agree to stay here for the full time needed, which will be 6 hours, until 4:00 pm, so nobody will leave until we all check in at the end. And (b), we all agree to not use our phones or devices until that time to limit outside communication and keep this as a safer space together. Do you agree?"*

It is often helpful to solicit an explicit agreement to stay, so that you can remind them of the agreement later if they have an urge to leave prematurely.

5. Invite a brief somatic awareness exercise

It is helpful to begin to shift the participant toward paying attention to their inner experience by using the exercise practiced in the preparation phase. This exercise should be approximately 10 minutes long. At the end of the exercise, encourage the participant to remain in that state of inner-directed attention as much as they can as they move toward the bed, take the medicine, and wait for it to take effect.

6. Provide the medicine

Provide the participant with the medicine. This may be an anxiety-provoking moment for some participants, so do not rush ingestion. Invite them to ingest it only when they are ready. Once they have taken the medicine, invite them to lie down on the bed, get comfortable, and put on their blindfold and headphones.

As the participant lies down, remind them of several guidelines:

- *Generally, the thing to do with what the medicine brings your way is to remain open and receptive to it instead of judging it or rejecting it. See if you can allow all the feelings, thoughts, and sensations to flow. If it ever gets overwhelming, remember that you have ways to resource yourself. And you can always ask me for support.*

- *Otherwise, I will remain mostly quiet and will not interfere in what's happening for you. I may check in briefly every so often to see how you're doing, but the session will be primarily between you and your unfolding inner experience. If there is something you are seeing or learning that you want to share, it would be best to save it and tell me about it later. You are always welcome to reach out to me for support if you feel you need it, but I encourage you to stay inside as much as possible.*
- *There may be times when it makes sense for you to move around, but generally it's most helpful to spend as much time as you can lying down, or sitting at times if you'd like. You can also ask me to change something about the room, like the temperature.*
- *You may see me writing something down in a notepad. That's just me taking notes on things you've said so we can remember them together during our follow-up sessions. I'll share these notes with you [you may actually choose to hand the participant your writing pad to show them that they will have full access to your notes]. This way, you don't have to try to remember all of what happens yourself. Also, you might see me using a tablet (or phone). This is only to adjust the music. I promise that I will not use it for any other reason and that I will be present here with you throughout the whole session.*

Once this is complete, suggest that they spend the rest of the waiting period turning their attention inward. This may be a good time to express to the participant one more time your faith in them and their capacity to bring themselves to an experience of healing. Offer a final moment of warm encouragement with a reminder that you are there for any support needs that arise.

Also, consider taking this opportunity to put your cell phone or other devices on airplane mode or "do not disturb" mode and ensure that you are sitting on your CUSHION (Chapter 4).

7. Support the participant's experience
After the participant has ingested the medicine, you may strive to cultivate a quiet, observing, compassionate presence. Consider angling your body so that your gaze is facing the same direction as the participant, perpendicular to the participant, or in another direction that avoids evoking the feeling that they are being stared at.

Specific advice on how to support the participant's experience is provided in the three sections that follow this agenda: "Basic Interventions," "Responding to Common Events That May Arise," and "Responding to Challenging Events That May Arise."

8. Check out with a short debrief and provide food
Once the required minimum number of hours have passed since ingestion of the medicine *and* the participant feels that they have mostly returned to a subjective baseline state, let them know that the session is coming to an end.

Provide food for the participant at this point. If done with intention, this act can communicate a kind of care that the participant receives very deeply. Your provision of nourishment after a challenging experience will likely help them to feel well-held in a vulnerable, fragile moment. Providing a wide variety of foods on a large, decorative serving plate may also signal a kind of abundance that offers a symbolic contrast to the various forms of scarcity that likely exist in a life impacted by depression. The food should continue the dietary restrictions observed prior to the medicine session and avoid any known food allergies of the participant. It is best to offer a tray of foods that are easy on the digestion, such as a tray of slices of fresh fruit (mangos, berries, orange slices) and other light foods (cashews, almonds, dates).

Once food has been provided, assess the participant's level of interest in discussing the content of their experience of the medicine. If they are feeling averse to this, allow them to refrain from doing so. Engage them minimally but enough to adequately assess their readiness for discharge. If they would like to discuss their experience, invite them to do so while advising them to retain their internal, embodied focus and to not rush back into their verbal, thinking mind. For participants who did not speak much during the session, give them more time than you would for someone who remained conversational throughout, as they might have "backlogged" material to express. Remain attentive to the fact that this moment may constitute a potent relational moment, as the effects of the medicine are likely to still be present in subtle ways.

Be sparse in providing reflections or interpretations. If asked to do so, let the participant know that you will do more of this during the integration sessions. The narrative telling should be mostly a "recap" of what unfolded. Stay with what happened—you can make sense of it together later on in integration. Explore the phenomena before jumping into meaning-making. If the participant seems overly concerned with interpreting or understanding what arose, gently encourage them to allow the material to remain unformulated for the remainder of the day. Take notes on any moments or internal phenomena that the participant references for use in the integration sessions.

Maintain a receptive, nonjudgmental presence that expresses a sense of genuine appreciation for what the participant experienced. If they are self-critical about how well they engaged in the medicine session, remind them that there is no way to do it "wrong." Invite them to bring that feeling to integration and assure them that you will do your best to help them benefit from whatever unfolded for them. If they apologize for any real or perceived relational ruptures that occurred, respond compassionately by assuring them that you are still very much committed to their treatment and are very open to exploring this dynamic further with them during integration. Limit this debrief to 10 minutes or so.

Instead of talking with the participant, you may offer arts and crafts supplies and encourage the participant to draw a mandala or use crayons, watercolors, or colored pencils to draw an image about what they experienced to keep for themselves. They can bring this to the integration session if they'd like.

It is likely to be helpful to invite the participant to do some light journaling in order to help them remember the most meaningful aspects of the session. You might say, "*When you get home, I invite you to give yourself some time to jot down any significant memories or impressions from the session, as these can sometimes fade quickly. It's okay if some aspects of your session aren't easy to remember. We'll review your experience during your integration sessions."* Advise them to refrain from writing excessively or trying too hard to make sense out of their experience that evening.

9. Attend to any persisting distress, dysregulation, or dissociation

Challenging emotional material, such as trauma memories, may arise during a medicine session and not get fully resolved by its end. In some cases, this activation can cause a significant level of distress that may lead you to feel concern about the participant's stability and readiness to leave. If so, be sure to devote sufficient time to supporting the participant's return to stability at the end of the session before letting them leave.

Your two primary goals in this scenario are to assess for suicidality and support the participant's capacity for containment and resourcing so that they can remain safe between now and the first integration session.

Throughout this process, honor the key trauma-informed principles of autonomy and empowerment. Give them ample time to debrief their experience, with full choice as to how much or how little they want to discuss. As they do so, ask whether they would find it helpful to adopt a posture of maximum physical comfort and restfulness (e.g., fetal position, many blankets). Give them permission to rest in whatever way feels right to them and to trust in what their body needs. Attend to any acute experiences of shame or embarrassment that are present. As much as is possible, allow the process of returning to unfold at their pace, and even provide them with reassurance that they will not have to leave until they feel ready.

If you have concerns about the participant's mental state, or if they show signs or symptoms that suicidality may be present, you should assess for suicidal thoughts, intent, plan, and behaviors. Some groups use a formal tool such as the brief form of the Columbia Suicidality Severity Rating Scale. However, in nonresearch settings, a simple set of questions about thoughts, plan, and intent from a skilled clinician is sufficient for assessing for current suicidality. Based on the participant's answers, provide them with the appropriate level of acute ongoing support.

Containment skills consist of practices that the participant can use to maintain stability between sessions. They include visualization exercises, embodied practices, journaling, and so on. Feel free to use any with which you or they are familiar. Ensure that the participant believes that the skill they have chosen will actually help them and that they feel as though it will be enough to support them between now and the next session. If they give any indication that they might need more support, help to ensure that they get this.

In addition, explore what other personal or social resources might support the participant in the interim. This conversation should have started during preparation (see Chapter 4 sections "Involving Other Providers" and "Involving Family Members or Loved Ones"), but it is advised that you revisit this plan to assess whether it still feels like it provides sufficient support for the participant. Make concrete plans as to how the participant will know it is time to access these supports and how they will do so.

During the first integration session you will assess again whether the participant needs any additional professional care or other forms of support. Before they leave, let them know this and express faith in their ability to continue stabilizing and healing with support from you and others in the coming days and weeks.

10. Remind the participant of next steps and ensure safe departure

Briefly remind the participant that you will be meeting again for an integration session. Encourage them to spend the evening in a calm, supportive environment. Remind them to minimize activity and to refrain from any unnecessary distractions (e.g., television, reading, work). Tell them that the effects of the medicine on sleep are unpredictable and that in addition to briefly journaling their experience, they should try to lie down and rest, even if they feel they cannot sleep.

The participant's readiness to leave safely requires that they show no signs of physical risk (vital sign stability, ability to stand and walk with coordination) or lingering psychological effects (e.g., strong perceptual distortions, abnormal thought processes, disrupted insight, affect, or mood). Remind the participant that they should not drive a vehicle for 24 hours after the initial administration of the medicine. Consider speaking briefly to the participant's companion to remind them of the degree of care and support the participant will need from them and the home environment.

MEDICINE SESSIONS: BASIC INTERVENTIONS

Really, all I felt from Jeff and Drew was kindness, and kind of a gentle but firm steering. There was one point where I just needed to get something expressed and Jeff just said, "Listen . . . just listen." What he meant was, "Be quiet, and listen." Well, why's Jeff bossin' me around? . . . Maybe for a nanosecond, I might've felt that . . . And then I thought, he's telling me this for a reason.
                                        —Caleb (Belser et al., 2017; Swift et al., 2017)

The following interventions are helpful go-to practices to have in your toolkit when supporting a participant through a medicine session. They do not capture the full spectrum of what might be supportive for a participant, but they reflect a strong base to begin from.

Quietly hold space with a CUSHION presence

For most of the session, this should be your default intervention. Sit on your CUSHION and strive to avoid FRAZZLE. Give the participant space to have an experience that is primarily between them and the medicine while remaining ready to greet them with an appropriate presence should they turn to you for support. Stay connected to your confidence in the participant's ability to bring themselves to healing without an excess of intervention. This is particularly true during a participant's first medicine session, which can, to some extent, be thought of as an introductory or "diagnostic" session that helps all parties get a sense of how the participant responds to the medicine. During the subsequent integration phase, you can collaboratively develop a sense of what additional support or intervention might be helpful next time based on this experience.

Gently guide them back toward their emotions or embodied experience

A participant's attention should be primarily directed toward what they are feeling in their emotions and in their body. If they indicate that they have become preoccupied with thoughts and ideas (e.g., telling you that their internal time has been spent cogitating or "figuring something out," speaking with you in a way that seems more "in their head" than "in their heart"), gently guide them back toward their emotional, embodied experience (e.g., "Can we check in to see what your embodied experience is like right now?"). If they have not indicated this, but you notice that they appear lost or distracted, you may invite them back toward their emotional, embodied experience (e.g., "Maybe now is a good time to check in with your feelings."). Attend to their sense of safety in doing so and guide them toward resources if needed.

Remind them about intentions

If a participant appears unfocused or distracted, it may also be helpful to remind them of the intentions they brought into their session (e.g., "Would now be a good time to explore your anger?").

Soften pathologization

A participant might pathologize an aspect of their experience during a medicine session (e.g., "I just want to get these stupid depressed thoughts out of my head." or "I need to stop feeling this anger!"). Gently ask them if they would be willing to try to allow that material be present instead of pushing it away. Briefly remind them that it may be most helpful to take an approach of "all is welcome" today. If appropriate, you may also encourage them to offer compassion or gratitude toward the part/thought/feeling that troubles them, as it may have served a valid protective function for them at some point.

Encourage slowness, curiosity, and empowerment around impulses

If a participant appears to be moving fast into challenging material and expresses fear or ambiguity about this (e.g., "I'm so scared, but I gotta look at it."), invite them to slow down and spend time with the part of them that is scared. In general, when a participant is battling with a part of themselves, invite them to call a truce with that part and get to know it. Remind them that they are free to take their time and choose what does and does not feel possible and helpful to explore.

Guide them toward resource (only if needed)

Psychedelic experiences can occasion very intense experiences for participants: grief, fear, and rage, along with behaviors such as sobbing, shaking, or yelling. Oftentimes, these experiences will be beneficial and therapeutic for them to have fully.

Other times, a participant will become so emotionally activated that they become distressed and dysregulated, which opens them to a risk of retraumatization (see "Trauma-Informed Care" section of Chapter 2). In these cases, you can intervene to help guide them back toward resource. You can use a range of interventions to do so. The following list is organized by ascending degree of invasiveness, so it will likely be best to first consider the earlier ones when intervening:

- Checking in with a simple question ("What's here for you right now?") or a reflection on how much they are struggling
- Inviting them to find their internal resources ("Can you find your strength?")
- Changing the music to something gentler
- Inviting them to use the self-regulation practice from the preparation phase
- Inviting them to focus on a safe point on their body (e.g., ears), preferably one that they previously indicated to you as safe
- Empowering them to "change the channel/lens"
- Inviting them to change their overall body position
- Empowering them to "bite-size" any challenging material present by engaging with a smaller portion of it (e.g., a specific image, sensation, etc.)
- Contacting a version of them (e.g., adult self, observer self) to bring it online (e.g., "Can we bring in the Josh from before who knows how good he is?")
- Inviting them to take off their eye pillow/headphones and sit up
- Supportive touch

Only intervene to guide the participant toward resource when they are clearly dysregulated. Be cautious about intervening upon any strong emotion, as this could arrest a therapeutic process and strengthen an existing tendency toward emotional avoidance. Before intervening, ask the participant whether they feel they need support or would prefer to continue the experience they are having unaided. Remember that the goal of resourcing is not to shut an experience down but to increase the participant's capacity to have it safely and fully.

When working with a participant over the course of multiple sessions, you may notice them naturally developing their capacity to regulate themselves with less support from you. You may also consider making this an explicit goal of treatment by gradually and explicitly shifting the locus of emotional regulation capacity from the interpersonal dynamic to within the participant.

Work with emotions

Once the participant is in contact with their emotions and well regulated, they should begin to explore, express, and deepen into them. Many times, this process unfolds without much support from you, though it may occasionally benefit from basic intervention, for example, when the participant is not aware of an emotion that is present or attempts to minimize their emotional experience.

Your support with emotions in a medicine session can take many forms that fit the needs of the participant. The following three-step conceptualization is offered as a rubric for understanding and supporting one of the most common paths this process can take. It draws from the teachings of EMBARK faculty member Adele Lafrance and her expertise in emotion-focused therapy.

1. *Help the participant name emotions with basic reflections.* If a participant is engaging with you verbally or nonverbally and appears to be experiencing an emotion, help them attend to it by offering a simple naming reflection (e.g., "It can be very scary/sad/etc."). Use core emotional language that can be easily understood (e.g., "You're angry.") rather than more complex ones (e.g., "You're disappointed."). You can also use nonsemantic affect words, like "yuck" or "ouch." If you notice that the participant appears to be experiencing an emotion while not engaging with you, refrain from offering a reflection.

2. *Encourage deepening and expression of emotions.* If a participant has indicated that they are feeling an identified emotion (e.g., "I just felt a little bubble of sadness when I said that."), encourage them to "stay with" that emotion and deepen their experience of it ("See if you can feel that sadness and, if it feels okay, let yourself go into it some more."). If they seem daunted, ask them if some kind of support (e.g., knowing that you are there, handholding) might help them feel safe enough to do so, while respecting the possibility that there may not be anything that helps them feel supported enough to deepen this emotion right now. For some participants, it may be helpful to encourage or give permission for any spontaneous expressions (e.g., growling, crying) that are normally not condoned. If helpful, you can make the sound first as a potent means of giving them permission to do the same.

3. *Invite curiosity about feelings under the feeling.* If you feel that this emotion may be a "secondary emotion" that covers over a "primary emotion," you could invite the participant to explore connecting with any other emotion that may be underneath the one they have been working with. For example, a participant's anger may represent a secondary or "reactive" emotion that they feel in response to a more tender, primary emotion, such as grief, shame, or fear. Once they have had a deep experience of the anger for some time, you could ask them, "Might there be another feeling under that anger?" If another feeling emerges, invite them to deepen, express, and explore that new emotion. You may also invite the participant to explore what unmet need drives the primary emotion (e.g., "What does that hurt need?"). If an answer arises (e.g., "love," "forgiveness"), explore whether they can move toward accessing an experience of that answer in themselves or in relationship with you ("What would it be like to forgive yourself?").

When working with emotions this way, remain attentive to the importance of the participant's contexts. Be attentive to the ways the participant's emotions—particularly anger—may be a rational response to the conditions around them, as this should influence the way you work with them. For example, if a participant feels anger toward an abusive partner or a sexist employer, it may be more appropriate to support them in using this anger as a catalyst for empowerment and self-protective action toward changing their contexts (see sidebar "Rejecting Anger Versus Empowered Anger").

Rejecting Anger Versus Empowered Anger

When working with anger, Dr. Adele Lafrance advises differentiating between two types of anger. The first, rejecting anger (e.g., "I hate you and never want to see you again."), is a secondary emotion that is often fueled by vulnerability, fear, grief, or shame. The participant should be encouraged to find the primary emotion underneath it. The second type, empowered anger (e.g., "This is not okay.", "I deserve more.", "I need space."), is a primary emotion that reflects healthy self-assertion and boundary-setting, and the participant should be helped to harness it rather than work through it.

Offer supportive touch

(See "Double Consent for Touch" section of Chapter 4 for important guidance on assessing consent for touch.) As discussed in Chapter 4, touch is thought to offer grounding, soothing, a sense of being accepted, and encouragement to deepen one's experience. It may help an anxious or dysregulated participant to settle themselves or coregulate with you. It may convey a sense of solidarity and support to a participant experiencing grief, or it could give a participant who feels alone or unlovable a reason to consider other possibilities. Some systems of somatic psychotherapy hold that touch may even provide "missing experiences" of care that were not available in the participant's early life. You may want to consider offering supportive touch (always using double consent) when the participant:

- Appears fearful
- Experiences strong grief
- Remains in a state of apparent struggle for some time
- Appears childlike or regressed
- Makes a bid for closeness, verbally or nonverbally

If offered in a mistuned or inappropriate way, touch can also be harmful or disruptive to a participant's experience. It is important to steer clear of this (see "Why Not Touch?" in Chapter 4 for review). Refrain from offering touch during moments in which the participant:

- Is engaged in a process from which touch would be distracting
- Appears to be learning to self-regulate their emotions without outside help
- Seems to be engaging in a traumatic enactment of a past abusive dynamic
- Is experiencing sexual feelings
- Is demonstrating paranoid or aggressive behaviors

Keep in mind that providing no touch or minimal touch may also create a therapeutic opportunity in that it may give the participant the opportunity to learn how to soothe or support themselves. A practice that some PAT practitioners have found helpful is the "WAIT" technique, which is an acronym that represents a question that might be helpful to reflect on: "Why am I talking/ touching?"

One helpful way to provide touch with minimal risk to a participant's autonomy is to let them know that you are leaving your open hand available for them to hold if and only if they would find that helpful (and if prior consent for handholding is present).

Periodically check in

Sometimes a participant is internally focused for long stretches, even hours. You may find it helpful to check in at times by gently asking how they are doing. This may be appropriate in moments when the participant is, for example, very still for over 30 minutes, appears to be struggling with challenging material for a while, displays concerning shifts in breathing patterns (e.g., no observable respiration), appears regressed or otherwise incapable of actively seeking support, and so on. As noted in the agenda, be sure to let them know ahead of time that you might check in with them occasionally so that the experience is not confusing.

Attend to your own internal experience

Your own emotions and embodied experience can be a helpful source of information about what is going on in the room. You may notice that something shifts or begins to feel "off" and could consider this information that may prompt a change in approach, such as changing the tone of the music or checking in with a participant who has been inward for a while. Or you could simply note it and discuss its relevance to the participant's treatment with your cotherapist, supervisor, or peers after the session. Importantly, this type of attunement is often unreliable and should be treated only as grounds for becoming curious, not as a source of truth or revelation about what is happening in the participant's experience.

Take notes

Record any participant statements or other events that may serve as helpful reminders during the integration sessions.

MEDICINE SESSION: RESPONDING TO COMMON EVENTS

This section offers guidance on how to respond to scenarios you will likely encounter at some point early in your work as a PAT practitioner. The suggested responses should not be seen as the be-all and end-all of how to intervene in these situations. You will likely develop your own preferred responses as you gain more experience. Still, it would be helpful to begin from this starting point and to give yourself the opportunity to connect with the internal logic that underlies these suggestions, as it reflects EMBARK's trauma-informed and ethically rigorous approach to PAT.:

If the participant experiences strong emotion and seeks support

Offer validation and a basic reflection. Encourage them to remain present to the content (e.g., "See if you can stay with it and see what's there."). If they express that the experience is intolerable, guide them toward resource with the interventions described in the "Basic Interventions" section in this chapter.

If the participant expresses strong positive beliefs

Examples: "No matter what, I am good." "I love my life." Assess whether or not they seem to expect a response. If they do not, it is not necessary to respond, and supportive silence is fine. If they seem to be looking for a response, respond in a way that is validating and encourages them to stay with the experience (e.g., "Sounds like you're learning."). Take note of these statements for potential use in the subsequent integration sessions.

If the participant expresses negative beliefs about themselves

Examples: "I'm worthless." "I can't change." Consider that this statement may be an implicit bid for support and respond accordingly. If their statement appears to solicit a response from you (e.g., "Am I loveable?"), respond genuinely and supportively (e.g., "Yes, you are."). In most cases, it will be best to then encourage them to stay with their inner experience of that belief or question rather than discussing it at length with you (i.e., guide them from the interpersonal search for answers to an intrapersonal search; e.g., "Maybe you can also look inside for that answer."). However, in some cases, a longer interpersonal exchange may be most facilitative for the participant (perhaps as a moment of relational repatterning) before they turn inward again.

If your clinical judgment leads you to believe that the participant has become stuck in a negative self-belief, it may be helpful to intervene in a way that encourages a mindful perspective on it. Statements that encourage a step back into an observer perspective (e.g., "Something difficult is happening for you right now, huh?") may help them move toward resolution. Refrain from offering these interventions excessively or prematurely.

If the participant appears to be avoiding challenging psychological material that has arisen

Some participants respond to the arising of challenging material by pushing it away. This may be a conscious effort, or it may occur outside of their awareness via restricting their breathing, tightening their musculature, or distracting themselves with idle thoughts or conversation with you. Sometimes, they may even appear to be engaging in behaviors that seem supportive of therapeutic outcomes (e.g., intentional breathing, positive self-affirmations, generating insights) but may actually be defending against affect.

Brief, simple interventions may be enough. A basic question about the participant's emotions (e.g., "What are you feeling?") may be enough to get them to connect more deeply with what is present. An empathic reflection about the difficulty they are experiencing with the challenging material (e.g., "It's so hard to feel what's here.") may also be facilitative. For a participant that is self-distracting, it may be helpful to gently remind them that it can be good to be open to any emotions that are present. Interventions that bring their attention to embodiment may also be helpful.

When intervening, be aware of giving off any appearance of colluding with the participant's sense that they are "failing" or somehow "doing it wrong." Demonstrate and encourage respect for any defenses/avoidance/protectors as beneficent self-protective strategies that may be playing an important part of their therapeutic process. Avoid pathologizing them or aggressively pushing past them.

If the participant is able to give voice to a self-protective strategy, perhaps with statements such as "I can't go there" or "It's too hard to feel that," affirm that it is important and good that they have identified and acknowledged that. Consider that it may be helpful to spend time deepening into and compassionately getting to know these protective elements as a focus for that moment of the medicine session ("Let's spend some time with the fear, just getting to know it."). Refrain from engaging them in a long conversation about the nature of the protective strategy. Simply turn their curiosity toward it and invite them to resume inward-focused exploration. Avoid saddling this exploration with the goal of making something happen. These protective elements may or may not resolve on their own after being given space to do what they are meant to do for a while.

If the participant attempts to engage you in conversation that resembles a talk therapy session

Use your clinical judgment and collaborative questioning to determine if this feels helpful for the participant. If it is likely to be more distracting to their internal process than helpful, respond to their comments in a way that is supportive but does not encourage further conversation. Remind them that they will have the chance to talk about it with you later ("This will be a good thing for us to talk about tomorrow.") and invite them to resume an inward focus when appropriate (e.g., "Maybe now's a good time to see what's happening inside; would you like to try that?"). It may be helpful to respond to what they are saying in a way that brings their awareness to their embodied and emotional experience of sharing it (e.g., "What's it like to hear yourself say that?"). If they worry about forgetting the details of their experience, suggest that they will likely remember the most important details later and that you can take notes if needed. If this bid for contact seems motivated by anxiety, support them in addressing this anxiety, perhaps by guiding them toward resource.

However, you should also consider that the participant's attempt to engage may also be an opening to an important relational moment. Use your clinical judgment and the participant's wisdom about what is right for them in making this determination.

During sustained interactions, remain attentive to the possibility that the participant is deriving the most significant benefit from the implicit dynamics and relational patterns that are present rather than the explicit content of the dialogue. This implicit level includes unspoken negotiations of trust, attachment, ability to seek and receive support, empathic mirroring, and so on. In other words, what is being said may be less important than how it is being said. For example, a participant may benefit most from their experience of successfully acting on the impulse to connect with you, expressing themselves in a more or less vulnerable fashion than usual, or struggling to fully accept the compassionate responses you give them.

Attend to your and their comfort with eye contact, physical proximity, and how they receive any statements of care you offer. Due to the heightened state of sensitivity and vulnerability that the participant is in, these factors are likely to be felt more strongly than they would be in a talk therapy session. Strive to offer consistent positive regard (without sacrificing genuineness and spontaneity) throughout the whole medicine session from within a CUSHION presence.

Your interventions during these relational moments should be less about narrative content and more attuned to the implicit relational and experiential dimensions of the content and the act of sharing it. For example, you can support a participant's attentiveness to their experience of sharing a story through basic reflections (e.g., "You were so alone that day.") or questions (e.g., "How does it feel to be talking about this?"). You could also invite them to feel into the quality of the interaction (e.g., "How is it to be sharing this with me?"). It may also be helpful to track for and reflect expressions of affect that are outside of the participant's awareness (e.g., "It looks like this is scary to talk about."). Interventions that challenge or interrogate the participant or invite insight, interpretation, and analysis (e.g., "Why do you think your parents thought you were worthless?") are likely to be less facilitative than those that support the participant in feeling contact with emotions and/or relational dynamics. Always keep in mind that a compassionate, nonjudgmental presence is key when attending to a participant who is implicitly asking to be seen or "witnessed" while doing something they consider risky, such as sharing a tender story or crying openly.

Sometimes, a participant may take the reins and explicitly ask for a moment of relational experimentation. They might want to engage with you in a new, transformative form of relating that is normally hard for them to access. For example, a shy or anxious participant may want to practice maintaining prolonged eye contact with you. During a medicine session, participants often get the sense that there is a window of opportunity or plasticity for "rewiring" their relational tendencies. This may allow them to reap greater therapeutic benefit from these relational experiments than they normally would. A request for a relational moment may present a significant therapeutic opening, as long as you use your clinical judgment to ensure that it is facilitated ethically and that the participant is given the chance to check in with any other parts of themselves that may be present and wanting to be attended to before a risky action. For instance, if a participant worries about feeling embarrassment or shame about vulnerable connection, it may be best to first listen to the deeper concern that is being communicated by that worry, rather than rushing past it.

If the participant experiences mild to moderate unpleasant somatic symptoms and seeks support

If the participant complains of nausea or somatic discomfort, try the following:

1. Provide explicit empathy, acknowledging their discomfort (e.g., "That sounds uncomfortable.").

2. Normalize that transient symptoms such as nausea, cramps, or headaches are common experiences for many people.
3. Encourage the participant to stay with the discomfort and view it as a potential source of therapeutic benefit (e.g., "Try to stay with the nausea and be open to what's there."), while recognizing the difficulty of doing so.
4. Encourage a self-regulatory breathing practice.
5. Optionally, offer the participant the emesis bowl to have nearby or hold in their lap as a way to manage the discomfort.
6. Offer the option to sniff an alcohol wipe, which may help alleviate nausea.
7. If the participant clearly expresses a preference for taking an antinausea remedy or analgesic for a headache (and a suitable one is available), consider administering antiemetic medication if you are authorized to do so.

A note about nausea: there is debate in the field regarding the therapeutic usefulness of transient nausea. While many practitioners readily administer medications such as ondansetron (Zofran) as needed or prophylactically to address nausea, some believe that nausea might have pro-therapeutic effects. Nausea can be psychogenic, and purging is regarded as part of a healing process in many ayahuasca and shamanic practices. In a psychedelic context, nausea is often seen as presenting an opportunity for the participant to engage with difficult psychological content in a different way with your abiding presence and support (Bogenschutz et al., 2018). For example, if the participant is holding the emesis bowl and dry heaving or vomiting into the bowl, this is sometimes called "bowl work," and once passed, this process often leads to profound relief for many participants (see Belser et al., 2017).

In psilocybin and MDMA research studies, most nausea is experienced as a transient and mild adverse event that is self-limiting, meaning it will pass or resolve without administering an antiemetic. However, respect participant self-determination and medical guidance. Be aware that nausea is highly stigmatized in many cultures, including perhaps your own. Be reflective about any dogmatic positions you may hold that may be motivated by personal biases or counter-transferences (e.g., your belief that the participant would do better to expel or purge, or alternatively, your need to save the participant from their fear of losing control associated with vomiting).

For returning participants who experienced significant nausea in previous sessions, discuss during preparation whether they found the nausea to contribute positively or negatively to their experience. Collaboratively decide whether they would prefer to take an antinausea medication (e.g., ondansetron) prophylactically this time.

If the participant requests physical contact

(See the "Double Consent for Touch" section of Chapter 4 for important guidance on assessing consent for touch.) Attend to the possibility that this request for physical contact may represent the participant taking a step toward many therapeutic outcomes: leaving isolation, reestablishing a sense of safety in connection, an increased willingness and trust in reaching out for help, and so on. Responding in a way that values both the risk and the growth inherent in their request can help them benefit from it. Responding in a way that undermines their sense of safety, autonomy, or worthiness of love may contribute to the harm caused by past traumas that diminished these capacities in the first place.

However, also consider the possibility that the touch being requested, while seemingly appropriate and nonsexual, may be part of an enactment of an abusive past dynamic. This determination can be made using your knowledge of the participant, your attuned sense of what is present in the dynamic, and a collaborative, nonshaming exploration of the request with the participant ("It is great that you want to connect. Before I give you a hand on your shoulder, can we take a moment to check in with all the parts of you that are here?"). If you feel that withholding the requested touch would benefit the participant more than providing it, gently decline their request with an assurance that it is born of a continuing sense of care for them and that you still want to be in relationship with them. Remain wholly present with them after declining until they indicate that they would prefer otherwise. Be sure to avoid acting rejectingly toward the participant or in a way that encourages them to feel ashamed of their request for touch. It may be helpful to keep in mind that any request for physical contact is motivated by a bid for connection, which is a fundamental need we all share.

If they request touch that is beyond what was agreed upon in the prior conversation about consent, first acknowledge the goodness (i.e., bravery, connectedness, etc.) of their request and your appreciation of it. Then, gently remind them that you made a promise to them that was born of your care for them and that you still want to be in relationship with them. Again, remain wholly present with them after declining until they indicate that they would prefer otherwise. Consider collaboratively coming up with another way to fulfill their request, such as having each of you hold the opposite ends of a string or ribbon.

If the participant complains that they are "stuck" or not feeling strong medicine effects

If this complaint arises, it is often enough to respond by either asking the participant what they are experiencing in their body or gently reminding them of the importance of attending to the flow of bodily sensations and their inner experience in general (e.g., "I wonder if now would be a good time to see what's happening inside/in your body."). Guide them toward patience and receptivity and avoid making them feel like something they are doing is wrong. Encourage them to listen more deeply to the music, which may deepen their experience of the medicine. Like most medicine session interventions, it is best to keep it brief.

If the participant continues to feel stuck and shows signs of tightness or restriction in their body, further intervention may be helpful. You can begin by asking them if they notice any movement that their body may "want" to do, such as flexing their feet, moving their hands, or placing their hands on their chest. If you notice any movement occurring (e.g., feet moving), call their attention to it. Invite them to experiment with pausing the movement for a minute, or alternatively, increasing its intensity a little bit. Ask them to remain attentive to what arises internally during these interventions.

Further light bodily practices may be helpful, such as guiding an activating breathwork exercise, holding or massaging the participant's hand or feet, or encouraging the participant to make small movements with their limbs to interrupt rigidity. It is important to suggest these interventions to the participant in a way that does not make them feel ashamed or embarrassed by their feeling stuck or that they have done something wrong. Present it all gently and avoid any indications that you are troubleshooting a problem (e.g., a furrowed brow).

If the participant still feels stuck after your intervening, help them accept and normalize this by encouraging them to stay with the "stuckness" as long as they need to. It might turn out to be a necessary "way station" they must pass through before experiencing more openness and flow in their embodied experience. Or they may spend the entirety of their medicine session in this stuckness. No matter the outcome, it is important not to collude (or appear to collude) with any feelings of failure the participant may hold or express. You should internally hold the possibility that they may experience stuckness for the full duration of the session and that this experience may still lead to benefit if integrated thoughtfully.

If the participant complains that they are "lost," despite feeling medicine effects

Normalize this experience first (e.g., "It's okay to feel lost."). Gently provide a simply stated reminder of their intentions (e.g., "Maybe now is the time to think about what has been hard about your relationship with your partner."). In any event, assure them that they are "where they need to be" and that they are not doing anything wrong. Refrain from excessively "troubleshooting" the situation. If there is any associated distress, consider verbally contacting it and guiding them toward resource.

If the participant wants to get up and move around the room

Participants may ask to express themselves in an embodied fashion during the medicine session by dancing, moving, pushing, clapping, and so on. Use your clinical judgment and knowledge of the participant to determine if this request is either a form of expression that is relevant to the therapy (e.g., a novel sense of liveliness that seeks physical expression) or a form of avoidance (e.g., distraction from challenging affect or physical symptoms). If movement may be therapeutic, allow them to do so. Perhaps change the music to a tempo that better matches their movement. You may also provide objects that facilitate expression, such as a pillow to punch or a piece of paper to tear in half. When you observe the initial impetus fading or the participant seems to enter a different subjective state, suggest that they return to lying down on the bed. If the movement seems to be avoidant, encourage them to "stay with" the experience they sought to avoid and/or the urge to get up and move or agree to allow them to move but limit its duration. Help them identify and explore any distress that may accompany this urge.

If the participant needs to use the bathroom

Ensure that the participant is able to walk safely to the bathroom, offering support if needed and remaining ready to calmly stabilize or catch them if they begin to fall. To reduce fall risk, you can make the environment safer by removing obstacles, ensuring good lighting, and installing safety devices such as handrails. If a participant who may normally urinate while standing is struggling to remain upright, suggest that they urinate while seated (e.g., "If it's hard to stand, feel free to sit."). Remember that the participant is still in a nonordinary state and that even a mundane activity such as going to the bathroom will still carry additional layers of meaning, such as struggles around autonomy, self-care, self-efficacy, and so on. Also, attend to the possibility that standing up suddenly, in addition to causing lightheadedness, may also "stir up" new psychological content.

If you need to use the bathroom

Do your best to wait for a moment in which your absence feels most clinically appropriate. If the participant is focused inward, it is most likely okay to briefly interrupt and say "I'll be right back." This is to avoid a scenario in which they hear you leave and do not know why you did. If they are engaged with you, let them know you will briefly step out. If they or you feel that your absence will be challenging, assure them that you will return, consider inviting them to pay attention to how your absence feels, and invite them to express anything they felt once you return, if they feel called to do so. Consider exploring this as a relational moment during the integration phase.

About rescue medications

In PAT, for most participants, common events and challenging events that arise are self-limiting and can be managed safely through the provision of skillful interpersonal intervention (Breeksema et al., 2022a). It is not uncommon for participants in psychedelic clinical trials to report experiences of transient psychological or emotional struggle often characterized by acute reactions of fear, confusion, panic, or paranoia (Belser et al., 2017). Many psychedelic clinical trial protocols permit the use of rescue medication (e.g., oral benzodiazepine for distress and agitation, antipsychotic medication for severe distress or thought disorder, antiemetic medication for nausea). However, in practice, their use is rare and avoided if possible.

When Should I Intervene?

It can be hard for a therapist to feel like they know when to intervene or not intervene during a PAT medicine session. The field of PAT is still in the early stages of developing an agreed-upon set of best practices. Dr. Adele Lafrance offered a helpful set of suggested markers for when intervention might be helpful during her presentation on the Affective–Cognitive domain:

- *Participant is battling with a part of themselves they feel they need to overcome.* Consider inviting them to explore how that part has tried and continues to try to help them or protect them from pain/harm.
- *Participant is experiencing a maladaptive emotion for an extended period of time* (e.g., shame, despair). After helping them to embody the state as fully as possible, invite them to explore which other emotion/s might be beneath the surface (e.g., empowered anger)
- *Participant anticipates postsession shame or regret* (e.g., "Boy, I'm going to feel stupid tomorrow."). Minimize the "shame hangover" by slowing down the process and inviting the participant to engage with these feelings in the present moment.
- *Participant feels pressured to do something they think is "right" but are conflicted about* (e.g., "Well, I don't wanna say this, but I guess this is the time to do it."). Encourage them to spend more time with the part of them that does not want to do it rather than jumping over it. The reintegration of this part is more important than confessing something. We never want them to fight any part of themselves.
- *Participant expresses uncertainty about "going somewhere"* (e.g., "I'm not sure if I should let myself feel it."). Invite them to pause and attend to the part of them that is hesitant; to get to know that part before moving ahead in one direction or another.

MEDICINE SESSION: RESPONDING TO CHALLENGING EVENTS

While they are mostly rare and, so far, uncommon in PAT clinical trials, you should be prepared to respond to a range of challenging in-session events. This section offers guidance on how to support participants in moments of distress.

You may notice that the interventions in this section sometimes involve a more directive approach than what is suggested in other sections. In moments of great distress or disorganization, you may be called upon to provide a sense of structure and forward momentum through the quality of your speech and presence that serves to move the participant through the storm. For example, rather than asking a highly distressed participant "would a breathing practice be helpful right now?" it may be better to simply say "breathe with me" and lead through example. Importantly, this shift in approach should not be applied to touch or used to override any consent agreements previously established.

If the participant experiences distressing somatic symptoms

Some participants undergo embodied experiences that may be startling to you and/or the participant. These may include intense physical tremors that involve part or all of the participant's body, vomiting or dry heaving (emesis basin should be brought forward), strong tingling sensations, convulsive contractions or tremors in the body, or large subjective fluctuations in body temperature. Unless the participant is showing signs of medical distress, it is advisable that you normalize and be supportive of these experiences. Almost always, these phenomena are not physically dangerous, and they have been hypothesized to sometimes contribute to therapeutic outcomes. Do very little to directly intervene during the experience; simply do whatever is required to keep the participant physically safe (e.g., removing objects from their vicinity) and assure them that you are attending to their well-being. If you are trained and competent in a trauma-informed somatic methodology that offers advanced techniques for supporting these forms of expression, they may be practiced here, within the guidelines of consent discussed above. If the participant experiences persistent distress and/or expresses that it is intolerable for them, you can guide them to resource with the interventions described in the "Basic Interventions" section above, such as inviting them to move or change the position of their body.

If the participant is restless or agitated

Provide empathy explicitly (e.g., "That sounds uncomfortable.") and normalize these feelings ("People sometimes have feelings of energy, or agitation, and that is okay."). A first set of possible therapist interventions is to encourage them to express their agitation vocally ("It's okay to yell or sing or hum, whatever feels right.") or physically ("You can move your legs and arms.").

In rare cases, a participant may move enough that they seem in danger of falling off the bed or appear to be ready to try to get up out of bed. To limit acute fall risk or risk of unintentional injury, remove obstacles and buffer the individual with pillows or cushions. To develop a sense of what might be most helpful, you may ask, "What is happening? Tell me about this movement." If agitation persists and you judge that the participant may harm themselves despite these interventions, consult with your team's qualified medical provider to discuss whether a rescue medication should be provided.

If the participant experiences intense paranoia

Occasionally, participants may experience pronounced distrust of real or imagined others, either present in the room or elsewhere. They may also express that they are seeing a threatening person, animal, or other entity. Some experiences of this sort subside without intervention. The first line intervention is to remind the participant of where they are ("You are in a therapy room. I am a therapist. You took a drug that makes you think differently. The effects will pass in two hours."). It may also be helpful to let them know that they are safe (e.g., "I do not want to hurt you. Let me know how I can help you feel safe."). If paranoia persists and escalates to agitation, guide them toward resource, skipping the first few items on the list provided in an earlier section and refraining from supportive touch. If the paranoia persists and may pose a heightened risk of harm, consult with your team's qualified medical provider to discuss whether a rescue medication (e.g., oral benzodiazepine) should be provided.

If the participant wants to leave before the end of the medicine session

Gently remind them that an agreement was made that they would stay for a set amount of time. Encourage them to be present and curious about their desire to leave. If they are anxious or agitated, identify this with them and consider inviting them to use self-regulation practices (e.g., breathing) to settle them.

If the participant urgently wants to use their phone during the medicine session

Some participants will insist that they need to contact a loved one or other outside party to talk to them during a session, often to express love, anger, suspicion, forgiveness, and so on. Gently remind them that an agreement was made to wait until later to use their phone. Invite them to use the session to focus on the feeling or concern they are having. If they worry about losing the thought or feeling they want to express, offer to make an audio or textual recording of it that they can send it later.

If the participant becomes dissociated

Dissociation refers to a defensive shutting down of emotions that a participant may use in response to intense emotions that arise. When this occurs, they may seem robotic or "blank." It is often difficult to encourage participants to leave a place of dissociation once they have arrived there. Instead, allow them to have this defense, and invite them to explore the dissociation and perhaps start a curious internal dialogue with it.

If the participant attempts to engage with you sexually

Respectfully remind them that you care about them, but you are there as their therapist ("I can feel that you care about me, and I care about you too. I'm here as your therapist, so what I can do is sit here with you and listen to you. Maybe you could try going back inside to feel these feelings?"). If the attempt to engage sexually arose while supportive touch was being offered, let the participant know that you will end the touch in a way that is nonshaming (e.g., "I want you to be safe to have all of your feelings."), and then do so. See the "If the Participant Requests Physical Contact" section in the "Responding to Common Events That May Arise in a Medicine Session" section above for more guidance.

If the participant discloses violent or homicidal intentions or demonstrates aggressive, violent, or disruptive behaviors

Follow your clinic or hospital's procedures for staff and participant safety. While there is no precedent for a participant to become physically threatening to a therapist in recent psychedelic clinical trials, if this did happen, the safety of all persons is paramount. When the participant is in a state of nonordinary consciousness, the first-line intervention is to verbally encourage the use of go-to self-regulation practices. Consider lowering the music and turning up the lights. The second-line intervention is to direct the participant to stop what they are doing, remain still, and reorient them ("Remember that you are here in this treatment room, and I am a therapist.") Maintain an awareness of the likelihood that this aggression is possibly the expression of a past trauma, so reorienting them to the present can be useful.

If a participant expresses any level of homicidal ideation or intent to harm another person, an immediate assessment is necessary. Refer to your previous therapeutic training in assessing violent feelings or intentions. Assessment of homicidality should follow these guidelines:

1. Determine if the participant harbors thoughts of harming anyone specifically and the nature of the harm.
2. Inquire about any history of violent behavior and its severity.
3. Evaluate if the participant has an actionable plan and means to execute it.
4. Identify who the participant wishes to harm, be it a generalized or specific target.
5. Encourage the participant to contact supportive individuals and suggest adaptive coping behaviors.

. 6. Perform a suicide risk assessment, as those with homicidal ideation have heightened suicide risk.

7. Document all assessments and actions taken.

8. If immediate risk is identified:
   - Ensure staff safety and call local security if available or 911 or active local emergency medical services.
   - Attempt to warn the endangered individual and document these efforts.
   - Elicit potential deterrents to the violent behavior.

A NOTE ON CHALLENGING EXPERIENCES

What I could for sure tell you and I remember was I noticed myself losing the firm grasp on sort of "me-hood." Like all the things that tether me to reality. My past, my relationships, my personality, everything that makes me feel like I have a soul if you will, or I have . . . I mean an individual were disintegrating and it was scary. I remember there is still a part left of me an observer part of me that said to himself "Gee, will you ever come back from this?" There was like that, as I was watching everything disintegrate away, there was the fearfulness that was kind of setting in of . . . everything is just sort of . . . everything . . . I was losing the ability to create rational thoughts. It was almost a descent into insanity and I watched that happen and it was scary, I guess, and it was all happening in my head. And while it was happening I suddenly was not again. I was far beyond the context of this room and this study.

—Dan (Belser et al., 2017; Swift et al., 2017)

"Challenging experiences" is a broad term that is often used to capture distressing events that arise during psychedelic treatment, including the events listed in the previous section and others: anxiety, fear, panic attacks, grief, worrying that one is "going crazy," worrying that one has experienced permanent damage to one's brain or personality, existential confusion, derealization, depersonalization, social disconnection, suicidality, vomiting, headaches, and pain. Other types of challenging experiences are described in more poetic or theological terms, like the difficult struggle, the dark night of the soul, encounters with the shadow, encounters with wrathful guardians of the gates of the mandala, experiences of ego death, visiting hell realms, and existential collapse (Barrett et al., 2016; Belser et al., 2017; Bouso et al., 2022; Breeksema et al., 2022b; Luke, 2023; McNamee et al., 2023).

There is currently insufficient evidence to come to any conclusive understanding of the clinical importance of challenging experiences that arise during psychedelic therapy. A refrain often heard in the field is that "hard experiences are the best experiences." However, this idea has been challenged by harm reduction advocates who have called attention to the lack of data supporting this notion and the various types of harm that could be done (and has been done) by facilitators who embrace it incautiously.

Researchers have looked at how challenging experiences have impacted the outcomes of people taking psychedelics in clinical trials and nonclinical settings. Generally, these studies have most often found that challenging experiences during a psychedelic experience either did not correlate or correlated negatively with improvements in primary measures of clinical improvement or well-being (Agin-Liebes et al., 2021; Davis et al., 2019; 2021; Fauvel et al., 2022; Garcia-Romeu et al., 2019; Gukasayan et al., 2022; Haijen et al., 2018; Nygart et al., 2022; Perkins et al., 2021; Roseman et al., 2019), though some have found a positive correlation (Carbonaro et al., 2016; Russ et al., 2019; Weiss et al., 2021). Periods of transient distress may serve as a necessary turning point in an unfolding process, as some participants describe moving from defensive resistance with feelings of fear, panic, and anxiety and surrendering or letting go into a deeper place marked by feelings of relief, meaning, wholeness, freedom, and affirmation (Belser et al., 2017).

Additionally, challenging experiences have often been found to predict how personally meaningful and/or spiritually significant participants feel their experiences were (Agin-Liebes et al., 2021; Barrett et al., 2016; Carbonaro et al., 2016; Davis et al., 2019; Gashi et al., 2021). To complicate things further, this sense of meaningfulness can often predict clinical benefit, even when the direct effect of challenging experiences on clinical indicators is not significant (Davis et al., 2019).

This ambiguous data may be the result of the ways challenging experiences have been measured. The studies cited above have mostly measured the degree of challenge a person experienced using the Challenging Experiences Questionnaire (CEQ; Barrett et al., 2016), which provides a combined score that measures a wide range of challenging experiences (e.g., grief, physical discomfort, paranoia). The rest of these studies used a single question that asks something akin to "How challenging was your experience?" (Kangaslampi, 2023). Both of these approaches risk conflating a broad set of challenging experiences into a single data point, which limits our understanding of what types of challenge may be helpful, unhelpful, or harmful. For instance, it may be that a participant benefits from a challenging experience of intense grief or shame that eventually resolves itself in a therapeutic way, while they would not benefit from feelings of paranoia toward their therapist or an overwhelming sense that they have been poisoned and are going to die. The current state of the evidence does not allow for this type of distinction. However, four studies have found that emotional breakthroughs can predict positive outcomes (Kangaslampi, 2023), which suggests a therapeutic role for strong, possibly challenging emotions, such as grief.

In the absence of decisive, evidence-based guidance, we recommend that you respond to challenging experiences by working collaboratively with the participant to determine what approach would most benefit them. Often, sufficient clarity will come from asking them whether they want to continue along the road they are going down or if they would like your support in going somewhere else. A participant's wisdom about their own process of healing can be your best guide to determining the most fitting clinical response to distress.

FOR CLINICAL TRIAL THERAPISTS: WHAT TO DO IF THE PARTICIPANT THINKS THEY GOT PLACEBO

As a study therapist, it may feel daunting to have a participant tell you, "I'm not feeling anything. I think I got the placebo." What will the two of you do together for the duration of the medicine session? The following suggestions may prove helpful in these moments.

Always remember that your role as a study therapist is to provide the same therapeutic care to the participant *regardless* of what condition they have been assigned to. It can be disappointing (or relieving etc.) for you as the therapist to consider the possibility that the participant in front of you got the placebo. However, be sure that this does not lead to a change in your presence or the interventions you use, as this would become a confounding factor in the research. The evaluation of the usefulness of the treatment should be left until the statistical analysis is conducted.

It may be helpful for you to remember that, in other randomized placebo-controlled studies of psychedelics, participants asked to indicate whether they thought they received the psychedelic or the placebo were incorrect in 10% of their judgments. In addition, study therapists can also be incorrect in their judgments about psychedelic or placebo, so rather than engage with the participant's judgment, it is preferable for the therapist to note that they were not told and do not know. If the participant believes they got the placebo and has feelings about it, explore those feelings and be cautious to neither join them nor invalidate their experience. Finally, remember that psychedelic medicines affect different people in different ways. A participant may say to you, "I'm not feeling anything." when in reality, they are experiencing alterations that they either do not consciously recognize or are choosing not to share with the therapists in order to maintain a sense of control.

If a participant states that they are not feeling the effects of the medicine:

Encourage them to remain present to the opportunity at hand rather than fixating on the question of whether they got the placebo or troubleshooting their experience. Instead, help them focus on the present moment in a nonjudgmental way. For example, you might invite them to relax back into their body as a way to recognize any subtle shifts that may be happening and/or to disrupt their ruminative thought processes. Consider offering to guide them in a breath-focused mindfulness practice or a full body scan if you feel competent in doing so. You may also invite the participant to contract each muscle as they focus on it and subsequently release it (progressive muscle relaxation). When offering any of these practices, do so in a way that signals spaciousness and a lack of pressure to make something happen.

Note that the medicine session is time that the participant has set aside time for their healing. If it would be helpful and supportive, consider reminding the participant that spending several hours in the care of one or more therapists may present opportunities for healing and growth with or without a psychedelic medicine. Invite them to make use of their time in a way that could benefit them, without eschewing the guidelines that all participants (medicine and placebo) are given (e.g., let the experience be primarily inner-directed, stay in a state of openness and receptivity to what is present internally).

Offer brief psychoeducation about the variability in timeline and character of the experiences of people who take psychedelic medicines. Each participant's timeline will differ due to a range of poorly understood physiological and psychological factors. Also, remember that subjective experiences of a psychedelic medicine are very variable across participants. For some participants, it may be very vivid, while for others it can be very subtle. One of the authors recalls a medicine session in which a participant felt they got "nothing," then woke up the next day to find that "their whole life had changed."

If the participant expresses disappointment, use discernment in exploring it. If a participant expresses disappointment, taken time to connect with that emotion. Offer your empathy and care, acknowledging the importance of that feeling. Consider that disappointment may sometimes reflect an enduring pattern of reactivity that they revealed in their preparation sessions. For example, they might feel often as though their life is out of their control, or they may carry an unhelpful amount of hope that that events in their life will magically fix everything. If you recognize this type of pattern, it may be worth exploring therapeutically. Conversely, there are times when a participant's disappointment will be a normal reaction to a situation that didn't turn out as they had wanted. Use your clinical judgment to determine whether their disappointment is tied to bigger life issues that would merit deeper exploration.

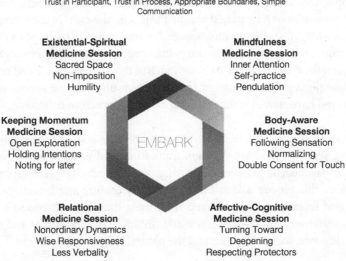

Figure 6.1. Medicine Session: Watch Words for Therapists

7

Integration Sessions

> *The universal challenge is to transform peak experiences into plateau experiences, epiphanies into personality, states into stages, and altered states into altered traits, or, as I believe Huston Smith once eloquently put it, "to transform flashes of illumination into abiding light."[1]*
>
> —Roger Walsh (2003, p. 4)

After a medicine session comes integration. You and the participant are now tasked with bringing whatever experience they had in their medicine session into their day-to-day life. Integration is where the rubber meets the road. As you have likely already surmised, it is a feat that requires a great deal of skillful effort from both you and the participant. However, the reward of a successful integration phase is a more enduring set of benefits that last long after treatment ends. Many PAT experts have emphasized that integration is the most important stage of treatment.

On the question of how to best conduct this task, the current consensus is a bit spottier. A wide range of integration approaches have arisen in recent years that differ in important ways. However, important points of agreement have thankfully begun to emerge, and these will form the basis for much of this chapter. Bathje and colleagues (2022) have done great work comparing and contrasting different approaches to integration and have arrived at the following excellent consensus definition:

> Integration is a process in which a person revisits and actively engages in making sense of, working through, translating, and processing the content of their psychedelic experience. Through intentional effort and supportive practices, this process allows one to gradually capture and incorporate the emergent lessons and insights into their lives, thus moving toward greater balance and wholeness, both internally (mind, body, and spirit) and externally (lifestyle, social relations, and the natural world) (p. 4).

[1] Quotation reproduced under a CC BY-NC-ND 4.0 license.

EMBARK Psychedelic Therapy for Depression. Bill Brennan and Alex Belser, Oxford University Press.
© Oxford University Press 2024. DOI: 10.1093/9780197762622.003.0008

In practice, this process will involve several nondrug sessions after each medicine session, in which you and the participant will engage in many, if not all, of the actions that make up this definition:

- "Making sense" of the participant's experience so that they feel like it has at least a tentative place in their understanding of themselves and the world, while avoiding any premature closing off of its unfolding meaning
- "Working through" and "processing" any psychological material that lingers on after the medicine session through focused therapeutic work with their emotional and embodied experiences
- "Translating" their medicine session experience into a response to their depression that introduces new capacities for healing and growth
- Encouraging "intentional effort" to actively disrupt the status quo of their life and introduce beneficial new habits and other changes derived from the medicine session
- Codeveloping "supportive practices" that can sustain and strengthen the participant in their integration efforts
- Helping them consider the ways their integration process might unfold in all spheres of their life, from the "internal" to the "external"
- As always, ensuring that the participant is supported to an appropriate extent for the degree of dysregulation or distress they may be experiencing

INTEGRATION: OVERVIEW

It can be helpful to group these activities into three overarching objectives: listening, goal-setting, and enacting. Integration always begins by listening for the things that are most salient and "alive" for the participant from their recent medicine session. They could be anything from a remembered vision to a new idea about themselves to a hard-to-name feeling lingering in their body. The process of listening will involve a deep dive into whatever is present for the participant by encouraging them to share their narrative, deepen into their emotions and embodiment, and draw on any other creative practices (e.g., art, poetry, journaling) that could help them get acquainted with the newly discovered capacities for healing and growth that they will work to carry forward.

This process of listening serves as both a means and an end unto itself. On one hand, the information it provides will inform goal-setting and enacting. But the act of providing a slower, more receptive space in sessions for the continued unfolding of the subtler effects of the medicine is also a crucial part of integration. These effects consist of quieter shifts in the participant's emotions and body that happen in the days following a medicine session, mostly outside of conscious awareness and without any effort beyond leaving space in one's life for them to occur. You will help the participant to balance active change work toward clear therapeutic goals with more contemplative practices that nurture these subtler shifts (e.g., spending more time looking inwards, being in nature, mandala work).

The second step of the integration process is goal-setting. It involves collaborating with the participant to explore how new capacities discovered in their medicine session could precipitate shifts in their life that impact their depression, culminating in the crafting of integration goals. Together you will explore the question of what new habits, behaviors, practices, and changes to their lived contexts support durable long-lasting benefit. (If the integration phase occurs between two medicine sessions, this goal-setting process will also focus on using the experience of the last session to inform the next.)

The goal-setting step is where you and the participant codetermine what the specific integration goals will be for the remainder of treatment. An integration goal can be thought of as a clear focus for the therapeutic work that will be done during the remaining integration sessions. For example, if the participant's medicine session experience led them to feel like they want to grow their capacity to connect with others, the rest of their time with you can explore and define ways to meet this goal. There can be multiple integration goals, though the number should remain manageable (one to three). A later section in this chapter provides suggested integration goals that are pertinent to depression, but you are encouraged to hew most closely to what naturally arises as a wise goal for the participant, whether or not it aligns with any of the suggestions.

Integration concludes with enacting these aimed-for changes in the participant's life. Together, you will develop concrete, actionable steps that they will take between sessions. Challenges will naturally arise, which you and the participant will troubleshoot together in the subsequent sessions. Setbacks need not be relapses. Although this process is generally linear, it is also recursive: participants will likely need to revisit earlier steps to reconnect with the felt sense and aliveness of the original capacities that arose in their medicine session as a continual wellspring of inspiration.

If it is a helpful metaphor, you can think of these three phases, respectively, as looking for sparks left by a bolt of lightning (listening), searching for kindling to fuel them (goal-setting), and sparking a fire hearty enough to be stoked and tended indefinitely (enacting).

The timeline of this process is likely to vary, though it is best to start soon after the medicine session. Most practitioners schedule the first integration session either the day after the medicine session or the day after that (with a phone or text check-in in the interim). Generally, two or three more integration sessions will follow the first on a weekly basis. However, more frequent sessions may be more supportive to a participant who had a difficult medicine session. As always, be ready to adjust your protocol to accommodate participant needs.

The goal of these sessions should not be complete integration of all of the material that arose during a medicine session. Due to their richness of meaning, many psychedelic medicine sessions take months, years, or perhaps the rest of one's life to fully integrate—longer than a time-limited course of treatment. This may be where contemplative practices reveal their importance. Your role in the more active aspects of integration is better thought of as helping the participant get to the point at which the remaining process of integration feels clear and achievable. You help them develop a sense of the changes they want to make, how they can make them, what to do when challenges arise—and then you take your hands off of the bike and let them ride off on their own.

INTEGRATION: AIMS

> *I am so much more able to do things that I wanted to do, and didn't feel I could, something always holding me back. Oh, I can't clean up that mess, it's just overwhelming to even look at. And now I can. And how am I going to lose all this weight? Well, I started, I just did. I really need new friends. . . . I made them.*
>
> —Edna (Belser et al., 2017; Swift et al., 2017)

This section lays out the specific aims that make up the process of listening, goal-setting, and enacting. It delineates these aims along two types of integration phase: interim and final.

For protocols with more than one medicine session, the interim integration phase is the nondrug sessions that occur between one medicine session and another. The final integration phase is the sessions that happen after the last medicine session of the treatment.

The therapist's aims for each integration phase can be found in the following table. Note that there are no set agendas for the sessions in the integration phase, as they are meant to be conducted flexibly, iteratively, and in a way that is responsive to what the participant brings forward from their medicine session.

INTERIM INTEGRATION PHASE	FINAL INTEGRATION PHASE
1. Debrief the participant's experience of the medicine session	1. Debrief the participant's experience of the medicine session
2. Identify new opportunities for healing and growth	2. Identify new opportunities for healing and growth
3. Address any lingering somatic or psychological concerns	3. Address any lingering somatic or psychological concerns
4. **(a)** Develop simple activities that help maintain contact with new capacities	4. **(b)** Develop integration goals and begin planning and enacting life changes that support them
5. Use challenges of the last medicine session to change the approach to the next	9. Treatment completion
6. Practice any interim preparatory skills that would be supportive	
7. Develop intentions for the next medicine session	
8. Conduct a relational check-in and reassessment of consent for touch-based interventions	

Note that both phases share the first four aims, as the interim and final sessions both involve debriefing and making meaning of the content that arose in the most recent medicine session. The emphasis on planning life changes (aim 4) is much greater in the final integration phase, comprising the bulk of the focus of its three sessions. The interim integration sessions instead devote much of their attention to four additional aims meant to help the participant prepare for the next medicine session. Final integration sessions also include a focus on concluding the therapeutic relationship.

Aim 1: Debrief the participant's experience of the medicine session

Generally, the first integration session in either integration phase should prioritize the participant retelling and reflecting upon their medicine session experience. First, invite them to share their psychedelic experience, *then* engage in sense-making and meaning-making later. The participant should be encouraged to debrief it in a self-directed way that focuses on what is most salient to them. Listen in an open, curious, and attentive way, prompting for more detail and disclosure when needed, with an ear out for which integration goals might best suit the participant's experience. This debrief should be allowed to unfold at its own pace and may take up the majority of the first integration session. The participant should not feel pressured to share any specific details of what arose if they would prefer to not discuss them.

In the debrief, the participant's own experience and meaningful interpretation of the medicine session should be given top priority. Only after they explore their own reflections and curiosities should you bring in observations of your own. When doing so, be careful not to impose your interpretations of events in a way that supplants those of the participant. Even if a participant seeks your interpretation of an event that was confusing to them, use your clinical judgment to decide if this would be in their interest. Consider that it may be more beneficial for them if you normalize the ongoing process of developing an understanding and gently guide them to stay with it until it resolves on its own, perhaps using mindfulness or somatic awareness-based interventions to help them "hold" the experience in a way that is less focused on effortful analytic interpretation. Remember that the participant is likely to still be somewhat suggestible during the first integration session, so your reflections may influence their sense of what occurred in a way that disrupts their sense of ownership of the experience. When you offer an interpretation, invite the participant to assess their own sense of its rightness.

During the interim integration phase, listen in the debrief for any difficulties that the participant experienced. This may provide information about how to adjust the approach that they take in the subsequent medicine session, as discussed in aims 5 and 6 for this phase. Also, listen for anything in their retelling that may indicate that a second session is not advisable (which is expected to be rare) or that other types of follow-up care might be needed.

Aim 2: Identify new opportunities for healing and growth

During the participant's debrief, listen for any indications that they have experienced any shifts in their lived experience that may support their healing. These shifts may take the form of new feelings, perspectives, attitudes, beliefs, embodied experiences, impulses, forms of awareness, and so on. A participant may have already identified and characterized these shifts as a new capacity for healing (e.g., "I feel a new kind of peace in my chest."). Others may have identified that they feel different in some way that they experience as positive but cannot articulate what opportunity for healing it could present (e.g., "When I went home, it felt really different to be around my family.").

In either event, it is likely to be helpful for you to help the participant to deepen their embodied, experiential connection to whatever shift they have experienced. You can use mindfulness-based or embodied interventions to do so. Gently explore this shift at the level of their lived experience and avoid becoming too analytical of it too quickly. In this process, gradually develop a sense of what new capacities for healing and growth this shift may represent, should they find a way to stay present to it. Once the new capacity has been clarified or even named, work with the participant to find a way to remain in touch with it.

It will likely be supportive to help the participant determine some small actions they can take or other changes they can begin making to remain in contact with these feelings by the end of the first integration session. For example, they may want to engage in an awareness practice that helps them continue to feel the openness to change they are feeling now. These actions can be preliminary ones that keep the ember alive until the second medicine session, which is likely to be when the more involved process of planning and implementing changes will naturally arise.

Aim 3: Address any lingering somatic or psychological concerns

Some participants may come to integration sessions experiencing lingering, uncomfortable somatic or psychological effects from the medicine session. These may include emotional lability, emotional sensitivity, intense emotions (e.g., fury), mood alterations, headaches, fatigue, bodily tension, pains, mild tremors, psychomotor agitation, or a sense that psychological material is "stuck" in a specific part of their body (Mithoefer et al., 2017; Rucker et al., 2022).

In all such events, the participant's safety should be the paramount concern. Consult with medical staff if there is any reason to believe that a participant might be experiencing a physical symptom of medical import. If they are experiencing any enduring symptoms of psychiatric concern (e.g., suicidality, depersonalization, derealization, possible manic or psychotic episode), ensure that they are given appropriate support. See the section entitled "Integration: Responding to Serious Adverse Outcomes" later in this chapter for more guidance.

In situations that have been determined to not present safety concerns, work with the participant to address these phenomena therapeutically during the integration sessions. This work should begin in the first session. Normalize their experience as something many participants have experienced and let them know that you will work with them to get them the support they need until it has resolved. See the section entitled "Integration: Responding to Challenging Events That May Arise" later in this chapter for more guidance.

Aim 4a: Develop simple activities that help maintain contact with new capacities (interim integration phase)

In an interim integration phase, there is less of an emphasis on cultivating new habits and making enduring life changes than in the final integration phase. The approach to integration in an interim phase should prioritize helping the participant enter the second medicine session with the same open, exploratory attitude that they brought into the first session. Too much emphasis on the concrete business of planning and enacting life changes at this point may detract from this. You should thus keep any movement toward making changes in balance with the importance of remaining open, receptive, and "in process" before the next medicine session.

Toward this end, it may be more supportive to continue to help the participant come up with simple activities that may help them stay in touch with the new capacities identified in aim 2: journaling, mindfulness practice, more time for contemplation, refraining from (or reducing) any habitual behaviors that may detract from the capacity, and so on.

Still, opportunities for making more substantive changes may arise spontaneously and present themselves during an interim integration phase. A participant may communicate that they have progressed through the stages of change and are now ready to take action. If this occurs, support them in doing so, using the suggestions in this chapter.

Aim 4b: Develop integration goals and begin planning and enacting changes that support them (final integration phase)

The final integration phase is the time to make a concrete plan with the participant to sustain gains posttreatment. Using the capacities identified in aim 2 as a basis, collaboratively develop specific integration goals that you and the participant will work toward for the remainder of treatment. Together, decide on which of these capacities are most likely to serve as durable new inroads to healing and growth and begin to develop a plan of action that will help them take hold in the participant's life.

These plans should generally be collaboratively set by the second integration session so that there is an opportunity to troubleshoot their barriers to the plan of action in the third integration session. It may also be helpful to troubleshoot any imagined difficulties prior to putting them into action. You may ask the participant to write down the plan themselves on a sheet of paper. Develop a relapse prevention plan that can be put into place and activated in the likely event that the participant finds themselves backsliding at some point. Finally, make sure that there is time in session to attend to any challenging emotions (fear, grief, or anxiety) that arise around the prospect of moving away from an old way of being.

Aim 5: Use challenges of the last medicine session to change the approach to the next (interim integration phase)

Spend time exploring what, if anything, the participant found challenging or unproductive about their medicine session. Debriefing these experiences will inform the preparation work done in this phase leading up to the next medicine session. Challenges may include:

- Difficulty remaining relaxed and receptive
- Feeling uncomfortable with the intensity of emotion that arose
- Bodily discomfort, nausea, tension
- Experiencing paranoia or mistrust of you
- Discomfort with your interventions (e.g., supportive touch)
- Disturbing visuals
- Confusion, unsettled feeling, fear of losing control
- Dissociation or amnesia

Allow the participant to speak from their own experience first. Next, offer any observations or interpretations of your own. At all times, ensure that the participant is not made to feel as though these challenges represent failure on their part. Also, dissuade them from adopting the mindset that they will have failed in the next medicine session if these difficulties arise again. Frame the appearance of these difficulties as a natural part of the therapeutic process, perhaps by ascribing meaning to encounters with these phenomena using language from your preferred clinical orientation (e.g., framing defenses as protectors, wounded child parts, or maladaptive strategies that can be welcomed and worked with).

If the participant experienced significant distress during their medicine session and expresses fear or trepidation about the next one, be sure to give them an opportunity to explore whether or not they would like to continue treatment. Offer this option in a way that does not suggest that you would prefer them to stop, as they may experience this as rejecting.

Aim 6: Practice any interim preparatory skills that would be supportive (interim integration phase)

Once you have identified any difficulties that the participant had, help them further develop the skills that will help them navigate these or any other challenges that may arise. Revisit the skills taught in the preparation phase: self-regulation, somatic awareness, mindfulness, and cultivating a state of open receptivity.

Ask the participant whether they think it would be helpful to deepen their practice of these previously learned exercises or if they would prefer to learn a different way of supporting themselves during challenging moments. Build on their experience from the medicine session to learn about what helped them and what did not. Avoid presenting this return to a previously learned practice as the correction of a deficiency. Frame it as something that builds on prior successes and/ or grows their capacity to go deeper during their next medicine session. Refer to Chapter 5 to refresh your sense of the guidelines you can use to introduce skills that may be supportive in medicine sessions.

Aim 7: Develop intentions for the next medicine session (interim integration phase)

This aim is similar to the process of developing intentions in the preparation phase. All of the same guidelines regarding how to craft an intention and carry it into a medicine session still apply.

One important difference is that the participant will now have more of a sense of how their intentions may play out in a medicine session. Invite them to take this into account when developing their intentions for the second medicine session.

They may use new material that arose in their first medicine session to inform their intentions. For example, someone who had an important experience of accepting care from you during the medicine session may now set an intention to turn their attention to the relational aspects of their depression in the next medicine session.

Many second-time participants run the risk of approaching their next medicine session with an unhelpful cockiness. They may feel an inflated sense of mastery or certainty toward the coming experience. Help them to balance their heightened sense of knowing where their work is with a humble, "beginner's mind" approach and open receptivity to the full range of what may arise.

Aim 8: Do a relational check-in and reassessment of consent for touch-based interventions (interim integration phase)

Check in with the participant to see if any relational dynamics arose during or since the medicine session that would benefit from processing together. These dynamics may stem from a misattuned intervention, something about your presence during the session, an internal shift in the participant, or other relational factors. Invite the participant to speak freely about them, asserting the importance of doing so before the next medicine session. Refer to the section on the relational check-in in Chapter 5 for further guidance.

If any therapist–participant touch occurred in the medicine session, be sure to explore how this was for the participant during this phase. Encourage them to speak freely about how the touch was received. Give them the opportunity to change the extent of the consent they previously gave for touch-based interventions. If they decrease their level of consent, frame this as acceptable and likely evidence of a healthy ability to recognize their discomfort and set a boundary that prevents it from happening again. If they ask to increase their level of consent for the next medicine session, devote ample time to exploring this request. Consider that it may be indicative of a movement toward empowerment and a restored ability to seek support or closeness despite past experiences of neglect, rejection, or abuse. Also attend to other dynamics that might be present, including any transferences, enactments, or power dynamics that may have arisen or deepened during the medicine session and that may benefit from further collaborative inquiry with the participant before they become the basis for increased consent.

Aim 9: Treatment completion (final integration phase)

The final integration sessions should also devote adequate time to completion processes (sometimes called termination), such as attending to feelings about the conclusion of the relationship (if it is concluding), celebrating successes, and coming to a place of acceptance with challenges still to come.

In the penultimate session, be sure to mention completion and invite the participant to bring to the final session any feelings or reflections they may have about the course of treatment and the therapist–participant relationships that arose therein. You are encouraged to do the same thing. Devote at least 5 minutes of the final integration session to sharing these feelings and reflections. Stay in your CUSHION presence and speak honestly from the heart about what you admired about the participant's way of being in the medicine session—their courage, their openness, the strength of their emotions. Give them every opportunity to leave with a recognition of the impact and meaning of what they have done for their own process of healing.

INTEGRATION: GENERAL GUIDELINES

> *I'm—different. I'm there in a different way . . . I feel more contented and happy about my place in the world in all the things I'm doing. If you're not anxious, you're sleeping more, you feel more happy, you feel more contented, and you're drawing on things when you need them, if you find that you're feeling upset, you can draw back onto whatever you might need by just sitting and listening to a tape [of the psilocybin playlist] or meditate a bit . . . This is pretty dramatic for me. It's really big.*
> —Mary (Belser et al., 2017; Swift et al., 2017)

Integrating a psychedelic experience can often feel like a woolly process for all parties involved. There are some general principles that will be helpful to keep in mind.

Trust and prioritize the participant's wisdom about their needs. Follow the unfolding of the participant's therapeutic process as occasioned by the medicine. The new practices, habits, and other changes that the participant derives from their own intrinsic motivation are likely to be the ones that offer them the most enduring benefit. The suggested goals provided in this chapter are just that— suggestions. Many participants will exit a medicine session with their own clear picture of what their experience meant and what life changes follow naturally from it. Follow their lead.

Use creativity. The suggested goals in this chapter are geared primarily toward treatment outcomes and practices that have the strongest basis in the existing psychotherapy research literature. However, there exists a broad diversity of ways a participant could carry their medicine session forward in a therapeutic way. Boxing lessons, breathwork, better boundary-setting, body scan meditations— there are as many paths as there are travelers. You are invited to think broadly about practices that might support posttreatment benefit. For more examples of creative integration interventions, see Aixalà (2022) or Bathje and colleagues (2022).

ART AS INTEGRATION

Some patients may find that creating art is supportive of their integration process. Integration coach Daniel Shankin (2023) has delineated six possible ways art may help with integration:

- Facilitating self-expression
- Processing complex emotions
- Capturing and exploring insights
- Encouraging self-reflection
- Providing a sense of control over challenging medicine session experiences
- Fostering connection through sharing with others

For a moving account of how art can intersect with the therapeutic process in PAT, see the artist known as Swoon's (2019) talk at the Horizons Perspective on Psychedelics conference entitled "Unearthing the Medea: The Intersection of Art & Psychedelic Assisted Therapy" (available on YouTube).

Stay connected to the last medicine session experience. A common misstep that therapists make during integration sessions is inadvertently shifting their approach back toward something like therapy-as-usual once the afterglow of the medicine session has worn off. Participants use the sessions to discuss the frustrations of the day or something else they generally struggle with, and their therapist works with this material as they would in a standard therapy session. This is particularly common from the second integration session onward, once the last medicine session has faded into memory a bit. Remember that your role in integration is to support the participant in obtaining enduring benefit through new habits, practices, and other changes that are *inspired by their medicine session experience*. That is the heart of this process.

If you or they feel like they have lost the thread, find a way to help them regain it. Returning to state-dependent memories (especially psychedelic memories) can recatalyze motivation. The context or state in which information is learned becomes a part of the memory trace, and congruence between learning and recall states can enhance retrieval of the memory. For instance, you could recall key statements they made during the medicine session, guide them through a mindfulness or embodiment practice that rekindles the felt sense of the medicine session, or give them access to the music playlist from the medicine session as a way to revisit the felt experience of it between sessions. Otherwise, the process of cultivating new behaviors and making other changes will likely become less of an inspired, heartfelt process and more of a dry mechanistic exercise in figuring out what the participant "should do."

Respect the old ways. Refrain from pathologizing or aggressively discarding a participant's long-held maladaptive patterns of behavior. Whether or not they explicitly request it, they will likely benefit from the implicit knowledge that they can resume their old way of being if and when they need. So, resist the temptation to, for example, speak in a denigrating way about a participant's past shyness even if they do so themselves. Healing is frequently nonlinear, and even though they are currently feeling a strong commitment to being bolder in social situations, they should not be made to feel ashamed if they need to return to their old protective isolation from time to time.

Be concrete and specific. Plans that specify exactly how the participant will take change-oriented action will be more helpful than those that skip over the details. For example, if a participant decides they want to learn how to meditate, it would be better to help them develop a plan that sounds more like "I will go to the weekly class at the yoga studio near my apartment this coming Thursday" rather than a sparser plan like "I will go to a class." Considering inviting the participant to write this down themselves on a piece of paper, in the form of a specific, concrete action statement: "I will [behavior] starting on [time/place] for [duration/frequency]." The use of goal setting accountability websites may also be helpful for more regular long-term goals.

Encourage spaciousness, patience, and gentleness in the days after a medicine session, particularly after "big ones." Suggest to participants that they refrain from returning too quickly to a full schedule of responsibilities whenever possible and leave as much space as they can in their lives for the subtler processes of integration to unfold. An invitation to let go of their urgency to figure out the meaning of an experience may be very relieving, especially for people whose medicine session experiences may take longer to integrate—or may never feel fully integrated. For instance, participants whose experiences felt at odds with the core tenets of their worldview may need extra time to process the sense of "ontological shock" they're experiencing. Let them know that they are under no requirement to feel like they have everything resolved by the end of treatment. Participants who feel pressured into doing so are done a disservice and possibly even harm.

Craft goals that are attentive to cultural and structural factors. When coming up with integration goals, make sure they are in sync with the participant's social location. This includes assessing the cultural "fit" of any suggested plans you offer. It also entails an attentiveness to how realistic any planned changes are given the opportunities and limitations faced by the participant. If you are in a comparatively privileged social location, you are likely to overestimate the ease or safety of any suggested changes and underestimate the risk and potential downsides to the participant.

Give ample space to the closing of the relationship. Endings can be hard, especially for participants who have experienced painful losses before. If your relationship with the participant will come to an end when treatment concludes, anticipate that this may be a significant event for them that may have repercussions for their continued well-being. Despite the brevity of a course of PAT treatment, the relationship that forms between you and the participant can be surprisingly deep. A unique bond often arises when someone undergoes an experience as singularly meaningful as a psychedelic medicine session in the context of deep care and attentiveness.

Other times, the participant may not feel connected to you, and this may also be an important dynamic to discuss insofar as it reflects something about their relational style. Be sure to leave space for any feelings that are present around the relationship and its ending throughout all integration sessions—not just the final one. The subsequent section on challenging events" will further discuss how to contend with feelings of abandonment, neglect, and betrayal should they arise.

> *I always regret that I can't see them, you know, that I can't see them anymore. I wanted Jeff to be my therapist, but . . . that's not allowed and I understand that. That wouldn't be appropriate. But I miss them both.*
> —Augusta (Belser et al., 2017; Swift et al., 2017)

Ensure adequate posttreatment support. Another important aspect of ensuring a proper closure to treatment is helping the participant arrange the supports they need after treatment. Ideally, this should be a process that is ongoing throughout treatment (see Chapter 4), but it should be concluded to the satisfaction of all parties by the end of the final integration session. See the section on adverse outcomes in this chapter for further guidance.

INTEGRATION: SPHERES OF INTEGRATION

> *I feel like my priorities have changed. So many people are walking in a trance and we're living to be consumers. I'm talking like a hippie, but the hippies are right about so much stuff. I haven't taken much action yet, but working to accrue more money to have more possessions seems like a waste. It's worth noting that after having your eyes opened up, it can be tough acclimating back to this crazy world afterwards.*
> —Greg (Participant in Bathje et al., 2021)

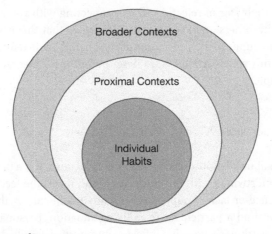

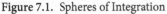

Figure 7.1. Spheres of Integration

Integration is a process that unfolds across the full breadth of a participant's lived world. In order for a participant to benefit fully from a medicine session experience, they sometimes have to put its outcomes in dialogue with the various contexts of their life so that the new green shoots of change are allowed to extend out as far as the roots of their depression. In EMBARK, participants are invited to explore the benefits that could come from change work across several spheres, including individual habits, proximal contexts, and broader contexts (Figure 7.1). The potential value of change in each sphere will be described in this section in a model that draws influence from liberatory and structurally informed systems of thought within psychotherapy, as well as Indigenous notions of reciprocity.

Sphere 1: Integration Within Individual Habits

For most participants, the postmedicine session state provides (a) an acute state of flexibility and openness to change and (b) increased access to capacities for healing and growth inside and around themselves. Taken together, these two qualities provide fertile ground for the cultivation of new habits that support the sustainment of these newly ascendent capacities. An important part of any course of integration will be working with the participant to take advantage of this moment of ripeness for making changes to old habits.

New habits can take many forms, including habits of behavior, thought, belief, emotional responsiveness, relating to others, and relating to oneself. What they all share is that they involve replacing an old, depressogenic facet of a participant's ingrained tendencies with an updated one drawn from their medicine session that supports continued movement away from their depression. For example, a participant who felt a strong sense of their own worth and goodness for the first time can train themselves to refer back to that moment, with increasing ease and automaticity, when the familiar cloud of self-loathing descends. Or a participant who overcame their fear of rejection when connecting with you can start to take similar risks with others and keep accruing evidence that this is something they can do. You can support the formation of new habits by listening, goal-setting, and enacting with your participant, as described in the "Integration: Aims" section of this chapter.

Sphere 2: Integration Within Proximal Contexts

The cultivation of new habits does not occur in a vacuum. It is a process of change that is deeply intertwined with the contexts around it and the feedback they provide. The presence or lack of supportive proximal contexts, or the most immediate settings around a participant (e.g., living situation, personal relationships, neighborhood, workplace, vocational field, communities, family dynamics, social groups or settings), will thus have a significant impact on their ability to sustain new habits posttreatment. Participants with unsupportive proximal contexts may benefit from directing some of their change work toward these contexts in order to turn them into a source of support rather than challenge.

Here is a clinical vignette: imagine a participant who has a spiritual experience during their medicine session and decides that further spiritual self-development may have a durable effect on their depression. During integration, they decide that they will cultivate a new habit by way of adopting a new, regular mantra meditation practice. However, this practice is set against by several elements in their lived context: their partner rejects it, their friends make fun of it, their job is at odds with the values inherent in it, and so on. The participant may feel as though they are trying to carry an ember through a windstorm, and their new habit of spiritual practice is not enough on its own. They may need to find a group or community that can help them keep the ember burning, or they may decide to gradually transition to a line of work more in sync with who they now experience themselves to be.

This distinction between individual habit change and proximal context change can be subtle, since individual habits play a big role in the creation and maintenance of proximal contexts. However, it is an important distinction to make for various reasons. For one, focusing on the need for proximal context change may help the participant avoid pathologizing the change they want to make. Many times, participants who come out of a medicine session with a new perspective or attitude may feel themselves to be out of sync with the norms of their family and friend groups or the culture of their workplace. This could lead them to feel insecure or even ashamed of the new capacities they are experiencing, even if they initially felt them to be desirable and healing. If you can help them to expand the locus of where change may be required—their contexts, not just them—it could help them feel more confidence in leaning into the new capacities and new habits they have developed in their treatment. This slight shift in clinical focus can send a supportive signal to the participant: maybe the changes you are trying to make will serve you better than adapting to the maladaptive status quo around you.

Collaboratively explore with the participant whether proximal context changes might be supportive of their posttreatment goals. When you do, be sure to avoid several pitfalls:

- Avoid engaging in "contextual bypassing," in which the participant is supported in avoiding the need for personal behavior change in favor of focusing exclusively on changing the contexts around them.
- Remain wary of setups and self-sabotage. Sometimes a participant will say it is really important that they make a change to their context that they have already told you is impossible. Be attentive to the possibility that the participant is enacting another kind of maladaptive pattern by assigning too much importance to a specific contextual change that is unlikely to happen. This could be an unconscious form of self-sabotage that will lead them to declare that their treatment was a failure.
- Do not lose sight of the fact that some changes might be impossible or unlikely, and the participant can end up disappointed and perhaps even harmed by their failure to effect such change. Shifting the locus of change outside of the participant's immediate control has risks. Avoid a disempowering focus.
- Even if a contextual change is achievable and clinically warranted, it may be disempowering for the participant to focus on this sphere. They may wish to focus entirely on changing their own behaviors as a way of feeling capable, strong, or powerful. Focusing on self-work could be the more beneficial strategy.
- Explore your own reactions to this idea of context change. Examine your own attraction or aversion to the idea that a participant's context is what needs to change. If you notice yourself "joining" with the participant in an excessive focus on contextual change, bring this to your supervisor and/or peers for further exploration. Also, be sure to reflect on the impact of privilege differentials between you and the participant when considering context change, as people vary greatly by social location in terms of how much they are able to change their contexts.

Sphere 3: Integration Within Broader Contexts

This third sphere represents the possibility that some participants' treatment benefit may be maximally supported by engagement with the broader contexts in which they find themselves. "Broader contexts" refers to the macrolevel conditions of the participant's life, which include all of the economic, political, and cultural elements that affect them and others. Examples include availability of housing and healthcare, impacts of climate change, pandemics, structural forms of discrimination, labor conditions, unemployment levels, trends in entertainment, or advances in technology—anything at the macrolevel that still has a substantive impact on individual well-being.

For example, in a large prospective study of lesbian, gay, and bisexual (LGB) people (N = 34,653), LGB people who lived in states that passed same-sex marriage bans had a 248% increase in generalized anxiety disorder. There were no effects for straight peers or LGB people in other states (Hatzenbuehler et al., 2010). Another study looked at the mental health impact of rising regional unemployment rates during the Great Recession of 2007–2009 and found a strong correlation with a rise in suicide rates in affected regions (Phillips & Nugent, 2014). These and many other studies have drawn a clear connection between what happens at the "big picture" level and the well-being of individuals.

There has been a slow turn in psychiatry and psychology toward recognizing the impact of these broader contextual factors on mental health. Still, psychotherapy practice has not kept pace with this process. When this type of "big picture" focus comes up, many therapists feel a reflexive urge to push it aside and refocus the work on the participant's personal material (Gerber, 1990, 1992). Sometimes they downplay these seemingly distant factors and focus on personal change ("Let's focus on what we can control."). As such, you may find this to be a challenging place to focus during a course of therapy.

In EMBARK, you are asked to reach beyond an individual level of analysis that is common in psychotherapy training. When developing and enacting integration goals, consider dimensions of the broader context—not only as contributors to depression, but as another potential target for actions that alleviate it. In integration, you are encouraged to remain open to the possibility that the participant would benefit from being in dialogue with the bigger picture of the world they live in, even if it may be hard to conceptualize concrete benefits.

This focus on the broader context is particularly germane to the practice of psychedelic therapy. Many participants have left their medicine sessions with an acute, deeply felt awareness of the broader contexts around them and the ways their lives intersect with them. Many have also felt strongly that in order for their integration process to feel truly complete, it must involve an emphasis on finding new ways to engage with and potentially change these broader contexts (Bathje et al., 2021). Remain open to the possibility that the integration process of the participant under your care would benefit from being in dialogue with the bigger picture of the world they live in.

Engagement with broader contexts may take a variety of forms. It could include engaging in collective organizing or activism, other forms of civic engagement (e.g., volunteering, hospice work), or joining an affinity group that provides a space for processing the more-than-personal dimensions of their medicine session experience (e.g., a group that gathers around a shared ancestral grief). The possibilities are vast.

The participant may emerge from the medicine session knowing exactly what they want to do, or they may feel a strong call to act on the broader contextual level but not yet know what action they will take. Give them an opportunity to explore possibilities during integration sessions with you. Respect the participant's autonomy by giving them full freedom to decide what form of engagement feels to them like the most natural outgrowth of their medicine session experience.

The main benefit to the participant of engaging with broader contexts may simply be that they are following through on their sense that doing so is something they must do. They may derive a sense of inner congruence from acting upon a deeply felt connection between themselves and the rest of the social and natural world. It is unnecessary to frame the value of this engagement in any other terms; it should be treated as an end unto itself. The field of psychedelic therapy is steadily awakening to the notion that integration is a process of change that ripples outward from ourselves, extending us through a series of expanding concentric circles around the limits of what we once thought of as "ours" (Keiman, 2023).

Still, there are a variety of notable potential benefits from this type of engagement that align with well-known psychotherapeutic goals. It may serve as a form of behavioral activation in that it gets them to commit to ongoing engagement in activities that may stimulate their interest and disrupt their isolation. It may also help them to come into alignment with their personal values by engaging in value-driven action. If they choose to take action as part of a group or collective, it may lead to greater socialization and more opportunity to form meaningful relationships. Also, their actions may bring them a sense of agency and empowerment through becoming a political actor in the world—an important level of human existence often overlooked in therapy. And, of course, there are also the benefits to individual well-being that would follow from any substantive change that the participant's work is able to bring about in the contextual conditions that adversely impact them.

As with the previous sphere, it is important to avoid potential pitfalls:

- Most importantly, it is never your role to foist this upon your participant if they are not inclined to do so. Trust their sense that their integration process would be better focused more locally.
- Be reflective about any bias you have toward rejecting or endorsing the value or importance of integration work in this sphere. As noted earlier, you may find it counterintuitive to focus on this sphere. However, you may also feel drawn to it in a way that leads you to pressure participants into engaging with it, perhaps rushing them past personal material. Reflect on your own urges, wants, beliefs, wishes, or feelings regarding the broader context that may be activated by seeing your participant engage with it.
- Refrain from trying to direct or shape the ways the participant engages with the broader context. If the participant chooses to bring their integration process into this sphere, the decision of what type of action this includes should be left up to them. Your role is simply to support the elaboration of any impulse that spontaneously arises in the participant.
- Also, ensure that the participant is not engaging in any form of "contextual bypassing," as discussed regarding the previous sphere. Their engagement with broader contexts should not be a substitute for actions in the other two spheres that contribute to their well-being. This broader

sphere is meant to expand prior notions of therapeutic change, not supplant them.
- A final note of caution: do not allow the seeds of false hope to take root. Making substantive changes to the broader contextual conditions of our shared world is an inherently slow process that sometimes takes generations. If a participant decides to put energy toward any form of systemic or structural change, ensure that they know that progress may be glacial and that they still feel that it would be beneficial for them to pursue it nonetheless.

[A psychedelic medicine session] requires a great amount of courage because you're going into a complete uncertainty with the intent to bring something back that is not only beneficial to the individual, but for future generations, for other people.
—Mike (Belser et al., 2017; Swift et al., 2017)

INTEGRATION: SUGGESTED INTEGRATION GOALS

This section's suggested integration goals outline how to work with a participant's medicine session experiences as a basis for sustained antidepressant benefits. The focus of this section is limited to goals supported by an evidentiary basis for the treatment of depression, so the list is far from exhaustive. These goals generally correspond to the mechanisms of change discussed in Chapter 3.

Keep this list in your back pocket and only draw from it when a participant's experience aligns with something on it (see Appendix D for help determining this). Also, recall that each participant's treatment should focus on a small set (one to three) of integration goals that are inspired by the most salient aspects of their medicine session experience. Generally, it is best to settle on what integration goals will be pursued by the second session so that there is enough time to enact them.

Suggested Integration Goals by Domain

Existential–Spiritual	• Nurture any interest in spiritual self-development that arose
Mindfulness	• Support sustained capacity for psychological flexibility and less reactive mental habits
	• Build upon any emergent capacity for self-compassion
Body-Aware	• Support any increases in embodiment as a basis for improved self-care and self-awareness
Affective-Cognitive	• Turn positive experiences of open receptivity into a sustainable new approach to emotions
	• Strengthen a new self-concept based on updated core beliefs

Relational	• Draw takeaways from any relational moments or dynamics that arose
	• Use feelings of connectedness or empathy to challenge isolation
Keeping Momentum	• Support the clarification and enactment of values that were felt as important

Existential–Spiritual: Integration

> *From when I was 17 until I did the study when I was 24, my spiritual life was like, dormant. I was going say dead. But just like dormant, it was non-existent. And this not only stirred that back up, it reassured me beyond doubt that there is a spiritual realm, and I need to be aware of it. It is an important part of my existence.*
> —Victor (Belser et al., 2017; Swift et al., 2017)

1. Nurture any interest in spiritual self-development that arose
Consider this goal if the participant:

Experienced any spiritual or mystical phenomena
Had any insights about meaning or purpose
Described any aspect of their experience as sacred or holy
Felt they learned something from God, their higher self, or other spiritual entities
Felt they came into their "truer" or "higher" self
Adopted a posture or position that may have indicated prayer or meditation
Expressed a sense of oneness or connectedness with all humanity

When participants experience existential, spiritual, or mystical phenomena in a medicine session, they may be inspired to make spirituality a higher priority in their lives. Support them in turning this inspiration into the impetus for an ongoing process of spiritual self-development.

Your exploration with the participant should be conducted in a humble, gentle, deferential way that respects the profundity and personal significance that these experiences most likely hold for the participant. Refrain from rushing to frame it in terms of its therapeutic utility, as this may be experienced as disrespectful, alienating, or secondary to their experience of its innate meaning. If they begin to focus exclusively on abstract topics such as the nature of reality in an intellectualizing way, then respectfully guide the participant back to the therapeutic importance of the experience. Consider questions such as, "If you were to live your life with this new perspective, what might change about your depression?"

If the insight they received was more of a wordless, felt sense of "knowing," encourage them to spend more time engaging with this feeling experientially, rather than trying to unpack it analytically. Rather than pressuring this felt sense to generate actionable ideas, invite the participant to sit with it, deepen into their experience of it, and perhaps see if they can put it "in dialogue" with their depression to see if the two lived experiences have anything to say to each other.

When considering what type of practice might sustain the participant in their spiritual self-development, it is worth considering some nuances in the literature on depression and spirituality. While most studies have found negative correlations between depressive symptoms and measures that assess spirituality, some have found positive correlations (Bonelli et al., 2012; Koenig, 2009). Two factors that have been suggested as possible differentiators between pro-depressive and antidepressive relationships to spirituality are the extent to which they foster rumination (Saunders et al., 2021) and the presence or absence of communal group involvement (Hastings, 2016). These may be important elements to keep in mind when deciding what spiritual practices might be most supportive for a participant.

When supporting this goal, be reflective about your own cosmological worldview. There are a number of nuanced ways that a therapist might unintentionally impose their own wishes or beliefs on the participant. Use language that matches the participant's expressed views (e.g., "God" versus "gods" versus "Spirit"), refraining from introducing your own perspective whenever possible, reminding them that your role is to support their process of understanding rather than give them your understanding. Stay attentive to the likelihood that the participant remains in an increased state of suggestibility. Any suggestions you offer may have an outsized influence that could divert them from their own process of discovery. Whenever a participant invites your perspective on any spiritual questions that arose for them, engage with them in a thoughtful, collaborative way that is attentive to power dynamics and whatever motives of yours may be present.

Be mindful of any friction that may be present between this new experience and the participant's prior religious background. If either of you notice a dissonance between their new and old ideas about spirituality, invite the participant to reflect on this without any pressure to resolve any dissonance. Assess whether the participant feels distressed by this dissonance and, if helpful, explore what resources might support them in contending with it. If it would be helpful, explore the pros and cons of developing practices within their prior religion as opposed to adopting a new one.

Finally, take care to avoid the pitfall of "spiritual bypassing." This term refers to a tendency to use spiritual ideas and practices to avoid facing difficulties in other spheres of one's life, such as the psychological or interpersonal spheres. For participants struggling with depression, spiritual bypassing may manifest in a belief that they will no longer feel depressed as long as they adopt a certain spiritual worldview, practice, and so on. Gently open a space in the treatment for considering that this may be an "afterglow" period. All spiritual paths involve periods of challenge.

Suggested approaches:

- Supportive counseling
- Spiritual evocation, a motivational interviewing-based approach (Miller et al., 2008)
- SERT-integrated psychotherapies, or adaptions of EBTs that incorporate spiritual, existential, religious, or theological elements (Palitsky et al., 2023)
- Existential psychotherapies
- Meaning-centered psychotherapy

Suggested practices:

- Prayer
- Meditation
- Creating an altar in one's home
- Sacred dance
- Kirtan singing
- Honoring the dead
- Gratitude practice
- Cleansing practices (e.g., smudging)
- Ancestral work
- Earth-based or elemental practices
- Service work

Mindfulness: Integration

I have a restored ease with life. The percentage of my life that I am able to be present in a moment has increased dramatically.
                                                     —Dan (Belser et al., 2017; Swift et al., 2017)

2. Support sustained capacity for psychological flexibility and less reactive mental habits
Consider this goal if the participant:

Experienced a kind of mental "quiet" or "calm" or "stillness"
Felt a sense of "mental freedom" or "liberation"
Gained more insight into or a new vantage point on their mental processes
Gained more control over their thoughts and feelings
Felt forgiveness or compassion toward themselves or someone else

During a medicine session, participants may experience freedom from their automatic mental behavior, such as rumination, reactive emotions, cravings, or other maladaptive impulses. This freedom may manifest in a variety of ways: a sense of inner stillness or calmness, an interruption of their habitual rumination, a new awareness of the automatic workings of their mind, an increased ability to take a step back from these workings and make more considered decisions about how to respond to them, or a general sense of "mental freedom" (Watts & Luoma, 2020, p. 95). In any event, they may feel like they have reached the shore of a churning sea.

Elements of these experiences may persist to some extent after the medicine session has ended. The participant might present in the first integration session with statements like "The chaos inside my head stopped for a while," "I have so much more control over my mind," or "I could see thoughts forming and could decide whether I wanted to pursue them or not." If this is the case, the integration sessions could be used to support these participants in using these experiences as the basis for cultivating a lasting relationship with their mind that is more mindful, flexible, and in control. Doing so may help them to gain leverage over any rumination, emotional reactivity, or automatic negative self-beliefs present within their experience of depression.

The interventions and practices brought in to support this goal would benefit from including a few key elements:

- Exercises or practices designed to deepen their experience of the new mindful or flexible mental state they have arrived at in order to build their relationship to it.
- Exercises that sustain and entrain their ability to access their new adaptive mental state when needed.
- Psychoeducation and/or collaborative discussion on how to apply their new capacity to their experience of depression.
- Development of an understanding of the functional value of the participant's maladaptive mental behaviors (e.g., exploring what purpose their rumination serves) to get a sense of what more adaptive behaviors could supplant them.
- Support in adopting new, adaptive mental habits that can replace the old, maladaptive ones. These may include self-regulation practices, forms of self-distraction, willful adoption of alternative adaptive thoughts, or seeking help from go-to support people.
- Respect for any discomfort around an increase in psychological flexibility. Attend to the possibility that some participants who experience a new degree of mental freedom may find it challenging. Remember that their old mental habits served a purpose for them. It may be helpful to assure them that they retain the ability to use any old coping strategies, should they decide to do so.
- Crafting a specific relapse prevention action plan. For example, a participant may use their more flexible, mindful state to recognize when they are experiencing a recurrence of ruminative thoughts. Once identified, they can then enact their action plan by replacing this automatic mental behavior with something else.

Suggested approaches:

- Acceptance and commitment therapy (ACT; Hayes et al., 2012)
- Dialectical-behavioral therapy (DBT; Linehan, 2014)
- Mindfulness-based cognitive therapy (MBCT; Segal et al., 2012)
- Rumination-focused cognitive behavioral therapy (RFCBT; Watkins, 2016)

Suggested practices:

- Mindfulness practices
  - Those focused on developing observer consciousness
  - Urge-surging exercises (e.g., that found in Bowen et al., 2010)
  - Changing radio stations (e.g., that found in Forsyth & Eifert, 2016)
- Meditation
- Breathing practices
- Self-regulation practices
- Journaling

3. Build upon any emergent capacity for self-compassion
Consider this goal if the participant:

Experienced a kind of mental "quiet" or "calm" or "stillness"
Gained more insight into or a new vantage point on their internal mental processes
Gained more control over their thoughts and feelings
Had an emotional opening
Had an experience of self-forgiveness
Shifted away from a narrow, critical sense of themselves
Felt forgiveness or compassion toward themselves or someone else
Gave themselves love or care, perhaps through self-touch

It is common to hear participants recount medicine session experiences of offering compassion or forgiveness to themselves for past mistakes, persistent shortcomings, or inherent human imperfections. For some, compassion is offered to one or more young, wounded parts of their psyche from a newly embodied core or adult self. These experiences of self-compassion often represent a novel stance toward oneself that breaks with years of shame and self-judgment. These experiences often feel like a great unburdening and are accompanied by an appropriately strong sense of relief or similar emotions. The question is how best to support them in developing their ability to bring compassion to themselves on an ongoing basis.

The approach that you take to working toward this integration goal will likely vary based on whether the participant experienced the self-compassion as global (e.g., "I realized I am loveable just as I am.") or offered to parts (e.g., "I saw the little child part of me that's always been afraid to connect with people, and I gave it the love it never got."). Here are some possible interventions:

- Spend time deepening and exploring the feelings associated with the experiences of giving themselves compassion and receiving that compassion from themselves. Frame this as a kind of experiential anchor to which they can return to remember what the experience of self-compassion feels like. It can also help them strengthen their ability to inhabit the adult part of them that is capable of giving compassion.
- Explore any challenges or fears they have had in the past around self-compassion and discuss what they might do if and when these arise again. This should include an exploration of what, if any, aspects of the participant's contexts may make it hard for them to be compassionate toward themselves (e.g., exposure to racist messaging in media or growing up in a homophobic, rejecting family of origin).
- Ask when they feel most self-compassionate. Encourage them to notice any skills or abilities that support their exercise of self-compassion. Honor them and consider strengthening them with new practices.
- It may be helpful to draw from Gilbert's (2009) six skills of compassion when doing this:
  - *Imagery:* Were there any images that arose (or that can be accessed now) that feel like they capture the experience of self-compassion?
  - *Attention:* What did the participant attend to that supported self-compassion? (e.g., their positive qualities)
  - *Feeling:* What did it feel like to experience self-compassion?
  - *Sensation:* What was it like in their body when they were being self-compassionate?
  - *Behavior:* Were there any actions the participant took that enabled self-compassion? Or were they able to experience any of the behaviors during the medicine session as self-compassionate acts, and if so, what was this like?
  - *Reasoning:* What was the style of thinking about oneself, others, and the world that facilitated self-compassion?
- Invite continued dialogue between their adult self (there are various nomenclatures, for example, higher self, observer consciousness, inner intelligence) and the part/inner child/self-state that received compassion. This communication could be verbal, embodied, and/or through other continued expressions of care.
- Provide psychoeducation and/or collaborative conversation about how self-compassion might help them with their depression, especially the role of negative self-beliefs in depression.
- Be attentive to the possibility that their adoption of compassion as a one-size-fits-all strategy for life may not work. Some situations require other adaptive emotions, such as anger channeled into assertive action, as well as healthy boundary-setting (e.g., with an abusive partner or in

exploitative work conditions). Help them explore the outcomes they imagine will occur if they adopt a more compassionate or forgiving stance toward these elements of their proximal or broader contexts.

Suggested approaches:

- Compassion-focused therapy (Gilbert, 2009)
- Internal family systems (IFS)
- Psychodynamic approaches (e.g., Malan & Coughlin Della Selva, 2007)
- Supportive counseling

Suggested practices:

- Metta meditation (Woolfe, 2023)
- Compassionate mind training (Gilbert, 2009)
- Compassionate imagery (Gilbert, 2009)
- Self-compassion breaks
- Inner child work
- Writing a compassionate letter to oneself as if written to a struggling friend
- Compassionate self-touch

Body-Aware: Integration

What's so funny is that nobody can really see it but yet for me everything has changed. It's really odd how that is. But it's subtle so it's not dramatic so it's like when you're participating in something or doing something, like I've taken up some activities and just as I'm doing them I'm . . . different. I'm there in a different way.

—Brenda (Belser et al., 2017; Swift et al., 2017)

4. Support any increases in embodiment as a basis for improved self-care and self-awareness
Consider this goal if the participant:

Felt alive or energized
Felt like they could feel or understand new things about their body
Listened to a bodily feeling that ended up leading them somewhere
Touched themselves lovingly or curiously
Had a lot of discomfort in their body
Vomited, gagged, dry heaved, wretched, or made choking sounds
Felt "lighter" or "younger" after a challenging moment
Looked or spoke differently in a way that seemed positive (e.g., "lit up")
Trembled, shook, made jerky movements, contorted their face, or vocalized

Some participants exit a medicine session feeling like their relationship with their body has somehow shifted. Often, this shift leaves them feeling more aware of, reconnected to, or simply "in" the body. In the first integration session, these participants might say, "I can feel my body in a way that I couldn't before," or "I can't believe how much there is going on in there," or perhaps "I feel so much more alive." Some participants may lack the language to describe this. If a participant speaks generally about feeling more "connected" or "alive," it may be necessary to inquire directly about whether they are feeling that way in their body.

For some participants, their postmedicine experience of embodiment could be marked by an abiding sense of vitality or wellness. The desire to maintain this state may become a source of intrinsic motivation to maintain a healthier relationship with their body that would benefit their struggle with depression. This new relationship may consist of a number of new behaviors, such as changes in diet and exercise, reduced neglect of medical conditions, more attention to their sexuality and associated needs, or more energy devoted to various forms of vital self-enjoyment. These behavioral changes can relieve depressive anhedonia.

Some participants have "wake-up call" experiences: they had more unpleasant sensations, such as an acutely intensified recognition of how exhausted, stressed, or physically unwell they have been. Some may experience feelings of bodily toxicity that they see as related to past unhealthy behaviors (e.g., substance use, insufficient self-care). If the participant is willing to do so, these wake-up call experiences provide motivation to address root causes and make new habits in life toward physical health.

In both cases, the shifts in embodiment experienced by the participant can become the inspiration for improved self-care. They can be leveraged to enhance the participant's body awareness, a key factor in sustained self-care improvement. If embodiment is part of their treatment journey, help them to use it to better identify and adaptively respond to depression-relevant internal states.

Some general guidelines for interventions in support of this integration goal:

- Respond compassionately to any challenging embodied experience that arose for the participant. Even if it can be worked with to become something supportive of their healing, acknowledge first that it was likely a stressful experience to undergo. Be attentive to the possibility that the presence of such feelings may also indicate the presence and activation of trauma memories.
- Devote ample time to listening to any shifts in the participant's embodiment that resulted from the medicine session. This is a valuable way to build a connection to these new states so that they can be revisited when needed. Some specific practices might include:
  - Giving the participant time in the session to savor and describe in detail any feelings they experience as positive.
  - Asking them to respond to depressogenic causal factors from within their embodiment of these new feelings (e.g., "From here, what would you do about the kind of workload you've been facing?").

- Consider providing psychoeducation about the wisdom of the body:
  - Somatic sensations are a good source of information about one's well-being and needs.
  - Aversive feeling states often show up in the body before they show up in the mind.
  - If left unaddressed, these aversive feelings may lead to a depressive state.
  - Remaining aware of one's bodily state can help to respond to signals in a more adaptive way that minimizes depressive symptoms.
- Develop a self-care plan that can be enacted in response to noticing aversive states. This plan may include specific self-regulation practices, distraction activities, or predetermined support people the participant can call.
- Participants often have a lot of shame and disgust for their own bodies. Support the participant in exploring any elements of their contexts or culture that have contributed to these feelings about their body. Assess what changes, if any, would be a necessary part of their healing. Refrain from dismissing or underestimating the impact of cultural messaging about bodies and how these impacts are likely to differ greatly across social locations.
- Whenever discussing the participant's body, always remain highly respectful. Continually assess their comfort level, use their chosen language, and attend to your own counter-transferences toward the body.

Suggested approaches:

- Somatic or experiential psychotherapies (e.g., hakomi, sensorimotor psychotherapy, focusing)
- Motivational interviewing
- Supportive counseling
- Dialectical behavioral therapy (DBT)
- Emotion-focused therapy (EFT)
- Dance movement psychotherapies
- Psychoeducation on the relationships between diet, exercise, and depression
- Sex therapy
- Awareness exercises from mindfulness-based relapse prevention approaches

Suggested practices:

- Exercise
- Dance
- Yoga
- Qigong

- Tai chi
- Embodied self-care practices
- Workshops that facilitate embodiment
- Visiting a nutritionist
- Embodied peer activity groups (e.g., exercise classes)

Affective–Cognitive: Integration

I feel feelings more deeply than before. I actually feel richer, like I'm a richer person—that I'm a more understanding person, that I even am not so hard on the person that I've always been the hardest on, which is myself . . . . I try to look a little deeper when I have negative feelings or thoughts about someone or something, so I try to see more into what is there. I feel the experience really gave me that.

—Augusta (Belser et al., 2017; Swift et al., 2017)

5. Turn positive experiences of open receptivity into a sustainable new approach to emotions
Consider this goal if the participant:

Had a strong emotional opening
Had an experience of emotions that previously felt "off-limits"
Overcame their fear of a challenging thought or feeling
Had a moment of struggle followed by a moment of relief or peace
Came away with a new view of themselves or felt they know themselves better
Gained more insight into or a new vantage point on their mental processes
Required the use of a grounding or self-regulation technique

It is common for participants to have a strong emotional opening in their medicine session. For many, it may have been a rare or even unprecedented experience that may take some work to integrate into their lives. For some, it may have felt cathartic or liberating, while others might have found it unnerving or embarrassing. In any event, as long as they do not feel they were harmed by the intensity of the emotional experience they had, then it could come to serve as proof that they might be able to feel more going forward and become less reliant on emotional avoidance as a coping strategy.

For participants who felt uncomfortable in some way about experiencing or expressing strong emotions, there is likely to be great benefit in exploring and addressing this discomfort. It likely reflects something important about the motives underlying the participant's emotional avoidance: a fear that they will drive you away, fear of destroying themselves or you, and so on. Exploring these motives may even bring them into contact with a core belief that is relevant to their depression (e.g., "If I open up, I am bound to be rejected.").

Work compassionately with any newly unearthed parts of their psyche that have been protectively dampening their emotional life, possibly through parts work or inner child work. Instead of pathologizing emotional avoidance, frame it as a strategy that was helpful in their past and may still be helpful at times. Then work to grow the participant's ability to elect other emotional strategies.

The intent of this integration goal is to help participants grow their willingness and capacity to experience their emotions more deeply. Consider the following guidelines when working on this goal:

- Allow adequate time for exploring any content associated with the emotions that were expressed, rather than simply treating it as an opportunity to develop a new skill. If they felt grief, invite them to discuss what they grieved for. If they felt anger, explore what made them angry.
- Deepen into their experience of the emotion, with specific attention paid to how it was for them to stay with the feeling (e.g., Did it feel easy? Challenging? How so?). Explore and normalize any moments of dissociation or disengagement that occurred or any attempts to use these strategies.
- If needed, revisit whatever psychoeducational approach was used during preparation to describe the potential value of remaining open and receptive to emotional material.
- Develop a specific plan for how the participant will engage differently with their emotions going forward. This should include practices that will help them build their capacity for recognizing emotions, attending to them without avoidance, and regulating their distress levels to ensure that the experience remains tolerable.
- If helpful, also consider working on the participant's capacity to notice, name, and attend to feelings in session. For those who struggle with alexithymia, this may be an important step.
- Always be sure to value the functional importance of the participant's emotional avoidance. Make sure they know that your work with them is not trying to take this away from them. Avoidance will remain in their repertoire to be deployed when needed.
- Attend to the ways the participant's social location may impact their relationship to their emotions. Be respectful and inviting toward any cultural norms around emotional expression. Also, be mindful of the fact that people who experience racist or gendered social dynamics may have more of a valid self-protective reason than those who do not to reduce the degree of emotionality they experience (e.g., "Boys don't cry."). Refrain from pushing them to a degree of expression that could have negative consequences for them given their social location and contexts.

Suggested interventions:

- Emotion focused therapy (EFT; Greenberg & Watson, 2006)
- Psychodynamic approaches
- Affect-focused psychodynamic psychotherapy (McCullough & Magill, 2009)
- Affect phobia therapy (Osborn et al., 2015)
- Internal family systems (IFS)
- Cognitive behavioral therapies
- Supportive counseling
- Dance movement therapies

Suggested practices:

- Artistic or creative expression
- Expressive arts therapy
- Freeform, expressive dance practices
- Journaling
- Continued weekly psychotherapy
- Mindfulness practice

6. Strengthen a new self-concept based on updated core beliefs
Consider this goal if the participant:

Had a strong emotional opening
Had an experience of emotions that previously felt "off-limits"
Overcame their fear of a challenging thought or feeling
Had a moment of struggle followed by a moment of peace
Came away with a new view of themselves or felt they know themselves better
Feels they came into their "truer" or "higher" self
Came away with a new view of themselves or know themselves better
Feels forgiveness or compassion toward themselves or someone else

Many medicine sessions include moments in which a participant is able to "work through" a maladaptive emotion by uncovering the more adaptive emotion underneath it. For instance, a participant may come to realize that the anger they have long felt is a secondary reaction to a deeper sense of shame they have been avoiding. Once this happens, the deeper set of needs can be acknowledged, and the process of getting them met can begin.

Most often, this process also involves an unearthing of depressive core beliefs that are associated with the primary emotion: "I am inadequate," "I am a failure," and so on. Part of the process of healing then involves addressing these core beliefs through a reconsideration of their validity in light of any corrective experiences. These experiences might occur in the participant's internal experience of the medicine or in their relational experience with you. It is a cognitive process of updating one's self-concept that often begins in the medicine session but can be expressly integrated in the sessions that follow.

To illustrate, a participant in this moment might feel something like the following toward themselves: "I've spent so much of my life acting like I'm happy alone, but I see now that I've just been afraid that, if I were to reach out, no one would respond because I'm unlovable. But I don't think that's true anymore." Your work is to help this person understand what life might look like in light of this new truth. The essence of this integration goal is to support the participant in reflecting on, consolidating, and acting upon a sense of self that has begun to disentangle itself from depressive core beliefs.

Some guidelines for interventions include:

- Allow ample time and space in sessions for the participant to become acquainted with or reformulate a new self-concept, new beliefs, and associated emotions. Consider slowing the process down to stay with these elements rather than jumping ahead to setting goals and planning action. If helpful, use mindfulness or other experiential exercises to do so.
- Attend to the possibility that the participant's ongoing relationship with you might play an important role in the continued reorganization of their self-concept. For instance, the care you demonstrate might be taken in by them as information in support of their lovability.
- Remain attentive to the likelihood that the process will not be linear and that negative self-beliefs will return periodically, both in sessions and in the participant's life. Normalize this for them as part of the process.
- If helpful, address other aspects of the participant's cognition that might make it hard to maintain their less depressogenic self-concept, such as any forms of habitually distorted thinking they engage in. A cognitive restructuring approach may be helpful.
- Use your clinical judgment to determine when it might be supportive to create an action plan that will help to consolidate the participant's self-concept.

Suggested approaches:

- EFT (Greenberg & Watson, 2006)
- Supportive counseling
- Cognitive behavioral therapies
- Existential psychotherapies
- IFS

Suggested practices:

- Daily self-affirmations
- Writing a personal mission statement

- Creative expression
- Writing a letter to oneself

Relational: Integration

Interviewer (Belser): What insights or new understandings did you gain?
Edna: That people can genuinely care about you—even though they really
aren't your loved ones and they are not your good friends—still they really,
you know, they would miss you if something bad happened to you. And when
they say, "how are you doing?" they really mean that. And when they say,
"Oh you look great, and I'm so glad you are doing well" they mean that. To
be able to accept that, I think, to accept that people love me. That I'm worthy
of being loved. The insight that I do belong here.
                                    —Edna (Belser et al., 2017; Swift et al., 2017)

7. Draw takeaways from any relational moments or dynamics that arose
Consider this goal if the participant:

Solicited or received support from therapists
Expressed any feelings toward therapists
Shared a significant relational moment with therapists
Solicited or received any touch from therapists
Required the setting of a relational or physical boundary
Experienced an interpersonal rupture in their relationship with the therapist
Required the use of a grounding or self-regulation technique

If any significant relational moments arose between you and the participant during the medicine session—such as an instance of connected conversation, provision of support, use of touch, a moment of prolonged eye contact, or any other moment that felt meaningful—it is important to debrief them and attempt to draw learnings from them during integration. Similarly, if you or the participant felt that they noticed any relational dynamics arising during the medicine session, such as frustration, power plays, or strong camaraderie, it would be beneficial to explore these openly as well.

Actively attending to these relational elements through metacommunication about the therapeutic relationship may help the participant solidify any relational repatterning that occurred. It is also important to proactively address any points of misunderstanding, confusion, discomfort, or other sense of being wronged. Failure to do so may reinforce feelings of abandonment, mistrust, shame, and so on, which may in turn reinforce maladaptive self-beliefs or relational patterns. If any rupture occurred during a medicine session, small or large, the participant should be given a chance to speak to their experience of it, and an attempt should be made to repair it during integration.

Pay particular attention to any instances in which the participant asked you for care, appeared to accept and feel grateful for care, or seemed like they wanted care but refrained from asking for it. What was happening for them? Did anything about it feel good? What, if anything, was challenging about it? How was this different than their typical reaction to care? What learning or hopes for the future are they taking away from it? How will they remember it and use some aspect of that memory as an "experiential anchor" they can bring themselves back to in the future?

When working on this goal, consider the following guidelines:

- If the participant does not bring up any relational moments or dynamics on their own and you think that this conversation needs to happen, open the topic yourself, noting the potential therapeutic value that could come from this conversation.
- If it feels awkward or uncomfortable for the participant to revisit a relational moment with you, attend to these feelings. They may represent the resurgence of an old relational pattern.
- If they experienced any challenges during the relational event, refrain from pathologizing this and honor it as a reflection of an old self-protective strategy. Explore these challenges and any core beliefs that may be informing them.
- Invite the participant to share about their experience in as much detail as they can. Ask them about the impulses, fears, self-talk, micro-emotions, and other phenomena they remember noticing.
- Remind the participant that they have not lost the option of responding to future relational moments in a way that reflects their old style. The choice between this and the new approach they used during the medicine session remains theirs. What is new is that they have a choice. Perhaps explore how they imagine their future interactions would be from within each of the two perspectives.
- Before moving away from a relational moment, let the participant check in with themselves to see if there is anything else that moment wants or needs from either of you (e.g., a reminder that you care about them after discussing a tense moment). This is particularly true after attending to a rupture.
- Remain aware of what is coming up in your own emotional reactions as you discuss a relational moment and seek peer consultation or supervision if helpful.
- Ask if anything about the relational moment was at odds with any cultural or contextual norms the participant may hold. If this is the case, explore the tension inherent between these norms and any new relational approaches the participant wants to make.

Suggested approaches:

- Relational psychodynamic/psychoanalytic approaches
- Attachment-based psychotherapy

- Supportive psychotherapy
- IFS
- Intensive experiential-dynamic psychotherapy (IEDP)
- Group therapy

Suggested practices:

- Experimenting with new approaches in relationships
- Various workshops that give practice in consciously relating
- Metta meditation

I felt more self-love and feeling of love for humanity very deeply. It's the first time I ever really felt like I was part of the world instead of separate from it.
—Erin (Belser et al., 2017; Swift et al., 2017)

8. Use feelings of connectedness or empathy to challenge isolation
Consider this goal if the participant:

Solicited or received support from therapists
Expressed any feelings toward therapists
Shared a significant relational moment with therapists
Solicited or received any touch from therapists
Felt forgiveness or compassion toward themselves or someone else
Expressed a sense of oneness or connectedness with all humanity
Made remarks about a loved one or a general desire to have better
  relationships

Some participants will come away from their medicine session with newfound feelings of connectedness or empathy. They may be aware of this shift and experience it as a strong desire to connect with others. It may show up as an unformulated feeling of openness that may require some support from you to "unpack" and understand. For some participants, these feelings may be accompanied by grief or embarrassment for all of the time they were more isolated and closed off from people. In any case, working with these feelings can help a participant lean more into their relational life as a source of support and enlivenment that helps alleviate their depressive symptoms.

Work toward this goal may benefit from the following suggestions:

- Elicit the participant's description of this experience and spend ample time naming and deepening this new state of being. If needed, help them to clarify their experience and put it into words. Encourage them to attend to any easeful, pleasant, or challenging feelings that are present in their body when they are connected to these new feelings. Frame this as a form of anchoring that will help them find their way back to this state in the future.

- Once the new feeling of connectedness, openness, or empathy has been named and embodied, spend some time looking out into the world with the new lens it provides. Ask them what it suggests about how to live their life, set their priorities, and so on. Put it in dialogue with their more closed, disconnected way of being. Explore which beliefs about themselves and the world it confirms or disconfirms. Name and explore any fears or worries that arise in this exercise.
- Consider using the therapist–participant relationship as a forum for exploration and experimentation with these new feelings. Explore how it feels to embody a new sense of connectedness or openness in relationship with you.
- If the participant has not done so already, invite them to explore how these new feelings could be supportive in addressing their feelings of depressive withdrawal, aloneness, social isolation, or relational estrangement.
- When the participant seems ready, help them think through and plan a new set of behaviors that follow naturally from this more connected or empathic state of being.
- Help them to anticipate relapses into a less open, connected way of being. Plan for how they will respond when this occurs.
- Attend to cultural or contextual norms in the relational moment.

Suggested approaches:

- Group therapy
- Relational psychodynamic/psychoanalytic approaches
- Attachment-based psychotherapy
- Supportive psychotherapy
- IFS
- IEDP

Suggested practices:

- Peer support groups
- Ongoing integration groups
- Volunteering and activism
- Prosocial activities (Taylor et al., 2017)
- Metta meditation
- Letter writing

Keeping Momentum: Integration

It has made me more aware that I cannot just live for material stuff and success.

—Adam (Belser et al., 2017; Swift et al., 2017)

9. Support the clarification and enactment of values that were felt as important
Consider this goal if the participant:

Said anything in session about wanting to make changes or live differently
Came away with a new view of themselves or felt they know themselves better
Felt they came into their "truer" or "higher" self
Came away with a strengthened desire to make some sort of change
Looked or spoke differently in a way that seemed positive (e.g., "lit up")
Came away with a strong sense of personal purpose, even if hard to put
   into words

Some participants will emerge from a medicine session with a felt sense that something has fundamentally shifted or changed about what is important to them. This kind of shift can often be helpfully framed in the language of values. And values can be worked with as the basis for meaning-making and linked to new actions that give rise to a less depressed life.

Some participants will have an experience of reconnecting with long lost values. For example, a participant who comes out of a medicine session saying, "I can't believe I haven't picked up a guitar in years when music used to be so important to me." may be reconnecting with their occluded value of creativity.

Other participants may experience a reordering of their values, with one or more newly ascendant values rising to the top. They may say something like, "I am ready to live my life without fear." after connecting with the value of courage or adventure. If you took notice of any such statements during the medicine session (or in the first integration session), it may be helpful to support the participant in clarifying what value or values have become active in them and using these as the basis for value-driven action.

The following suggestions may be helpful to consider when supporting a participant in working toward this outcome:

- Give the participant a good amount of time to reengage with the experience that changed how they relate to their values and priorities.
- Watch out for the possibility that what was originally a deeply felt experience of a personally important value has become a "should" or a self-critical sense of obligation to be a particular way. To use dynamic language, beware the overactive super-ego. If either of you sense that this has happened, return to the original experience using mindfulness-based or embodied practices to reconnect with its felt importance.
- If a participant has connected with values that fall within one of the other domains (e.g., spirituality, connectedness, self-expression), read the goals in that domain for further guidance on how to turn them into the basis for action.

- When planning actions, be specific ("I will play guitar in the hour after dinner three nights a week.") rather than general ("I will play guitar more."). Also ensure that planned actions are realistic. Consider delineating them in phases (e.g., "One hour a day for three months, followed by two hours a day for three months.").
- Actively plan for predictable setbacks. Troubleshoot any difficulties that the two of you can foresee. How might their depressive symptoms derail their intended actions? Also consider slowing down to see how other, quieter parts of themselves feel about the plan of action.
- Consider using a worksheet to create a written version of the action plan—perhaps one that allows them to track their progress.
- Spend time discussing any friction that they imagine this plan of action will encounter in their contexts—cultural, social, structural, and so on.

Suggested approaches:

- Motivational interviewing
  - The values card sort activity (Miller et al., 2001)
- Acceptance and commitment therapy
  - Valued living questionnaire (Wilson & Groom, 2002)
- Supportive counseling
- Coaching-style approaches

Suggested practices:

- The sky is the limit! Think broadly and collaboratively with the participant about the full spectrum of activities that may help them enact their values.

INTEGRATION: WORKING WITH DISAPPOINTING MEDICINE SESSION EXPERIENCES

I feel like somehow I failed because I did not get a favorable result and feel shame in discussing it. I think this shame comes from the fact that I shut down and did not let the medicine work. This in turn makes me feel a bit hopeless or too difficult a case for the medicine but I know this is just my insecurities and fundamental belief that I am not worthy.
—Participant (Evans et al., 2023)

As noted at the start of the chapter, integration is the process of bringing the participant's medicine session experience into their life. So, what do you do if that experience was nothing to write home about?

A disappointing session can happen for a variety of reasons that are poorly characterized as of now. From what is currently known, they include each participant's unique metabolism and drug absorption properties, variability in the alkaloid content of naturally occurring plant medicines (e.g., psilocybin-containing mushrooms), the potency and purity of the drug, a participant's psychological openness to the effects of the medicine, putative self-protective mechanisms in the psyche that decided that today was not the day, and so on. In a double-blind randomized clinical trial, it may also mean that the participant received the placebo. In any event, it is important to retain your clinical equipoise and provide the same degree of care to the participant as you would if they had a profound experience—particularly when working on a clinical trial. The following suggestions may be helpful in working with a participant who feels as though they do not have much to integrate.

- **Hold space for disappointment.** Even if you devoted adequate energy to setting realistic expectations for treatment, disappoint may still arise. Allow them to express this disappointment and refrain from any poorly attuned attempts at reframing the situation (e.g., "This may have been exactly the kind of experience you needed"). If they give you lemons, do not make lemonade with platitudinous statements. Instead, enter empathically into the grief and anger that make up disappointment.

  If you get the sense that disappointment is present but not articulated, consider the use of a question that invites more challenging feelings they have about the treatment. Participants may be invested in the idea that you wanted them to have a great, healing experience; communicate openly that they do not have to hide their disappointment from you. At the same time, refrain from joining with them in any kind of implicit agreement that their treatment has been a failure. Regard their disappointment as valid and meaningful but not reflective of any predetermined conclusions about treatment outcomes. Also, consider working with their disappointment therapeutically, as it may be an entrée into depression-relevant beliefs about themselves or the world. Even if you do conceptualize their disappointment as a global tendency of theirs, never lose track of the here-and-now validity of their disappointment about the present situation.

- **Invite and amplify anything that did occur.** As noted in the earlier section regarding possible placebo sessions (Chapter 6), even a medicine session without active medicine can be an opportunity for rest, reflection, and receiving support from one or two therapists for 4–8 hours. The participant may have found something about their experience to be therapeutic or meaningful. For example, a participant may have reached an important conclusion about themselves or their depression, or they may have spent the day meditating and feeling more embodied than they have in a long time. Either of these events could be the basis for treatment benefit if worked with in the integration sessions and beyond. Of course, many disappointed participants will have already discounted this possibility, leaving it up to you to raise the possibility.

- **Balance an integration approach with therapy-as-usual.** To an even greater extent than usual, integration with these participants may tempt you to treat the integration sessions as standard talk therapy sessions, as opposed to sessions that work with content that arose during the medicine sessions. If there is no such content to work with, still attempt to focus these sessions on changes that the participant hopes to make in their behaviors or lived contexts based on their experience of treatment. In a clinical trial, this will help to ensure a maximal degree of similarity between the therapeutic approach taken across the control and experimental conditions.

- **Explore relational dimensions that arose.** Providing several hours of devoted therapeutic care and attention is an intensive therapeutic intervention in and of itself and may have been a significant relational event for the participant. Consider exploring how it was for them to receive this care and whether their experience may hold implications for their relationships outside of treatment.

- **Minimize participant shame.** Above all, ensure that the participant's disappointment does not lead to any lasting harm to them. Explore any feelings of shame, failure, or hopelessness and work to ameliorate them as much as possible before the end of treatment. Try to prevent this disappointing treatment experience from reinforcing any maladaptive self-beliefs or precipitating any suicidality.

INTEGRATION: RESPONDING TO CHALLENGING EVENTS

The following day I could not talk to anyone. I felt mute and shy and completely self-conscious. I kept thinking that I did not belong, I don't belong anywhere.

—Participant (Evans et al., 2023)

Integration, even in the best circumstances, can be a demanding journey for participants, encompassing a variety of challenges. These can range from grappling with unhelpful beliefs after the medicine session, enduring emotional instability for days or weeks, dealing with feelings of shame or embarrassment about their conduct during the session, to managing an intense urge to overhaul their lives. They may also face disappointment in treatment outcomes, strain on close relationships due to the treatment, feelings of abandonment, neglect, or betrayal at the end of treatment, and the resurgence of "recovered memories."

Many of the challenging events described in this section are likely to be the result of difficult unresolved psychological material getting churned up in the participant's medicine session. As such, the participant will likely respond well to working skillfully with this material as you would with similarly difficult events in traditional psychotherapy. Assess the participant's capacity for working with this material and incorporate the use of self-regulation skills as needed. Discuss the participant's sense of how much and what kind of support would be best for them and help them find a way to obtain it.

If they are willing, invite the participant to spend time in session paying guided attention to any emotional or embodied experiences that may be present. A variety of somatic awareness or mindfulness techniques may be applied here, so long as they help the participant (a) turn their attention inward, (b) attend to how the material is showing up in their experience, (c) encourage any spontaneously arising forms of expression, and (d) allow latent psychological meaning to arise. Working with the material may facilitate its integration and may help to reduce its intensity. Remain humble and responsive, as working with subacute psychedelic sequelae is an area in which our understanding of possibilities for effecting therapeutic outcomes is still very much developing.

Resourcing is key: generally, suggest to any struggling participant that they engage in activities that they find nourishing or supportive. Give them encouragement to do the things that they find most grounding and centering. Help them understand that doing so may be an important part of a prolonged and unfolding healing process. Appendix A provides a list of possible suggestions, though it is advisable that they draw from their own sense of what is resourcing for them.

Participant exits medicine session with an unhelpful belief. Sometimes, a participant's lingering concern may be a counter-therapeutic idea that they developed during the medicine session. They may have experienced something that confirmed their sense of hopelessness ("I realized that I'm always going to be depressed.") or badness ("I saw my depression as punishment for things I've done."). If they present such a belief, remain respectful of the strong subjective veracity it likely holds for them and explore the process by which it arose. Encourage them to hold it lightly with curiosity, rather than adopting it uncritically. Consider exploring what is underneath their willingness to believe this idea so readily. Interventions that treat it like a maladaptive core belief may be helpful, particularly expressive interventions that elicit, explore, and transform associated emotions. Resist the urge to correct the participant by reinterpreting what they experienced during the medicine session, as this will likely not be effective and may negatively impact the therapeutic alliance. If a counter-therapeutic idea arises in the first medicine session, suggest that the participant bring this idea to the next medicine session for further exploration.

Participant is emotionally labile for days or weeks after a medicine session. This is an outcome that will most likely run its course without any corrective intervention. The top priority is to ensure that the participant feels they have adequate resources for getting through it. These resources may include psychotherapeutic or psychiatric support, peer support, support from loved ones, and calling upon internal resources. If the participant is distressed by this lability, encourage them to use whatever nonharmful means they have at their disposal to support themselves, including all of the aforementioned resources in addition to their fa-vored self-care practices. Consider that this may not be the time to encourage them to "stay open." Communicate that it is sometimes okay to employ their go-to nonharmful defensive strategies (e.g., distracting themselves, shutting down, iso-lating). The participant may be better served by allowing themselves to err on the side of containment and self-protection for a limited period. Be attentive to any situational or structural factors in the participant's life that may further necessi-tate the use of existing defenses (e.g., a workplace that does not allow for lability).

Shame or embarrassment about medicine session conduct. Some participants may feel embarrassment or shame about something that arose during the medicine session in your presence. They may have expressed themselves in a bold, unprec-edented way while under the influence of the medicine and are now experiencing interpersonal discomfort in the integration sessions. They may have attempted to disrobe or urinated in their bed. Remain attentive to the possibility of overt or covert feelings of shame about whatever transpired and work with it relationally.

An urgent desire to make big changes in one's life. Some participants exit a med-icine session with a strongly felt edict for change. They may want to file for di-vorce, quit their job, or make other "big moves" that they feel will help them live a less depressed or more fulfilling life. It is advisable to suggest a more gradual ap-proach and to caution them against making any such changes in the days or weeks after a medicine session. Participants may be experiencing a resurgence of a long-neglected facet of themselves—a desire to be free, a strongly independent streak—that, perhaps because it was dormant for so long, is now exerting an outsized influence on their decision-making. While you should encourage them to get to know this new facet, it is important to explain that the other facets—defenses, pragmatic thought, compromises, responsibilities—will likely come back online in the near future and possibly lead the participant to regret any rash action they took. There is no hard-and-fast rule as to how long of a waiting period to suggest. Work with them to postpone action until you both feel that they have returned to their subjective baseline.

Depressive episode following disappointment with treatment outcome. This may occur when treatment is either ineffective or fails to live up to the participant's hoped-for level of effectiveness. In clinical trials that do not use a crossover de-sign, this may also result from being assigned to the placebo group. It is essential to manage posttreatment disappointment, as depressed participants who saw psy-chedelic treatment as their last hope may become prone to feeling neglected or betrayed, or to suicidality. As discussed in the chapter on the preparation phase (Chapter 5), minimizing disappointment begins with managing pretreatment ex-pectations and contending with unrealistic beliefs about psychedelic therapy.

During the integration phase, you may be called upon to hold space for tre-mendous disappointment in the context of a spike in depressive symptomatology. You may have to hold the hope for continued healing while also honoring the fact that the participant is currently inconsolable. Suicidality should be assessed, and a safety plan should be in place and revisited as needed. With participant consent, invite their support people into the conversation about how they are holding their disappointing treatment outcome. When it feels appropriate and possible, advocate for using the integration sessions as you would in the absence of disappointment: to make pro-therapeutic changes in the participant's life. For suggestions on how to do so, see the section in this chapter entitled "Integration: Working With Disappointing Medicine Session Experiences."

Stress put on the participant's close relationships due to treatment. When people change, their relationships are often strained to accommodate new roles and ways of being. There are a number of ways a participant may feel changed by their treatment that could put a strain on their close relationships, causing them to feel alienated or isolated. They include personality changes, revamped value systems, or a new perspective on how they want to live their life. If a participant shows up to integration complaining of relational stressors, there are a few ways you can help. You may encourage them to find a way to sit with the tension in the short term without taking any immediate actions (e.g., breaking up with a partner). You may help them develop a sense of how to discuss these changes with their loved ones. You could also help them connect with groups or communities that could provide a space in the participant's life for nurturing these nascent aspects of themselves, which might take the pressure off of existing relationships. There are a number of peer- and professional-led integration groups available online with which they could connect.

Participant feels abandoned, neglected, or betrayed at the end of treatment. Some participants may feel an acute sense of loss when their relationship with you ends. The closure of a relationship that was home to intense vulnerability and openness supported by ample therapeutic care may be understandably hard for participants who generally lack this type of relationship in their lives. It may lead to an enactment in which past relational traumas and losses become activated and the risk for deepening the harm associated with them becomes heightened. The most effective way to mitigate this possibility is to attend to it throughout treatment by being clear about the limits of the therapeutic relationship from the outset, especially in a time-limited treatment. Proactively discuss any dynamics of dependence that either party has noticed arising. To minimize the participant's sense of being "dropped" at the end of treatment, work diligently to ensure that they have the ongoing support they need and that a "warm handoff" occurs with their existing or new providers. Devote sufficient time in the integration sessions to working with these emotions, understanding their connection to prior experiences of loss, and developing the participant's sense of what positive experiences of their relationship with you they can take with them. Consider letting them know from a genuine place in yourself how much the relationship has meant to you and what you will take with you from it as well. Ensure that they leave treatment with a sense of what goals they might want to bring to their next treatment.

Resurgent, "recovered memories." During a medicine session, participants will occasionally experience images depicting a past instance of abuse or mistreatment of which they were previously not aware. They may be shocked by this revelation, especially if the perpetrator was someone they had long trusted. They may ask you to confirm for them that this could be the case, or they may already be convinced by the experience they had. In any event, it is crucial to communicate to them that while some research suggests that "recovered memories" are of comparable accuracy to "continuous memories" (Dalenberg, 2006), there is no guarantee that what they experienced in the medicine sessions as "memories" are in fact accurate reflections of the past. The visions produced by psychedelic medicines are rarely perfect replays of historical events.

Although it is possible the experience may point to specific events, it is often the case that they are "mythopoetic," or not plainly factual though they may hold a deeper, less obvious meaning. Nevertheless, be open to the possibility that past physical or sexual trauma did in fact happen; one can believe the client's experience without knowing historical facts. It may be helpful to relate these visions to the participant's dreams, which reflect and convey important things but do not need to be taken at face value. This is important to communicate in order to prevent harm being done to the participant's relationship with the person who appeared in their visions. Invite them to hold the vision with curiosity and a willingness to continue feeling into it so that its true message may eventually become manifest.

INTEGRATION: RESPONDING TO SERIOUS ADVERSE OUTCOMES

> *I collapsed into a severe, almost catatonic depression. I could not even tell my husband that I was having suicidal ideation. I reached out to my therapist for integration sessions once and when he did not reply, I fell further into the abyss of hopelessness and despair. I went through the motions of existing, grateful that my busy schedule held me accountable for staying alive, but I did not see the point. This lasted over 2 months.*
>
> —Participant (Evans et al., 2023)

While most challenging events that may arise after a medicine session (such as those detailed in the previous section) can be worked through with appropriate support from you and/or the participant's outside therapist, other outcomes may require a higher level of intervention. This section details some of the adverse outcomes that often rise to the point of becoming a psychiatric concern. Although the events in this section are rare, they are serious and reflect a need for additional support.

Persistent dysregulation, often due to resurgent traumatic material. A participant who came in contact with traumatic material during a medicine session may continue to experience a range of symptoms for days, weeks, or even longer after the session. These include intrusive memories or flashbacks, difficulty sleeping, hypervigilance, panic attacks, severe anxiety, emotional flatness, avoidance of places or situations, isolation, dissociation, depersonalization, derealization, irritability, and mood disruptions (Bouso et al., 2022; Guthrie, 2021; Lutkajtis & Evans, 2023). While it is possible that these symptoms will resolve themselves on their own, it is likely that they will require additional support from you, other professionals, and/or the participant's loved ones in order to not lead to further deterioration.

Best practices for supporting this type of treatment outcome are still very much evolving. The suggestions in this section are drawn from the best evidence currently available on what has been helpful for participants who experience persistent dysregulation (Aixalà, 2022; Evans, 2023b; Evans et al., 2023). You are advised to remain up to date on this literature, as ongoing research on the topic is slated to be published in the near future.

- *Self-care and spaciousness:* Encourage the participant to allow themselves as much rest and spaciousness as they can. Invite them to engage in restful and rejuvenating activities of their choice, such as additional sleep, eating favorite foods, or going for long walks. Some participants who experienced these symptoms have found it helpful to engage in vigorous exercise.
- *Maintaining a regular schedule:* Suggest that the participant keep a consistent schedule, insofar as they can, as a way of cultivating a sense of stability and regularity in their life.
- *Containment:* Work with them to develop their containment skills to increase their capacity for emotional self-regulation between sessions. As much as possible, develop and activate the participant's sense of capacity and self-efficacy for maintaining some degree of equilibrium.
- *Arrange social support:* Ensure that these support people can be reasonably counted on to be responsive to the participant's needs. Consider providing the support people with psychoeducation about trauma if the participant consents and feels that this would be helpful.
- *Communication with other providers:* For participants who see a psychiatrist or weekly therapist, this type of scenario may benefit from a conversation between you and that other provider (with the participant's consent) to communicate important information to them.
- *Referrals to additional providers:* It may be beneficial to refer the participant to a specialist with relevant expertise, such as a trauma specialist, a psychiatrist, or a somatic therapist with training in working with trauma. There are differing opinions on the approach that should be recommended. Some practitioners advise referrals to providers who can help the participant better contain their symptoms, such as a psychiatrist or a cognitive behavioral therapist. Others see these symptoms as an incomplete experience that must be completed through another depth-oriented methodology, such as holotropic breathwork or somatic experiencing. It is currently unknown how to determine whether one or the other approach is advisable.
- *Additional sessions:* Consider scheduling additional integration sessions with them, either between the originally scheduled sessions or after

their intended end date. If they are concerned about the added financial burden, either offer the sessions for free (perhaps framing them as part of the same course of treatment) or find another way to ensure that this hurdle does not prevent them from receiving needed care. If your relationship with the participant must end before these symptoms fully resolve themselves (e.g., in a clinical trial), it is still your responsibility to ensure that they receive suitable ongoing care.

- *Attend to shame:* Be aware that many participants who revisit traumatic material in a medicine session experience significant shame. Notice whether a participant feels shame or embarrassment about anything that happened while they were reexperiencing a trauma and, if so, normalize this for them. Explore the relational dimensions of these feelings (e.g., how they imagine it changed your perception of them, imagined interpersonal consequences, etc.) when the participant feels that this would be welcome and supportive.

- *Avoid dogmatic interpretations:* Common dogmas participants have encountered include "the medicine gives you what you need" or "trust the process." Participants in distress have reported that they find statements like this particularly unhelpful and upsetting (Evans, 2023b). An honest acknowledgement that there is no way to know for certain how and why these symptoms are occurring, or whether they will ultimately bring something good, may be a more helpful tack.

- *Meaning-making:* Leave room in the participant's recovery process for making meaning of what they are experiencing, as this is often a key element to regaining a sense of control and normalcy. In addition to engaging in this process with you, they may find it supportive to journal, make art, or educate themselves to weave together a narrative.

- *Exposure:* Once the participant has demonstrated a capacity for containment, consider whether a process of gradual exposure therapy in their sessions with you or another provider would be a helpful way to defuse the intensity of traumatic memories. One exposure-based approach could be to invite them to gradually increase their experience of any traumatic memories associated with their current symptoms, perhaps through a process of retelling a trauma narrative on a regular basis. You could also invite them to set aside 30 minutes each day to allow themselves to experience their current symptoms more intensely, or invite them to really call to mind their worst fears (e.g., being like this forever, going crazy) for a delimited period of 30 minutes to gradually disempower those fears (Aixalà, 2022). Once a participant demonstrates improvement, another form of exposure that has been recommended is the "prescription of relapses" (Aixalà, 2022), in which the participant intentionally sets aside a full day when they will choose to let their symptoms worsen in order to further gain control over them.

- *Rerealization:* Some participants who experience derealization have found it helpful to make a practice of repeating to themselves "this is real" throughout the day.
- *Hope and acceptance:* Work with participants to restore their sense that what they are experiencing may not last forever.
- *Peer support:* Connecting with others who have been through similar experiences is something that many participants have found immensely helpful. Provide them with peer-support resources to give them an opportunity to share stories with those who have come before them.

Hallucinogen persisting perceptual disorder (HPPD). As many as 4.5% of recreational psychedelic users experience lasting changes in their visual perception after the drug effects have worn off (Kurtom et al., 2019). Most often, these aftereffects are transient (less than 2 weeks) and do not have a serious adverse impact on the user (Baggott et al., 2011). However, those who experience longer-term distress and impairment as a result of these visual alterations are often diagnosed with HPPD. This diagnosis is more likely to develop in psychedelic users with a prior diagnostic history of anxiety disorders (Irvine & Luke, 2022). Notably, the visual aspect of this condition is often accompanied by anxiety, panic symptoms, depersonalization, and derealization (Prideaux, 2023a). There is at least one documented case of this condition developing in a contemporary PAT trial participant (Prideaux, 2023b), so you may encounter it at some point in your practice.

Although best practices are still evolving in this understudied area, the following suggestions may help you in supporting a participant who is experiencing persistent visual distortions. If the participant has been experiencing distortions for less than 2 weeks:

- *Abstinence from further medicine sessions:* If a participant experiences any visual alterations that last more than 48 hours, it would be best to refrain from administering another psychedelic medicine to them, as this might worsen the condition and extend its duration. Also encourage them to avoid cannabis or other psychoactive substances.
- *Normalization:* Let them know that it is very common to experience visual distortions for a week or two after a medicine session and that this experience most often resolves itself. This may help to reduce any acute feelings of anxiety or panic they are feeling in the first days of the visual distortions.

If the participant continues to experience symptoms beyond 2 weeks, your work with them should focus on reducing any comorbid anxiety, depression, catastrophic thinking, or fixation on the distortions. Although there is little you can do that will reliably lead to reduction in the visual distortions themselves, you can work with the participant to help the condition become less emotionally stressful, which is anecdotally thought to sometimes result in improvements in the condition itself. Some techniques that have been found to be helpful for reducing

HPPD-related anxiety (Perception Restoration Foundation, 2021; Prideaux, 2023c) include:

- Progressive muscle relaxation
- Exposure-based approaches to triggers that activate HPPD
- Cognitive reframing of the visual distortions to reduce fixations on possible consequences
- Emphasizing self-care and spaciousness
- Healthy sleep, exercise, and other basic hygiene habits
- Psychoeducation on the condition
- Working toward acceptance and patience
- Working on any stigma associated with living with a drug-derived condition

Psychiatric deterioration: suicidality, psychosis, or mania. Although rare, some PAT participants have experienced significant psychiatric deterioration after a course of treatment (Evans et al., 2023; McNamee et al., 2023). If you suspect that a participant is experiencing suicidality, psychosis, or mania to a degree of severity that undermines their safety, escalate their case to a higher level of care rather than attempting to alleviate these symptoms within their treatment with you. Contact any family members or other providers for whom you have consent to contact and inquire as to whether this has happened before and, if so, what has been most helpful (e.g., medication, hospitalization).

If it is the first time a participant has experienced such symptoms, there may be more of a temptation to wait to see if they resolve on their own or even to frame them as part of their treatment. While it is possible that what is emerging could be a kind of spiritual emergency or other transformative process with the potential for a positive outcome, consider the intense degree of support the participant will need for weeks or months in order to safely arrive at such an outcome. Most practitioners are simply not equipped to provide a sufficiently safe and supportive container for a prolonged expansive experience. Even if you feel that something may be lost be involving medical providers whose approaches will likely try to diminish the experience, more would be lost if the participant is allowed to harm themselves or others.

In summary, integration in psychedelic therapy is a crucial process, often considered the most important stage of treatment by many experts. As a therapist, you'll work with your participant to ensure they've landed on their feet and have what they need to incorporate their experiences from the medicine session into their daily life.

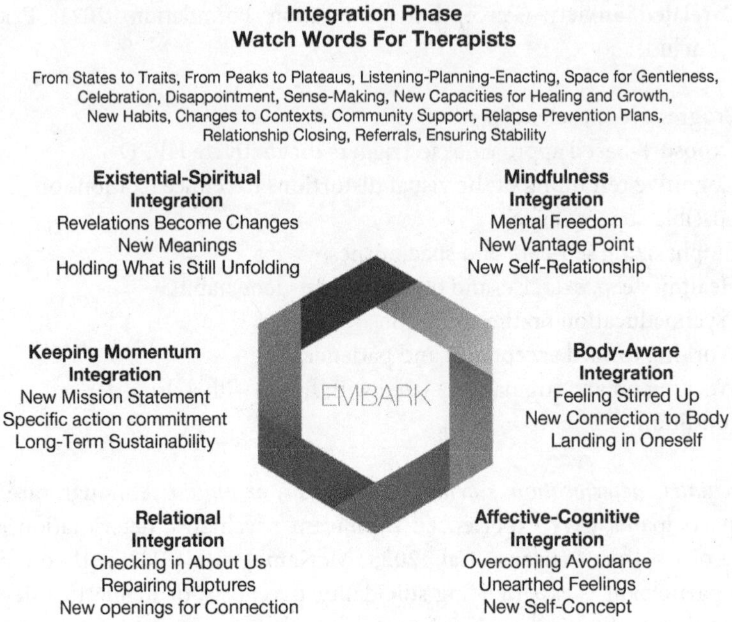

Integration Phase
Watch Words For Therapists

From States to Traits, From Peaks to Plateaus, Listening-Planning-Enacting, Space for Gentleness,
Celebration, Disappointment, Sense-Making, New Capacities for Healing and Growth,
New Habits, Changes to Contexts, Community Support, Relapse Prevention Plans,
Relationship Closing, Referrals, Ensuring Stability

Existential-Spiritual
Integration
Revelations Become Changes
New Meanings
Holding What is Still Unfolding

Mindfulness
Integration
Mental Freedom
New Vantage Point
New Self-Relationship

Keeping Momentum
Integration
New Mission Statement
Specific action commitment
Long-Term Sustainability

EMBARK

Body-Aware
Integration
Feeling Stirred Up
New Connection to Body
Landing in Oneself

Relational
Integration
Checking in About Us
Repairing Ruptures
New openings for Connection

Affective-Cognitive
Integration
Overcoming Avoidance
Unearthed Feelings
New Self-Concept

Figure 7.2. Integration Phase: Watch Words for Therapists

8

Bringing It Home and Carrying It Forward

As we experience a resurgence of interest in psychedelics, we can again fantasize about a different future.

—Erika Dyck, PhD (2021)

Congratulations on reaching the conclusion of the important, intense, and meaningful path of supporting someone through a course of psychedelic-assisted therapy (PAT)! Give yourself plenty of time to rest and reflect on all that transpired. If it is given the space it deserves, we have found that this can be immensely rewarding work that brings the therapist into regular contact with the ground of their own being. We, the authors, wish you all that you need to continue this work in a spirit of service and support for those whom you will support and the countless others whose lives and well-being are intertwined with theirs.

Throughout this book, we have aspired to provide a comprehensive guide to how to skillfully practice the rich art of psychedelic therapy. The detailed instructions provided are built upon the best available evidence about what makes psychedelic therapy efficacious in the treatment of depression. The approach in this book was developed upon a careful review of well-regarded clinical protocols and other literature in the field. Its ethical stances derive from a deep consideration of harms that have already occurred in the field, the experiences of those most harmed, and expert perspectives on minimizing further harm that have been put forth. As you read this book and practice within the EMBARK approach, we hope you feel it was imbued with the thoughtful and heartfelt consideration that we intended.

It is in this spirit that we close with a nod to the future we envision for EMBARK and the broader field of psychedelic therapy research.

EMBARK Psychedelic Therapy for Depression. Bill Brennan and Alex Belser, Oxford University Press.
© Oxford University Press 2024. DOI: 10.1093/9780197762622.003.0009

FUTURE DIRECTIONS FOR EMBARK: CULTIVATING CURIOSITY AND COLLABORATION

It is our hope that EMBARK will prove helpful to you as a clinician and to researchers looking to develop and refine psychedelic therapy approaches. We have intended the architecture of the six clinical domains and four care cornerstones (6 + 4) to provide a testable and extensible theoretical and clinical approach.

We outline below a number of future directions to mature the approach and to answer lingering scientific and clinical questions. As part of EMBARK's open-source ethos, we welcome you to take up some of these ideas and run with them or consider a collaboration with us. Here are some potential future directions for EMBARK:

1. **Multisite randomized controlled trials (RCTs):**
   To gain a more comprehensive understanding of EMBARK's efficacy, we plan to coordinate multisite phase 2b/3 RCTs, involving a broader range of settings and populations.
2. **EMBARK certification program:**
   - At the University of Washington, Lenox Hill Hospital, and at three sites sponsored by Cybin, we have already trained five cohorts of EMBARK facilitators.
   - In response to the growing demand for well-trained psychedelic therapists, and to address this training bottleneck, we intend to extend EMBARK's scope to include comprehensive training programs for therapists.
   - In the future, we are exploring the development of a broader training program, including an EMBARK certification program for therapists, emphasizing knowledge sharing and capacity building.
3. **Adaptation for other psychedelic medicines:**
   - How might EMBARK be adapted for use with other psychedelic substances such as DMT, LSD, MDMA, and ketamine? As we openly source EMBARK to the clinical community, we invite collective exploration of this potential.
4. **Broadening therapeutic contexts:**
   - How might EMBARK be applied in other therapeutic settings such as group psychedelic therapy and couples psychedelic therapy? We welcome research to investigate these possibilities.
5. **Inclusion of diverse populations:**
   - EMBARK seeks to serve all who might benefit. How might it be adapted in affirming ways to best support people of color, LGBTQIA+ participants, and other communities? How might it be adapted by, with, and for these communities to address sexual, gender, and racial minority stress processes? We invite collaborative input into this essential discussion.

6. **Education and professional development:**
   - As part of EMBARK's open-source principle, we hope this book and future work with EMBARK will inform the development of other training programs for psychedelic practitioners.
   - We realize there is a need for better continuing education about psychedelic therapy, so we are currently exploring the feasibility of offering CE and CME accredited courses. If you are interested in acquiring CE/CME credits in a future EMBARK training for clinicians, you may sign up to be notified here: https://www.centerforbreakthroughs.com/embark

7. **Public education:**
   - We are considering creating a layperson's guide to EMBARK to enhance public understanding of the principles, processes, and potential benefits of psychedelic therapy.

8. **Research collaborations:**
   - Collaborative efforts with various research organizations, university partners, and psychedelic organizations are essential for the ongoing development and adaptation of EMBARK.

In line with our commitment to scientific curiosity, we pose several important questions for future investigation:

- **Determining treatment efficacy:** If EMBARK proves efficacious for depression, how might we tease apart the benefits attributable to the therapy, the psychedelic medicine, and their combination? A factorial design RCT or dismantling trial could provide insights into this complex interplay, though there are ethical and methodological challenges.
- **Evaluating psychological mechanisms:** The 12 proposed mechanisms of change in the EMBARK model are based on our current understanding of psychedelic therapy and depression, but our understanding of these processes is still evolving. These mechanisms are hypotheses that need to be tested and validated in future research.
- **Therapy duration:** How many sessions of therapy are needed? Longitudinal RCTs with various amounts of therapy could help determine optimal durations and frequencies.
- **Exploring dose effects:** Could EMBARK be effective with psycholytic doses (lower doses) of psychedelic substances? A clinical trial to evaluate psycholytic doses, rather than psychedelic doses, combined with thoughtful therapy could be promising. This approach would be aligned with a long history of psycholytic psychedelic therapy in Europe and also with emerging practices using ketamine-facilitated psychotherapy at low to moderate doses to facilitate talk therapy.
- **Therapist dynamics:** Can EMBARK be effectively delivered by a single therapist, or is a dyadic approach necessary, and for whom? Comparisons of patient outcomes in RCTs with these differing configurations could provide valuable data.

- **Comparisons with other therapies:** How does EMBARK fare against other leading psychedelic therapies, such as those based on ACT? Direct comparison trials would be required to explore this question.
- **EMBARK in different contexts:** How might adaptations of EMBARK benefit people in multiple contexts: psychedelic retreats, legal or decriminalized settings, or for broader healing and self-development? How might it be used "for the betterment of well people," as Bob Jesse asks (Pollan, 2015)? Longitudinal observational studies and qualitative research in these settings could provide valuable insights.

With these possible future directions, we extend an open invitation to researchers, clinicians, and the broader community to join us in shaping the future of EMBARK, driven by a spirit of scientific curiosity, collaboration, and learning together.

THE ROAD AHEAD FOR PSYCHEDELIC THERAPY

We hope that EMBARK and its emphasis on sound, ethical care will have an impact on the way PAT is practiced as it continues to take its place in our world. Our work, our research, and our personal experience have all confirmed for us that there is a tremendous amount of good that could come from a wise integration of psychedelic medicines into our kit of healing practices.

Still, the integration of psychedelic therapies into Western biomedically oriented psychiatry will require more than just the creation of a new therapy model. It will require a broader appraisal of the fit between two paradigms and a reckoning with any points of tension that arise when attempting to unify them.

We conclude this book with a consideration of just a few of these tensions. We will focus on those that have particular relevance to us as practitioners. They point to tensions between existing notions of care and the vision of care that seems implicit in the experiences engendered by psychedelic medicine.

It has often been asked, How do *psychedelic therapy practices* have to change to make them fit the existing molds of Western psychiatry and conventional medical care. However, we must ask the converse question: How do *we* have to change in order to properly hold the transformative experiences that psychedelic medicines offer us?

FROM TREATING SYMPTOMS TO HEALING THE WHOLE PERSON

> *It was an intense, intense struggle, and that's where it became medicinal because it allowed that struggle to happen. It didn't coat it. It wasn't an antidepressant . . . it brought it all out.*
>
> —Mike (Belser et al., 2017; Swift et al., 2017)

At present, the lion's share of the funding, research, and popular enthusiasm about psychedelics has gone toward the project of developing them into FDA-approved psychiatric medications. Success on this path will require demonstrating that they have efficacy in treating discrete psychiatric indications, such as MDD or obsessive–compulsive disorder. Many providers hold nuanced views of how psychedelic treatment will be translated. However, for some, the end goal of this vision is retrofitting psychedelic medicines into our existing pharmacopoeia, giving them a place alongside more conventional drugs. Save for some differences in administration protocols, psychedelics will be assimilated into the existing medicalized paradigm of treating psychiatric disorders by reducing their associated symptoms.

Is this paradigm, as it currently stands, the most suitable home for the therapeutic potential of psychedelic medicines? Certainly, we have seen dramatic reductions in symptoms following PAT treatment within a psychiatric framework. This fact should not preclude the possibility that there are aspects of this paradigm that are at odds with what psychedelic medicines have to offer.

Psychedelics may reduce symptoms, but they do not do so neatly. Traditional psychiatric medications work in a targeted way, aiming to reduce symptoms through a direct alleviatory process. Psychedelic medicines elicit nonordinary experiences that can be lured toward antidepressant outcomes, but which could open many other doors of the psyche in a way that is largely outside of the control of provider and participant alike. What lies behind these doors is often outside of the purview of a medical treatment paradigm. The experiences that arise often gesture toward a different, broader set of possibilities for engaging with the determinants of one's suffering that is only secondarily interested in reducing mood-related symptoms.

We have seen this in our work with participants. Many of them leave a medicine session heavy with a new, uncomfortable realization about themselves. Others may leave with the woeful conviction that everything about their life needs to change, along with the acute agony that accompanies this belief. For these and other participants, it often seems as though their encounter with psychedelic medicine provided less of a cure for their symptoms and more of an initiation into the work of their life. This may result in some immediate relief from their symptoms. But it may not. Even in cases where the psychedelic treatment does provide relief, a participant may experience this as secondary to a kind of beleaguered gratitude for finally being shown the path ahead of them (Noorani, 2020).

To accommodate this more expansive picture of what a beneficial outcome may look like, the field of PAT may find it helpful to incorporate less of a *treatment* paradigm and more of a *healing* paradigm (King, 2023). The difference in these terms is more than just semantic. Healing is a notion that looks beyond symptom reduction toward a more expansive kind of well-being that values wholeness and eudaemonic flourishing. It includes elements not often found in a treatment paradigm, such as self-knowledge, authenticity, living in alignment with one's purpose, and capacity for experiences of awe or deep meaningfulness. A healing orientation is more open to seeing an individual's struggles as a meaningful part of their longer process of becoming who they are instead of a burden to be dispelled. It is a paradigm that has more resonance with the schools of psychotherapeutic thought that have historically had less of a relationship with medicine and psychiatry—humanistic, existential, transpersonal, —than the more solution-oriented psychotherapies, such as cognitive behavioral approaches.

This recommendation is not meant to devalue the utility of PAT conducted within a treatment paradigm. For many participants, this orientation will be more aligned with their needs. However, others may be better served by a broader approach to psychedelic therapy that ventures beyond the usual purview of symptom reduction, entering into a deeper engagement with the complexity of the human experience. To do so would require an approach that is better equipped to emphasize and support the complex, unpredictable experiences that these medicines can engender. Such an approach would give both participants and their therapists more latitude to appreciate the richness and mysteriousness of what their experiences offer instead of zeroing in on symptom reduction.

In writing this book, we strove to incorporate this broad view. We see EMBARK's integrative, multidomain model as an important step toward a healing paradigm, though we recognize its origins as a model for clinical trials that emphasize psychiatric symptom management. We hold a hopeful belief that the conceptual breadth of EMBARK will allow future iterations of the model to embrace a deeper healing orientation.

We recognize that we are not alone in advocating for more of a healing orientation to psychedelic therapy. Many in the field trust that the more stringently medical phase we are in will open the door to a diversity of orientations going forward. We sincerely hope that this is the case and that our field is collectively able to accommodate the demand that these medicines seem to be making on us and our notions of what it is that PAT can offer participants (Cheung et al., 2023).

MORE HANDS TO HOLD US

> *The danger with psychedelics is that, after the "transformative cosmic trip" you must now return to your customary world, the baffled glares and embarrassed silences about what you've been through. You are now set apart, no one understanding . . . . This is why we are seeing psychedelic subcultures growing online. People search out their kin.*
>
> —James Davies, PhD

In recent years, there has been a groundswell in psychedelic circles emphasizing the importance of community. It has sometimes seemed as though every new psychedelic article, conference presentation, or working group in the field has stressed the crucial roles that community can play in helping us hold and integrate psychedelic experiences. In a field full of wildly differing opinions, community has been one of the few points of consensus. We seem to have collectively determined that psychedelic therapy is something meant to be held by many hands.

Many people have found that their psychedelic experiences have pushed them outward toward community for one reason or another. After a profoundly positive session, they may feel a strong impulse to share the fruits of their experience with others. For someone who has had a destabilizing experience, there is no softer place to land than the hands of someone who has been through something similar. And when a journeyer feels inspired to integrate their experience through a commitment to everyday action, who better to help keep that momentum than a group of people who understand that particular kind of urgency? The impulse to somehow involve others seems to be common after many psychedelic medicine experiences (Noorani, 2020).

It is perhaps unsurprising then that PAT participants have often found community to be very supportive after treatment. Several organizations have arisen that have helped these communities form. They run the gamut from drop-in virtual meetings to longer commitments among a small group of fellow travelers. Their work has often been a real blessing to those in need.

Still, these groups remain distinct from the treatment itself. More often than not, the only linkage between treatment and community support comes in the form of referrals to these outside organizations. This is likely because our current models of psychedelic therapy—EMBARK included—have retained much of the individualistic notion of care that prevails in Western institutions of healing. In psychiatry and psychology alike, therapeutic care most often consists of carefully delimited interactions between a patient and their providers. Community may be seen as beneficial but, with few exceptions, it is something that patients do outside of treatment settings. This fractured approach is limiting.

What would it look like if community involvement were considered a more integral part of PAT treatment? It could look like many things:

- Emphasizing group therapy approaches in preparation and integration
- Devoting more effort to include participants' loved ones in the treatment process
- As part of integration, encouraging the creation of community-based relationships of accountability in support of ongoing integration practices
- Integrating technological treatment adjuncts (e.g., apps) with features that facilitate community support during and after treatment
- Creating broadly available forms of psychoeducation that increase our collective capacity to hold and support people who have gone through PAT
- Inviting past participants to come together to provide their collective input on aspects of treatment
- Broadening the focus of integration to ask participants how their process of integrating their experience could involve loved ones and other people more generally (see Chapter 7)
- Building communities of practice for PAT practitioners to provide them with the kind of deep camaraderie, support, and feedback that enables them to do this work ethically and sustainably

Each of these suggestions is a way to shift the container of care we are placing around psychedelic medicines toward a greater embrace of community. This shift can guide us in crafting approaches to psychedelic therapy that resonate with the recurring longing of participants to walk their therapeutic path in the companionship of others.

Of course, opening the door to community also opens the door to added risks. We must tread carefully, acknowledging the diversity and complexity of what is referred to as "community." While many find strength and healing within their community, some encounter rejection, discrimination, or worse. Additionally, harmful forms of community have been known to develop around the use of psychedelic medicines. This is perhaps due to the confluence of several factors: the dissolution of boundaries, heightened suggestibility, and a pull toward community. Integrating community into PAT requires a proportional increase in prudence and vigilance. However, greater integration of community into treatment may serve a protective function as well, in that it makes it easier to discern when a participant's desire to connect could be dangerous or harmful.

Accommodating the impulse toward community within our models of care may be another way for us to make them a better home for psychedelic medicines (Noorani et al., 2023). Such a change would do justice to the many participants whose treatment experiences seem to cry out to be held by a bigger container. Our approaches to psychedelic therapy would be well served by making space for the primal desire for shared experiences and mutual understanding awakened by these medicines.

TILLING THE SOIL

> *Human history suggests that without a social vessel to hold the wine of revelation, it tends to dribble away . . . . That's the next research question, it seems to me: What conditions of community and practice best help people to hold onto what comes to them in those moments of revelation, converting it into abiding light in their own lives?*
>
> —Huston Smith, PhD

One idea that has remained present in psychedelic discourse since at least the 1960s is the notion that psychedelics can change the world. It is a thought that has taken on many different forms to fit the era, but the central thrust is that if enough people experience psychedelic medicines, something will gainfully shift in our collective approach to the problems that plague us, from climate change to police brutality. The staying power of this idea may be explained by its inherent attractiveness—namely, that we can overcome the worst impulses in the human condition, not through concerted effort, but by simply letting psychedelics change our minds.

While any sober analysis would reject the more extreme versions of this idea, a more grounded variation on this theme has begun to make its way into our models of integration. A growing chorus in the field has come to see the integration work of psychedelic therapy as fundamentally embedded in the structural and collective dimensions of a participant's life. In this view, inspired participants could see engagement in efforts to change the collective conditions that influence their well-being as part of how they integrate their experiences. EMBARK adapts this concept with its Collective Care cornerstone and its instruction to therapists to view integration as a process unfolding on individual and contextual levels (see Chapter 7). These ways of channeling the transformative power of psychedelics toward collective change could be seen as using psychedelics, not to change the world in as radical a way as some would hope but to maybe move the needle on it ever so slightly.

In this closing section, we highlight a different facet of the relationship between psychedelics and societal change. What if our focus shifted: instead of asking how psychedelic experiences could change the world, we might ask How could we change the world to support psychedelic experiences?

We pose this as a thought experiment. Consider the experience of a participant leaving their first medicine session and reentering their life in a densely populated coastal city in the United States. It is likely they have just had one of the most meaningful, spiritually significant experiences of their life. They feel transformed and are brimming with intrinsic motivation to give this newness the space in their life they feel it deserves. But when they depart for home, what awaits them?

- Financial pressures to return to their job less than 48 hours after they come down
- A lack of personal days they can use to get out of that obligation
- Employers, coworkers, and loved ones who would take issue with their decision to take a day off anyway
- A lack of religious contexts that could provide a respectful home for their experience
- A lack of shared cultural stories that could offer an interpretive framework for the experience
- A small, noisy apartment that does not allow for the rest and spaciousness that their therapist told them to adopt
- Cultural expectations to be responsive to texts and emails at all times, which undermine their ability to focus enough to stick with their integration goals
- A lack of noncommercial public spaces that would support their efforts to connect more with others
- No green spaces within walking distance that could nourish a deeply felt pull toward nature
- Increasing crime rates due to recent cuts in social program spending, which turns their commute into an experience that favors guardedness and hypervigilance
- Travel options that include a failing, underresourced public transit system or congested highways

They are up against a lot. To revisit a metaphor from the chapter on integration, they may feel as though they are trying to keep an ember alive in a hurricane. Their therapist can try to work with them in integration to make whatever changes they can in these unsupportive contexts. But many of them will likely prove to be beyond their reach. Despite its initial brilliance, this is an ember that might go out.

Could it be that the wish for psychedelic therapy to change the world gets it backward? From this example, it seems more as though the world might be the first thing that needs to change. Only then could this participant expand into the way of being that their encounter with a psychedelic medicine seemed to invite them into. This reframing may paint a more realistic, though less appealing, picture of the relationship between psychedelics and social change.

In doing so, it also brings us back to the central question of this chapter: what changes will we have to make to realize the full promise of psychedelic medicines? From here, the required changes appear to be far-reaching. Beyond updating our notions of healing or bringing more community into treatment, it seems as though psychedelic therapy would also be best served by a reformed set of social conditions that prioritize our expansion into the fullness of who we can be.

This is no small feat. Its immensity should be sobering. We present it here as part of this thought experiment as a challenge to lazy notions of what it would mean to become a society that lives in resonance with psychedelic medicines. The bulk of the change work is up to us, as it always has been. As practitioners who believe in the work we do, it is especially incumbent upon us to become advocates, not just for psychedelic medicines, but for the more far-reaching changes required to realize their (and our) full possibilities.

BON VOYAGE

In parting, we honor your sincere interest in psychedelic-assisted therapy and your intention to step into this meaningful work. Your decision to make *EMBARK Psychedelic Therapy* a part of your journey down that road touches our hearts in a very real way. We look forward to continuing on this path with you all as companions.

Personal Care for the Therapist

When I was a beginning practitioner, it often took me two or three days to recover from a session. So of course that has a lot of ripples into your life and uh, makes resourcing so important, make self-care so important. If you're not careful, it can affect your life in so many ways . . . . I think in this work, we just need so much support. We need solid self-care practices that work. I have a team of people who attend to me, basically. I have a craniosacral practitioner. I have a therapist I see every week. It takes a team of people to sustain this.

—Psychedelic guide (Brennan et al., 2021)

With the long hours, devoted presence, and openheartedness that psychedelic practice demands, it can be very demanding on a therapist. Diligence in personal care is one way to mitigate the stress and burnout that this can cause. This appendix contains a list of suggested practices for personal care activities from which you can choose practices that are supportive for you. Of course, you are encouraged to use any other practices that you know work for you. However, leave room for the likelihood that this work may make additional demands on you relative to your traditional therapy practice, which may require additional personal care practices.

Before listing these suggestions, it is important to note the potential pitfalls of emphasizing self-care for oneself when it is inappropriate to do so. If you are feeling burnt out, overstressed, or vicariously traumatized by your clinical work, consider the possibility that you are either overworked, underresourced, or both. If this is the case, the suggestions on this list may not be sufficient to ameliorate these feelings. If at all possible, consider reducing your workload. It can be easy to assume that psychedelic clinical work places little burden on the practitioner because they may spend most of the time in medicine sessions sitting quietly. However, this work can burden and overwhelm practitioners in subtle ways. Remember the "spheres of change" discussed in Chapter 7 and consider the possibility that your work or proximal contexts and/or your relationship to them are what need to shift in order to bring relief. We recognize that this may not always be possible, but remaining open to this perspective may help to prevent an unhelpful exclusive focus on personal care as a solution.

PRACTICES TO CONSIDER ON AN ONGOING BASIS

- Personal therapy
- Meditative practice
- Clinical supervision
- Peer consultation
- An active, supportive social life
- Healthful diet
- Exercise
- Yoga
- Massage/bodywork
- Metta or compassion-focused meditative practice to ground yourself in compassion

SUGGESTIONS FOR BEFORE A MEDICINE SESSION

- Give yourself adequate time to enter into a CUSHION presence, possibly through meditative practice.
- Eat a healthy and filling meal that will keep you full for hours without making you feel sluggish.
- Do some grounding exercises that help you feel stable and secure in your body and your role.
- Check in with your body and its needs, perhaps using a body scan meditation.
- Stretch or do yoga to facilitate a day of sitting, possibly in a prolonged static position.
- Check in with your hopes and expectations for the session and the participant to ensure that they are realistic and grounded in service to the participant's needs.
- Take a moment to increase your awareness of how you are and what you are "bringing in." If you notice any of your own needs showing up (e.g., for love, affection, recognition), attend to them before session to avoid unwittingly asking the participant to do so.

SUGGESTIONS FOR DURING A MEDICINE SESSION

- Pay attention to your body's signals and respond appropriately.
- Check in periodically with your sense of how comfortable you are with your posture and position in the room and realign if necessary during an appropriate moment.
- Whenever possible and appropriate, take a moment to return to mindfulness.

- Use subtle grounding exercises (e.g., feeling your feet or your seat on the ground) to return to feeling solid in your body and role.
- PAT practitioners often feel that they have somehow taken in an emotion that a participant has kept out of awareness. Notice whether you feel as though you are "holding" any psychological material that would be better held by the participant, and intentionally decide to let it go.

SUGGESTIONS FOR AFTER A MEDICINE SESSION

- Do not rush to return to ordinary life. Allow yourself a gentle return to your other affairs, just as you would encourage for a participant.
- Engage in a ritual that marks the transition back to ordinary life, such as going for a walk around the block, having a cup of tea, or thanking your ancestors for their support.
- Smudge with sage or other cleansing plants that feel more culturally relevant to you.
- Avoid the urge to eat or drink unhealthily to alleviate stress or exhaustion.
- Engage in a movement practice, such as dance or exercise.
- Do some grounding exercises.
- Spend time connecting with water, earth, or fire (elemental work).
- Spend time attending to what personal material was stirred up during the session that you might bring to other relationships.
- Debrief with a peer.

PREPARATION PHASE

- Build a rapport characterized by trust, connectedness, and empowerment
- Learn about the participant's experience of depression
- Continue to assess participant suitability and informed consent for treatment
- Explain elements of the treatment
- Explore consent for supportive touch
- Develop the intentions that the participant will bring to the medicine session
- Identify and build upon participant skills that may be supportive during the medicine session:
  - Emotional self-regulation
  - Attending inwardly to feelings and somatic sensations
  - Meeting all that arises with open receptivity

MEDICINE SESSION (REQUIRED)

- Prepare the space.
- Provide the medicine.
- Provide mindful, compassionate attention, even when the participant is focused internally.
- Maintain appropriate boundaries.
- Ensure participant safety and well-being.
- Supportively listen to the participant's first impressions as the medicine wears off.
- Ensure that the participant departs from the session safely.

MEDICINE SESSION (AS NEEDED)

- Encourage the participant to remain open and receptive to material that arises.
- Respond to participant needs or concerns.
- Provide relational support and care when appropriate.

- Remind the participant of their intentions if they become unfocused.
- Take notes of significant statements or themes that arise for the participant.
- Provide supportive, consensual touch when appropriate.
- Respond appropriately to challenging events that may impact participant well-being.

INTERIM INTEGRATION	FINAL INTEGRATION
1. Debrief the participant's experience of the medicine session	1. Debrief the participant's experience of the medicine session
2. Identify new opportunities for healing and growth	2. Identify new opportunities for healing and growth
3. Address any lingering somatic or psychological concerns	3. Address any lingering somatic or psychological concerns
4. (a) Develop simple activities that help maintain contact with new capacities	4. (b) Develop integration goals and begin planning and enacting life changes that support them
5. Use challenges of the last medicine session to change the approach to the next	9. Treatment completion
6. Practice any interim preparatory skills that would be supportive	
7. Develop intentions for the next medicine session	
8. Conduct a relational check-in and reassessment of consent for touch-based interventions	

Working Within the EMBARK Domains Cheat Sheet

Domain	General mechanisms	Preparation goals	Medicine session goals	Integration goals (as relevant)
Existential–Spiritual	Spiritual self-development Mystical experiences	Create the conditions for experiences of existential and spiritual content to arise	Create a space that is respectful of the sacred	1. Nurture any interest in spiritual self-development that arose
Mindful-ness	Freedom from rumination A more flexible identity Greater compassion for oneself	Help the participant learn how to attend to their internal experience and to soothe themselves if needed	Model and encourage a mindful, self-compassionate presence	2. Support sustained capacity for psychological flexibility and less reactive mental habits 3. Build upon any emergent capacity for self-compassion
Body-Aware	Embodiment and enlivenment Somatic trauma processing	Develop the participant's ability to tune in to the wisdom of the body	Help the participant stay present to their embodied experience	4. Support any increases in embodiment as a basis for improved self-care and self-awareness
Affective–Cognitive	Transforming emotions and updating core beliefs Increased acceptance of emotions	Invite the participant to remain open and receptive their emotions and self-beliefs	Support the participant in welcoming and exploring emotions that arise	5. Turn positive experiences of open receptivity into a sustainable new approach to emotions 6. Strengthen a new self-concept based on updated core beliefs
Relational	Relational repatterning Increased interpersonal openness	Build a relationship that conveys safety, acceptance, and empowerment	Provide a container of ethical, compassionate care that could support relational repatterning	7. Draw takeaways from any relational moments or dynamics that arose 8. Use feelings of connectedness or empathy to challenge isolation
Keeping Momentum	Building motivation for beneficial new habits and other life changes	Begin instilling the importance of making posttreatment changes	Listen for and record statements of motivation or intention to make life changes	9. Support the clarification and enactment of values that were felt as important

Choosing Suggested Integration Goals

Integration goals to consider as needed.

Did the participant...

	1. Nurture any interest in spiritual self-development that arose	2. Support sustained capacity for psychological flexibility and less reactive mental habits	3. Build upon any emergent capacity for self-compassion	4. Support any increase in improved self-care and self-awareness	5. Turn positive experiences in embodiment as a basis for	6. Strengthen a new self-concept based on updated core beliefs	7. Explore any relational moments or dynamics that arose on interpersonal insight or change	8. Use feelings of connectedness or empathy to challenge isolation	9. Support the clarification and enactment of new post-medicine values
...experience any spiritual or mystical phenomena?	y								
...have any insights about meaning or purpose?	y								
...describe any aspect of their experience as sacred or holy?	y								
...feel they learned something from God, their higher self, or spiritual entities?	y								
...adopt a position that may indicate prayer or meditation?	y								
...express a sense of oneness or connectedness with all of humanity?	y							y	
...feel they came into their "truer" or "higher" self?	y						y		y
...feel a wordless sense of wisdom or knowing?		y							
...experience a king of mental quiet, calm, or stillness?		y	y						
...experience a sense of mental "freedom" or "liberation?"		y							
...gain more insight into or a new vantage point on their mental processes?		y	y		y				
...gain more control over their thoughts and feelings?		y	y						
...come away with a new view of themselves or know themselves better?						y	y		y
...feel forgiveness or compassion toward themselves or someone else?		y	y				y	y	
...give themselves love or care, perhaps through self-tough?			y						
...have a strong emotional opening?			y			y	y		
...have an experience of self-forgiveness?			y						
...shift away from a narrow, self-critical sense of themselves?			y						
...feel alive or energized?					y				
...feel like they could feel or understand new things about their body?					y				
...listen to a bodily feeling that ended up leading them somewhere meaningful?					y				
...touch themselves lovingly or curiously?					y				
...have a lot of discomfort in their body?					y				
...vomit, gag, dry heave, wretch, or make choking sounds?					y				
...feel "lighter" or "younger" after a challenging moment?					y				
...look or speak differently in a way that seemed positive (e.g., "lit up")?					y				y
...tremble, shake, make jerky movements, contort their face, or vocalize?					y				
...have an experience of emotion that previously felt unknown, hidden, or "off-limits?"						y	y		
...require the use of a grounding or self-regulating technique?						y		y	
...overcome their fear of a challenging thought or feeling?						y	y		
...have a moment of struggle followed by a moment of peace?						y	y		
...solicit or receive support from therapists?							y	y	
...express any feelings toward therapists?							y	y	
...share a significant relational moment with therapists?							y	y	
...solicit or receive any touch from therapists?							y	y	
...require the setting of a relational or physical boundary?							y		
...experience an interpersonal rupture in their relationship with the therapist?							y		
...make remarks about a loved one or a general desire to have better relationships?								y	
...come away with a strengthened desire to make some sort of change?									y
...say anything about wanting to make changes or live differently?									y
...make any mention of priorities or values?									y
...come away with a strong sense of personal purpose, even if hard to put into words?									y

REFERENCES

Abramson, H. A. (1966). LSD in psychotherapy and alcoholism. *American Journal of Psychotherapy, 20*(3), 415–438.

Aday, J. S., Davis, A. K., Mitzkovitz, C. M., Bloesch, E. K., & Davoli, C. C. (2021). Predicting reactions to psychedelic drugs: A systematic review of states and traits related to acute drug effects. *ACS Pharmacology & Translational Science, 4*(2), 424–435.

Aday, J. S., Skiles, Z., Eaton, N., Fredenburg, L., Pleet, M., Mantia, J., ... & Woolley, J. D. (2023). Personal Psychedelic Use Is Common Among a Sample of Psychedelic Therapists: Implications for Research and Practice. *Psychedelic Medicine, 1*(1), 27–37.

Agin-Liebes, G. (2020). *The Role of Self-Compassion in Psilocybin-Assisted Motivational Enhancement Therapy to Treat Alcohol Dependence: A Randomized Controlled Trial.* Dissertation, Palo Alto University.

Agin-Liebes, G., Haas, T. F., Lancelotta, R., Uthaug, M. V., Ramaekers, J. G., & Davis, A. K. (2021). Naturalistic use of mescaline is associated with self-reported psychiatric improvements and enduring positive life changes. *ACS Pharmacology & Translational Science, 4*(2), 543–552.

Aixalà, M. (2022). *Psychedelic integration: Psychotherapy for non-ordinary states of consciousness.* Sante Fe, NM: Synergetic Press.

Akers, B. P., Ruiz, J. F., Piper, A., & Ruck, C. A. (2011). A prehistoric mural in Spain depicting neurotropic Psilocybe Mushrooms? *Economic Botany, 65*(2), 121–128.

Alagna, F. J., Whitcher, S. J., Fisher, J. D., & Wicas, E. A. (1979). Evaluative reaction to interpersonal touch in a counseling interview. *Journal of Counseling Psychology, 26,* 465–472.

Aldworth, B. (2019). Gender equity in cannabis and psychedelics. *MAPS Bulletin, 29*(1), 54–55. https://maps.org/news/bulletin/gender-equity-in-cannabis-and-psychedelics-spring-2019

Alyn, J. H. (1988). The politics of touch in therapy: A response to Willison and Masson. *Journal of Counseling and Development, 66,* 432–433.

American Psychiatric Association. (2013). *Cultural Formulation Interview.* American Psychiatric Association. Retrieved from https://www.psychiatry.org/File%20Library/Psychiatrists/Practice/DSM/APA_DSM5_Cultural-Formulation-Interview.pdf

Anderson, B. T., Danforth, A., Daroff, R., Stauffer, C., Ekman, E., Agin-Liebes, G., ... & Woolley, J. (2020a). Psilocybin-assisted group therapy for demoralized older long-term AIDS survivor men: An open-label safety and feasibility pilot study. *EClinicalMedicine, 27*, 100538.

Anderson, B. T., Danforth, A. L., & Grob, C. S. (2020b). Psychedelic medicine: Safety and ethical concerns. *The Lancet, 7*(10), 829–830.

APA (2006). APA presidential task force on evidence based practice. *American Psychologist, 61*, 271–285.

Arnovitz, M. D., Spitzberg, A. J., Davani, A. J., Vadhan, N. P., Holland, J., Kane, J. M., & Michaels, T. I. (2022). MDMA for the treatment of negative symptoms in schizophrenia. *Journal of Clinical Medicine, 11*(12), 3255. https://doi.org/10.3390/jcm11123255

Aronovich, A. (2020, September 22–24). *Ayahuasca as relational medicine: Intimate encounters at the frontiers of liquid modernity.* Interdisciplinary Conference on Psychedelic Research, Haarlem/Amsterdam, The Netherlands.

Backman, I. (2022, May/June). Revived interest in psychedelic therapies. *Medicine@ Yale.* https://medicine.yale.edu/news/medicineatyale/article/revived-interest-in-psychedelic-therapies/

Bacorn, C. N., & Dixon, D. N. (1984). The effects of touch on depressed and vocationally undecided clients. *Journal of Counseling Psychology, 31*(4), 488–496. https://doi.org/10.1037/0022-0167.31.4.488

Baggott, M. J., Coyle, J. R., Erowid, E., Erowid, F., & Robertson, L. C. (2011). Abnormal visual experiences in individuals with histories of hallucinogen use: A web-based questionnaire. *Drug and Alcohol Dependence, 114*(1), 61–67.

Barber, G. S., & Dike, C. C. (2023). Ethical and practical considerations for the use of psychedelics in psychiatry. *Psychiatric Services, 74*(8), 838–846.

Barnes, J. (2022). *Opinion: Current psychedelic therapies use flawed models of the mind— it's time for relational therapy.* HealingMaps. https://healingmaps.com/opinion-current-psychedelic-therapies-use-flawedmodels-of-the-mind-its-time-for-relational-therapy/

Barnes, J., & Briggs, S. (2021). Relational psychotherapy and psychedelic treatment. MIND Foundation blog. https://mind-foundation.org/relational-psychotherapy.

Barrett, F. S., Bradstreet, M. P., Leoutsakos, J. M. S., Johnson, M. W., & Griffiths, R. R. (2016). The challenging experience questionnaire: Characterization of challenging experiences with psilocybin mushrooms. *Journal of Psychopharmacology, 30*(12), 1279–1295.

Barrett, F. S., Johnson, M. W., & Griffiths, R. R. (2015). Validation of the revised Mystical Experience Questionnaire in experimental sessions with psilocybin. *Journal of Psychopharmacology, 29*(11), 1182–1190.

Bathje, G. J., Fenton, J., Pillersdorf, D., & Hill, L. C. (2021). A qualitative study of intention and impact of ayahuasca use by Westerners. *Journal of Humanistic Psychology,* https://doi.org/10.1177/00221678211008331

Bathje, G. J., Majeski, E., & Kudowor, M. (2022). Psychedelic integration: An analysis of the concept and its practice. *Frontiers in Psychology, 13*, 824077.

Becker, A. M., Holze, F., Grandinetti, T., Klaiber, A., Toedtli, V. E., Kolaczynska, K. E., ... & Liechti, M. E. (2022). Acute effects of psilocybin after escitalopram or placebo pretreatment in a randomized, double-blind, placebo-controlled, crossover study in healthy subjects. *Clinical Pharmacology & Therapeutics, 111*(4), 886–895.

Beiner, A. (2021). Who's in charge of psilocybin? Chacruna. https://chacruna.net/who_owes_psilocybin.

Belser, A. B. (2018). *The psychedelic mystical experience.* Talk presented at Colloquium on Psychedelic Psychiatry, 2018, Stockholm, Sweden [video]. www.youtube.com/watch?v=BE80piBCdNs

Belser, A. B. (2019, July). *A queer critique of the psychedelic mystical experience.* Queering Psychedelics Conference [video]. https://www.youtube.com/watch?v=0RBS57JiTms&feature=emb_imp_woyt

Belser, A. B., Agin-Liebes, G., Swift, T. C., Terrana, S., Devenot, N., Friedman, H. L., ... & Ross, S. (2017). Patient experiences of psilocybin-assisted psychotherapy: An interpretative phenomenological analysis. *Journal of Humanistic Psychology, 57*(4), 354–388. https://doi.org/10.1177/0022167817706884

Belser, A. B., & Field, M. (2022). Other Eligibility Considerations Assessment. Unpublished instrument.

Belser, A.B., & Keating, A. (2022). A queer vision for psychedelic research: Past reckonings, current reforms, and future transformations. In A, B. Belser, C. Cavnar, & B. C. Labate (Eds.), *Queering psychedelics: from oppression to liberation in psychedelic medicine* (pp. 3–12). Synergetic Press.

Bennett-Levy, J. (2019). Why therapists should walk the talk: The theoretical and empirical case for personal practice in therapist training and professional development. *Journal of Behavior Therapy and Experimental Psychiatry, 62,* 133–145.

Bird, C. I. V., Modlin, N. L., & Rucker, J. J. H. (2021). Psilocybin and MDMA for the treatment of trauma-related psychopathology. *International Review of Psychiatry, 33*(3), 229–249.

Bogenschutz, M. P., & Forcehimes, A. A. (2017). Development of a psychotherapeutic model for psilocybin-assisted treatment of alcoholism. *Journal of Humanistic Psychology, 57*(4), 389–414.

Bogenschutz, M. P., Forcehimes, A. A., Pommy, J. A., Wilcox, C. E., Barbosa, P., & Strassman, R. J. (2015). Psilocybin-assisted treatment for alcohol dependence: A proof-of-concept study. *Journal of Psychopharmacology, 29*(3), 289–299. https://doi.org/10.1177/0269881114565144

Bogenschutz, M. P., Podrebarac, S. K., Duane, J. H., Amegadzie, S. S., Malone, T. C., Owens, L. T., ... & Mennenga, S. E. (2018). Clinical interpretations of patient experience in a trial of psilocybin-assisted psychotherapy for alcohol use disorder. *Frontiers in Pharmacology, 9,* 100. https://doi.org/10.3389/fphar.2018.00100

Bogenschutz, M. P., Ross, S., Bhatt, S., Baron, T., Forcehimes, A. A., Laska, E., ... & Worth, L. (2022). Percentage of heavy drinking days following psilocybin-assisted psychotherapy vs placebo in the treatment of adult patients with alcohol use disorder: A randomized clinical trial. *JAMA Psychiatry, 79*(10), 953–962.

Bonelli, R., Dew, R. E., Koenig, H. G., Rosmarin, D. H., & Vasegh, S. (2012). Religious and spiritual factors in depression: review and integration of the research. *Depression Research and Treatment,* 962860. https://doi.org/10.1155/2012/962860

Bonson, K. R. (2018). Regulation of human research with LSD in the United States (1949–1987). *Psychopharmacology, 235*(2), 591–604.

Bonson, K. R., Buckholtz, J. W., & Murphy, D. L. (1996). Chronic administration of serotonergic antidepressants attenuates the subjective effects of LSD in humans. *Neuropsychopharmacology, 14*(6), 425–436.

Bouso, J. C., Andión, Ó., Sarris, J. J., Scheidegger, M., Tófoli, L. F., Opaleye, E. S., ... & Perkins, D. (2022). Adverse effects of ayahuasca: Results from the Global Ayahuasca Survey. *PLOS Global Public Health*, *2*(11), e0000438.

Bouso, J. C., Doblin, R., Farré, M., Alcázar, M. Á., & Gómez-Jarabo, G. (2008). MDMA-assisted psychotherapy using low doses in a small sample of women with chronic posttraumatic stress disorder. *Journal of Psychoactive Drugs*, *40*(3), 225–236.

Bowen, S., Chawla, N., & Marlatt, G.A. (2010). *Mindfulness-based relapse prevention for the treatment of substance use disorders: A clinician's guide*. Guilford Press.

Breeksema, J. J., Kuin, B. W., Kamphuis, J., van den Brink, W., Vermetten, E., & Schoevers, R. A. (2022a). Adverse events in clinical treatments with serotonergic psychedelics and MDMA: A mixed-methods systematic review. *Journal of Psychopharmacology*, *36*(10), 1100–1117.

Breeksema, J. J., Niemeijer, A. R., Krediet, E., Vermetten, E., & Schoevers, R. A. (2020). Psychedelic treatments for psychiatric disorders: A systematic review and thematic synthesis of patient experiences in qualitative studies. *CNS Drugs*, *34*, 925–946. https://doi.org/10.1007/s40263-020-00748-y

Breeksema, J. J., Niemeijer, A., Kuin, B., Veraart, J., Kamphuis, J., Schimmel, N., ... & Schoevers, R. (2022b). Holding on or letting go? Patient experiences of control, context, and care in oral esketamine treatment for treatment-resistant depression: A qualitative study. *Frontiers in Psychiatry*, *13*, 2716.

Breeksema, J. J., & van Elk, M. (2021). Working with weirdness: A response to "moving past mysticism in psychedelic science". *ACS Pharmacology & Translational Science*, *4*(4), 1471–1474.

Brennan, B. (2020, July 3). *The revolution will not be psychologized: Psychedelics' potential for systemic change*. Chacruna. https://chacruna.net/the-revolution-will-not-be-psychologized-psychedelics-potential-for-systemic-change/

Brennan, W., & Belser, A. B. (2022). Models of psychedelic-assisted psychotherapy: A contemporary assessment and an introduction to EMBARK, a transdiagnostic, trans-drug model. *Frontiers in Psychology*, *13*, 866018.

Brennan, W., Jackson, M. A., MacLean, K., & Ponterotto, J. G. (2021). A qualitative exploration of relational ethical challenges and practices in psychedelic healing. *Journal of Humanistic Psychology*. https://doi.org/10.1177/00221678211045265

Brennan, W., Kelman, A. R., & Belser, A. B. (2023). A systematic review of psychotherapeutic elements in psychedelic clinical trials: Current reporting practices and rationale for increased consideration. *Psychedelic Medicine*. https://doi.org/10.1089/psymed.2023.0007

Brewerton, T. D., Wang, J. B., Lafrance, A., Pamplin, C., Mithoefer, M., Yazar-Klosinki, B., ... & Doblin, R. (2022). MDMA-assisted therapy significantly reduces eating disorder symptoms in a randomized placebo-controlled trial of adults with severe PTSD. *Journal of Psychiatric Research*, *149*, 128–135.

Buchanan, N. T. (2021). Ensuring the psychedelic renaissance and radical healing reach the Black community: Commentary on culture and psychedelic psychotherapy. *Journal of Psychedelic Studies*, *4*(3), 142–145.

Byock, I. (2018). Taking psychedelics seriously. *Journal of Palliative Medicine*, *21*(4), 417–421.

Calder, A. E., & Hasler, G. (2022). Towards an understanding of psychedelic-induced neuroplasticity. *Neuropsychopharmacology*, *48*, 104–112.

Carbonaro, T. M., Bradstreet, M. P., Barrett, F. S., MacLean, K. A., Jesse, R., Johnson, M. W., & Griffiths, R. R. (2016). Survey study of challenging experiences after ingesting psilocybin mushrooms: Acute and enduring positive and negative consequences. *Journal of Psychopharmacology, 30*(12), 1268–1278.

Carhart-Harris, R. L. (2018). The entropic brain-revisited. *Neuropharmacology, 142*, 167–178.

Carhart-Harris, R. L., Bolstridge, M., Day, C. M. J., Rucker, J., Watts, R., Erritzoe, D. E., ... & Nutt, D. J. (2018a). Psilocybin with psychological support for treatment-resistant depression: Six-month follow-up. *Psychopharmacology, 235*(2), 399–408.

Carhart-Harris, R. L., Bolstridge, M., Rucker, J., Day, C. M. J., Erritzoe, D., Kaelen, M., ... & Nutt, D. J. (2016). Psilocybin with psychological support for treatment-resistant depression: An open-label feasibility study. *The Lancet Psychiatry, 3*(7), 619–627.

Carhart-Harris, R. L., Erritzoe, D., Haijen, E., Kaelen, M., & Watts, R. (2018b). Psychedelics and connectedness. *Psychopharmacology, 235*(2), 547–550.

Carhart-Harris, R. L., & Friston, K. J. (2019). REBUS and the anarchic brain: toward a unified model of the brain action of psychedelics. *Pharmacological Reviews, 71*(3), 316–344.

Carhart-Harris, R., Giribaldi, B., Watts, R., Baker-Jones, M., Murphy-Beiner, A., Murphy, R., ... & Nutt, D. (2021). Trial of psilocybin versus escitalopram for depression. *New England Journal of Medicine, 384*, 1402–1411. doi:10.1056/nejmoa2032994

Carhart-Harris, R. L., Kaelen, M., Whalley, M. G., Bolstridge, M., Feilding, A., & Nutt, D. J. (2015). LSD enhances suggestibility in healthy volunteers. *Psychopharmacology, 232*, 785–794.

Carhart-Harris, R. L., Leech, R., Hellyer, P. J., Shanahan, M., Feilding, A., Tagliazucchi, E., ... & Nutt, D. (2014). The entropic brain: A theory of conscious states informed by neuroimaging research with psychedelic drugs. *Frontiers in human neuroscience, 8*, 20.

Carhart-Harris, R. L., & Nutt, D. J. (2017). Serotonin and brain function: A tale of two receptors. *Journal of Psychopharmacology, 31*(9), 1091–1120.

Carhart-Harris, R. L., Roseman, L., Haijen, E., Erritzoe, D., Watts, R., Branchi, I., & Kaelen, M. (2018c). Psychedelics and the essential importance of context. *Journal of Psychopharmacology, 32*(7), 725–731.

Carr, S., & Spandler, H. (2019). Hidden from history? A brief modern history of the psychiatric "treatment" of lesbian and bisexual women in England. *The Lancet Psychiatry, 6*(4), 289–290.

Cavnar, C. (2018, November 15). Can psychedelic "cure" gay people? Chacruna. https://chacruna.net/can-psychedelics-cure-gay-people/

Celidwen, Y., Redvers, N., Githaiga, C., Calambás, J., Añaños, K., Chindoy, M. E., ... & Sacbajá, A. (2023). Ethical principles of traditional Indigenous medicine to guide Western psychedelic research and practice. *The Lancet Regional Health-Americas, 18*, 100410.

Chapkis, W., & Webb, R. J. (2008). *Dying to get high: Marijuana as medicine.* NYU Press.

Chapman, L. K., DeLapp, R. C., & Williams, M. T. (2014). Impact of race, ethnicity, and culture on the expression and assessment of psychopathology. In D. C. Beidel, B. C. Frueh, & M. Hersen (Eds.), *Adult psychopathology and diagnosis* (pp. 131–162). John Wiley & Sons.

Cheung, K., Patch, K., Earp, B. D., & Yaden, D. B. (2023). Psychedelics, meaningfulness, and the "proper scope" of medicine: continuing the conversation. *Cambridge Quarterly of Healthcare Ethics, 27*, 1–7.

Csordas, T. J., & Harwood, A. (Eds.). (1994). *Embodiment and experience: The existential ground of culture and self* (Vol. 1). Cambridge University Press.

Cuijpers, P., Reijnders, M., & Huibers, M. J. (2019). The role of common factors in psychotherapy outcomes. *Annual Review of Clinical Psychology, 15*, 207–231.

Cuijpers, P., Stringaris, A., & Wolpert, M. (2020). Treatment outcomes for depression: challenges and opportunities. *The Lancet: Psychiatry, 7*(11), 925–927. https://doi.org/10.1016/S2215-0366(20)30036-5

Curtis, R., Roberts, L., Graves, E., Rainey, H. T., Wynn, D., Krantz, D., & Wieloch, V. (2020). The role of psychedelics and counseling in mental health treatment. *Journal of Mental Health Counseling, 42*(4), 323–338.

Dakwar, E., Anerella, C., Hart, C. L., Levin, F. R., Mathew, S. J., & Nunes, E. V. (2014). Therapeutic infusions of ketamine: Do the psychoactive effects matter? *Drug and Alcohol Dependence, 136*, 153–157.

Dalenberg, C. (2006). Recovered memory and the Daubert criteria: Recovered memory as professionally tested, peer reviewed, and accepted in the relevant scientific community. *Trauma, Violence, & Abuse, 7*(4), 274–310.

Danforth, A. L., Grob, C. S., Struble, C., Feduccia, A. A., Walker, N., Jerome, L., ... & Emerson, A. (2018). Reduction in social anxiety after MDMA-assisted psychotherapy with autistic adults: a randomized, double-blind, placebo-controlled pilot study. *Psychopharmacology, 235*(11), 3137–3148.

Davidson, T. (2022). Psyched straight: the early life of LSD as a conversion therapy drug. In A. B. Belser, C. Cavnar, & B. C. Labate (Eds.), *Queering psychedelics: from oppression to liberation in psychedelic medicine.* Synergetic Press.

Davies, J. (2021). *Sedated: How modern capitalism created our mental health crisis.* Atlantic Books.

Davies, J., Pace, B. A., & Devenot, N. (2023). Beyond the psychedelic hype: Exploring the persistence of the neoliberal paradigm. *Journal of Psychedelic Studies.*

Davis, A. K., Barrett, F. S., & Griffiths, R. R. (2020). Psychological flexibility mediates the relations between acute psychedelic effects and subjective decreases in depression and anxiety. *Journal of Contextual Behavioral Science, 15*, 39–45.

Davis, A. K., Barrett, F. S., May, D. G., Cosimano, M. P., Sepeda, N. D., Johnson, M. W., ... & Griffiths, R. R. (2021). Effects of psilocybin-assisted therapy on major depressive disorder: A randomized clinical trial. *JAMA Psychiatry, 78*(5), 481–489. doi:10.1001/jamapsychiatry.2020.3285

Davis, A. K., Barrett, F. S., So, S., Gukasyan, N., Swift, T. C., & Griffiths, R. R. (2021). Development of the Psychological Insight Questionnaire among a sample of people who have consumed psilocybin or LSD. *Journal of Psychopharmacology, 35*(4), 437–446.

Davis, A. K., So, S., Lancelotta, R., Barsuglia, J. P., & Griffiths, R. R. (2019). 5-Methoxy-N, N-dimethyltryptamine (5-MeO-DMT) used in a naturalistic group setting is associated with unintended improvements in depression and anxiety. *American Journal of Drug and Alcohol Abuse, 45*(2), 161–169.

Dean, K. E., Long, A. C. J., Trinh, N., McClendon, J., & Buckner, J. D. (2022). Treatment seeking for anxiety and depression among Black adults: A multilevel and empirically informed psycho-sociocultural model. *Behavior Therapy, 53*(6), 1077–1091.

de Laportalière, T. T., Jullien, A., Yrondi, A., Cestac, P., & Montastruc, F. (2023). Reporting of harms in clinical trials of esketamine in depression: a systematic review. *Psychological Medicine, 53*(10), 1–11.

De Rios, M. D., & Katz, F. (1975). Some relationships between music and hallucinogenic ritual: The "jungle gym" in consciousness. *Ethos, 3*(1), 64–76.

Devenot, N., Seale-Feldman, A., Smith, E., Noorani, T., Garcia-Romeu, A., & Johnson, M. W. (2022a). Psychedelic identity shift: a critical approach to set and setting. *Kennedy Institute of Ethics Journal, 32*(4), 359–399.

Devenot, N., Tumilty, E., Buisson, M., McNamee, Nickles, D., & Ross, L. K. (2022b). *A precautionary approach to touch in psychedelic-assisted therapy.* Bill of Health. https://blog.petrieflom.law.harvard.edu/2022/03/09/precautionary-approach-touch-in-psychedelic-assisted-therapy/

Ditman, K. S., Moss, T., Forgy, E. W., Zunin, L. M., Lynch, R. D., & Funk, W. A. (1969). Dimensions of the LSD, methylphenidate and chlordiazepoxide experiences. *Psychopharmacologia, 14*(1), 1–11.

Doerr-Zegers, O., Irarrázaval, L., Mundt, A., & Palette, V. (2017). Disturbances of embodiment as core phenomena of depression in clinical practice. *Psychopathology, 50*(4), 273–281.

Doss, M. K., Madden, M. B., Gaddis, A., Nebel, M. B., Griffiths, R. R., Mathur, B. N., & Barrett, F. S. (2022). Models of psychedelic drug action: modulation of cortical-subcortical circuits. *Brain, 145*(2), 441–456.

Dos Santos, R. G., de Lima Osório, F., Rocha, J. M., Rossi, G. N., Bouso, J. C., Rodrigues, L. S., ... & Hallak, J. E. C. (2021). Ayahuasca improves self-perception of speech performance in subjects with social anxiety disorder: A pilot, proof-of-concept, randomized, placebo-controlled trial. *Journal of Clinical Psychopharmacology, 41*(5), 540–550. https://doi.org/10.1097/JCP.0000000000001428

D'Souza, D. C., Syed, S. A., Flynn, L. T., Safi-Aghdam, H., Cozzi, N. V., & Ranganathan, M. (2022). Exploratory study of the dose-related safety, tolerability, and efficacy of dimethyltryptamine (DMT) in healthy volunteers and major depressive disorder. *Neuropsychopharmacology, 47*(10), 1854–1862.

Dubus, Z. (2022). High dose psychedelic shock therapy with LSD and mescaline: The conversion treatment of a French doctor on two homosexual adolescents in the 1960s. In A. B. Belser, C. Cavnar, & B. C. Labate (Eds.), *Queering psychedelics: From oppression to liberation in psychedelic medicine* (pp. 59–64). Synergetic Press.

Dupuis, D. (2021). Psychedelics as tools for belief transmission. Set, setting, suggestibility, and persuasion in the ritual use of hallucinogens. *Frontiers in Psychology, 12*, 730031.

Dupuis, D., & Veissière, S. (2022). Culture, context, and ethics in the therapeutic use of hallucinogens: Psychedelics as active super-placebos?. *Transcultural Psychiatry, 59*(5), 571–578.

Durana, C. (1998). The use of touch in psychotherapy: Ethical and clinical guidelines. *Psychotherapy: Theory, Research, Practice, Training, 35*(2), 269–280. https://doi.org/10.1037/h0087817

Dyck, E. (2005). *Psychedelic psychiatry: LSD and post-World War II medical experimentation in Canada* [Ph.D. dissertation, McMaster University]. https://macsphere.mcmaster.ca/bitstream/11375/24416/1/dyck_erika_2005_phd.pdf

Dyck, E. (2008). *Psychedelic psychiatry: LSD from clinic to campus.* JHU Press.

Dyck, E. (2021). Can psychedelics promote social justice and save the world? Chacruna https://chacruna.net/social-justice-revolution-psychedelics/

Earleywine, M., Low, F., Altman, B. R., & De Leo, J. (2022). How important is a guide who has taken psilocybin in psilocybin-assisted therapy for depression? *Journal of Psychoactive Drugs, 55*, 51–61.

Eisner, B. G. (1964). *Psychedelics and people as adjuncts to psychotherapy*. Paper presented at the First International Congress of Social Psychiatry, London, England]. Betty Grover Eisner Papers, 1927–2002, Department of Special Collections and University Archives (Box 5, Folder 8), Stanford University Library.

Eisner, B. G. (1967). The importance of the non-verbal. In H. Abramson (Ed.), *The use of LSD in psychotherapy and alcoholism* (pp. 542–560). Bobbs-Merill.

Eisner, B. G., & Cohen, S. (1958). Psychotherapy with lysergic acid diethylamide. *Journal of Nervous and Mental Disease, 127*(6), 528–539.

Engel, L. B., Thal, S. B., & Bright, S. J. (2022). Psychedelic forum member preferences for carer experience and consumption behavior: Can "trip sitters" help inform psychedelic harm reduction services? *Contemporary Drug Problems, 49*(4), 356–368.

Ens, A. (2022). LSD and mescaline psychedelic conversion therapies in postwar North America. In A. B. Belser, C. Cavnar, & B. C. Labate (Eds.), *Queering psychedelics: From oppression to liberation in psychedelic medicine* (pp. 45–52). Synergetic Press.

Evans, J. (2023a, April 11). *Adam Aronovich on communitas, raving, and healing from healing*. Ecstatic Integration. https://www.ecstaticintegration.org/p/adam-aronov ich-on-communitas-raving

Evans, J. (2023b, June 6). Extended difficulties after psychedelic trips and what helps people deal with them. OPEN Foundation Online Events. https://open-foundation. org/events/online/

Evans, J., Robinson, O. C., Argyri, E. K., Suseelan, S., Murphy-Beiner, A., McAlpine, R., ... & Prideaux, E. (2023). Extended difficulties following the use of psychedelic drugs: A mixed methods study. *Plos One, 18*(10), e0293349.

Farchione, T. J., Fairholme, C. P., Ellard, K. K., Boisseau, C. L., Thompson-Hollands, J., Carl, J. R., ... & Barlow, D. H. (2012). Unified protocol for transdiagnostic treatment of emotional disorders: a randomized controlled trial. *Behavior Therapy, 43*(3), 666–678.

Fauvel, B., Kangaslampi, S., Strika-Bruneau, L., Roméo, B., & Piolino, P. (2022). Validation of a French version of the mystical experience questionnaire with retro-spective reports of the most significant psychedelic experience among French users. *Journal of Psychoactive Drugs, 55*(2), 170–179.

Fischer, F. M. (2015). *Therapy with substance: Psycholytic psychotherapy in the twenty first century*. Muswell Hill Press.

Flory, J. D., & Yehuda, R. (2022). Comorbidity between post-traumatic stress disorder and major depressive disorder: alternative explanations and treatment considerations. *Dialogues in Clinical NeurosciencE, 17*(2), 141–150.

Fogg, C., Michaels, T. I., de la Salle, S., Jahn, Z. W., & Williams, M. T. (2021). Ethnoracial health disparities and the ethnopsychopharmacology of psychedelic-assisted psychotherapies. *Experimental and Clinical Psychopharmacology, 29*(5), 539–554.

Forstmann, M., & Sagioglou, C. (2021). How psychedelic researchers' self-admitted sub-stance use and their association with psychedelic culture affect people's perceptions of their scientific integrity and the quality of their research. *Public Understanding of Science, 30*(3), 302–318.

Forsyth, J. P., & Eifert, G. H. (2016). *The mindfulness and acceptance workbook for anxiety: A guide to breaking free from anxiety, phobias, and worry using acceptance and commitment therapy*. New Harbinger Publications.

Fotiou, E., & Gearin, A. K. (2019). Purging and the body in the therapeutic use of aya-huasca. *Social Science & Medicine, 239*, 112532.

Friesen, P. (2022). Psychosis and psychedelics: Historical entanglements and contemporary contrasts. *Transcultural Psychiatry, 59*(5), 592–609.

Gable, R. S. (2004). Comparison of acute lethal toxicity of commonly abused psychoactive substances. *Addiction, 99*(6), 686–696.

Garcia-Romeu, A., Davis, A. K., Erowid, F., Erowid, E., Griffiths, R. R., & Johnson, M. W. (2019). Cessation and reduction in alcohol consumption and misuse after psychedelic use. *Journal of Psychopharmacology, 33*(9), 1088–1101.

Garcia-Romeu, A., Himelstein, S. P., & Kaminker, J. (2015). Self-transcendent experience: A grounded theory study. *Qualitative Research, 15*(5), 633–654.

Garcia-Romeu, A., & Richards, W. A. (2018). Current perspectives on psychedelic therapy: use of serotonergic hallucinogens in clinical interventions. *International Review of Psychiatry, 30*(4), 291–316.

Garel, N., Thibault Lévesque, J., Sandra, D. A., Lessard-Wajcer, J., Solomonova, E., Lifshitz, M., ... & Greenway, K. T. (2023). Imprinting: expanding the extra-pharmacological model of psychedelic drug action to incorporate delayed influences of sets and settings. *Frontiers in Human Neuroscience, 17*, 1200393.

Gashi, L., Sandberg, S., & Pedersen, W. (2021). Making "bad trips" good: How users of psychedelics narratively transform challenging trips into valuable experiences. *International Journal of Drug Policy, 87*, 102997.

Gasser, P., Holstein, D., Michel, Y., Doblin, R., Yazar-Klosinski, B., Passie, T., & Brenneisen, R. (2014). Safety and efficacy of lysergic acid diethylamide-assisted psychotherapy for anxiety associated with life-threatening diseases. *Journal of Nervous and Mental Disease, 202*(7), 513.

Gasser, P., Kirchner, K., & Passie, T. (2015). LSD-assisted psychotherapy for anxiety associated with a life-threatening disease: a qualitative study of acute and sustained subjective effects. *Journal of Psychopharmacology, 29*(1), 57–68.

Gelb, P. (1982). The experience of nonerotic contact in traditional psychotherapy: A critical investigation of the taboo against touch. *Dissertation Abstracts International, 43*(1-B), 248.

George, J. R., Michaels, T. I., Sevelius, J., & Williams, M. T. (2020). The psychedelic renaissance and the limitations of a White-dominant medical framework: A call for Indigenous and ethnic minority inclusion. *Journal of Psychedelic Studies, 4*(1), 4–15. doi:10.1556/2054.2019.015

Gerber, L. A. (1990). Integrating political-societal concerns in psychotherapy. *American Journal of Psychotherapy, 44*(4), 471–483.

Gerber, L. (1992). Intimate politics: Connectedness and the social-political self. *Psychotherapy: Theory, Research, Practice, Training, 29*(4), 626.

Gibbs, R. W., Jr. (2005). *Embodiment and cognitive science*. Cambridge University Press.

Gilbert, P. (2009). Introducing compassion-focused therapy. *Advances in Psychiatric Treatment, 15*(3), 199–208. doi:10.1192/apt.bp.107.005264

Gilbert, P., McEwan, K., Matos, M., & Rivis, A. (2011). Fears of compassion: Development of three self-report measures. *Psychology and Psychotherapy: Theory, Research and Practice, 84*(3), 239–255.

Goldhill, O. (2020, March 3). *Psychedelic therapy has a sexual abuse problem*. Quartz. https://qz.com/1809184/psychedelic-therapy-has-a-sexual-abuse-problem-3/

Goodman, M., & Teicher, A. (1988). To touch or not to touch. *Psychotherapy: Theory, Research, Practice, Training, 25*(4), 492.

Goodwin, G. M., Aaronson, S. T., Alvarez, O., Arden, P. C., Baker, A., Bennett, J. C., ... & Malievskaia, E. (2022). Single-dose psilocybin for a treatment-resistant episode of major depression. *New England Journal of Medicine, 387*(18), 1637–1648.

Goodwin, G. M., Croal, M., Feifel, D., Kelly, J. R., Marwood, L., Mistry, S., ... & Malievskaia, E. (2023). Psilocybin for treatment resistant depression in patients taking a concomitant SSRI medication. *Neuropsychopharmacology, 48*, 1492–1499.

Goss, K., & Allan, S. (2014). The development and application of compassion-focused therapy for eating disorders (CFT-E). *British Journal of Clinical Psychology, 53*(1), 62–77. doi:10.1111/bjc.12039

Grabbe, L., & Miller-Karas, E. (2017). The trauma resiliency model: A "bottom-up" intervention for trauma psychotherapy. *Journal of the American Psychiatric Nurses Association, 24*(1), 76–84. https://doi.org/10.1177/1078390317745133

Greenberg, L. S., & Watson, J. C. (2006). *Emotional-focused therapy for depression.* American Psychological Association.

Greer, G. R., & Tolbert, R. (1998). A method of conducting therapeutic sessions with MDMA. *Journal of Psychoactive Drugs, 30*(4), 371–379.

Greer, J. C. (2022, Autumn/Winter). The greening of psychedelics. *Harvard Divinity Bulletin.* https://bulletin.hds.harvard.edu/the-greening-of-psychedelics/

Griffiths, R. R., Hurwitz, E. S., Davis, A. K., Johnson, M. W., & Jesse, R. (2019). Survey of subjective "God encounter experiences": Comparisons among naturally occurring experiences and those occasioned by the classic psychedelics psilocybin, LSD, ayahuasca, or DMT. *PloS One, 14*(4), e0214377.

Griffiths, R. R., Johnson, M. W., Carducci, M. A., Umbricht, A., Richards, W. A., Richards, B. D., ... & Klinedinst, M. A. (2016). Psilocybin produces substantial and sustained decreases in depression and anxiety in patients with life-threatening cancer: A randomized double-blind trial. *Journal of Psychopharmacology, 30*(12), 1181–1197.

Griffiths, R. R., Johnson, M. W., Richards, W. A., Richards, B. D., Jesse, R., MacLean, K. A., ... & Klinedinst, M. A. (2018). Psilocybin-occasioned mystical-type experience in combination with meditation and other spiritual practices produces enduring positive changes in psychological functioning and in trait measures of prosocial attitudes and behaviors. *Journal of Psychopharmacology, 32*(1), 49–69. https://doi.org/10.1177/0269881117731279

Griffiths, R. R., Johnson, M. W., Richards, W. A., Richards, B. D., McCann, U., & Jesse, R. (2011). Psilocybin occasioned mystical-type experiences: immediate and persisting dose-related effects. *Psychopharmacology, 218*, 649–665.

Griffiths, R. R., Richards, W. A., McCann, U., & Jesse, R. (2006). Psilocybin can occasion mystical-type experiences having substantial and sustained personal meaning and spiritual significance. *Psychopharmacology, 187*(3), 268–292. https://doi.org/10.1007/s00213-006-0457-5

Grinspoon, L., & Bakalar, J. B. (1981). The psychedelic drug therapies. *Current Psychiatric Therapies, 20*, 275–283.

Grinspoon, L., & Doblin, R. (2001). Psychedelics as catalysts of insight-oriented psychotherapy. *Social Research, 68*(3), 677–695.

Grob, C. S., Danforth, A. L., Chopra, G. S., Hagerty, M., McKay, C. R., Halberstadt, A. L., & Greer, G. R. (2011). Pilot study of psilocybin treatment for anxiety in patients with advanced-stage cancer. *Archives of General Psychiatry, 68*(1), 71–78.

Grof, S. (1980) *LSD psychotherapy: Exploring the frontiers of the hidden mind.* Hunter House.

Gukasyan, N., Davis, A. K., Barrett, F. S., Cosimano, M. P., Sepeda, N. D., Johnson, M. W., & Griffiths, R. R. (2022). Efficacy and safety of psilocybin-assisted treatment for major depressive disorder: prospective 12-month follow-up. *Journal of Psychopharmacology, 36*(2), 151–158.

Gukasyan, N., & Nayak, S. M. (2022). Psychedelics, placebo effects, and set and setting: Insights from common factors theory of psychotherapy. *Transcultural Psychiatry, 59*(5), 652–664.

Guss, J. (2022). A psychoanalytic perspective on psychedelic experience. *Psychoanalytic Dialogues, 32*(5), 452–468.

Guss, J., Krause, R., & Sloshower, J. (2020, August 13). *The Yale manual for psilocybin-assisted therapy of depression (using acceptance and commitment therapy as a therapeutic frame).* https://doi.org/10.31234/osf.io/u6v9y

Guthrie, L. (2021). *A phenomenology of challenging psychedelic experiences: From relational trauma to relational healing* [Doctoral dissertation, Duquesne University].

Haijen, E. C., Kaelen, M., Roseman, L., Timmermann, C., Kettner, H., Russ, S., ... & Carhart-Harris, R. L. (2018). Predicting responses to psychedelics: a prospective study. *Frontiers in Pharmacology, 9,* 897.

Halman, A., Kong, G., Sarris, J., & Perkins, D. (2023). *Drug-drug interactions between classic psychedelics and psychoactive drugs: a systematic review.* medRxiv. https://www.medrxiv.org/content/10.1101/2023.06.01.23290811v2

Harris, R. (2023). *Swimming in the sacred: Wisdom from the psychedelic underground.* New World Library.

Hartogsohn, I. (2018). The meaning-enhancing properties of psychedelics and their mediator role in psychedelic therapy, spirituality, and creativity. *Frontiers in Neuroscience, 12,* 129.

Hastings, O. P. (2016). Not a lonely crowd? Social connectedness, religious service attendance, and the spiritual but not religious. *Social Science Research, 57,* 63–79.

Hasty, M. (2022, February 18). *MDMA commercialization with Joy Sun Cooper and James Acer from MAPS.* Psychedelic.support. https://psychedelic.support/resources/when-can-i-get-mdma-therapy

Hatzenbuehler, M. L., McLaughlin, K. A., Keyes, K. M., & Hasin, D. S. (2010). The impact of institutional discrimination on psychiatric disorders in lesbian, gay, and bisexual populations: A prospective study. *American Journal of public Health, 100*(3), 452–459.

Hayes, S. C., Strosahl, K., & Wilson, K. G. (2012). *Acceptance and commitment therapy: The process and practice of mindful change* (2nd ed.). Guilford Press.

Healy, C. J., Lee, K. A., & D'Andrea, W. (2021). Using psychedelics with therapeutic intent is associated with lower shame and complex trauma symptoms in adults with histories of child maltreatment. *Chronic Stress, 5,* 24705470211029881.

Herman, J. L. (1998). Recovery from psychological trauma. *Psychiatry and Clinical Neurosciences, 52*(S1), S98–S103.

Herzberg, G., & Butler, J. (2019, March 13). *Blinded by the white: Addressing power and privilege in psychedelic medicine.* Chacruna. https://chacruna.net/blinded-by-the-white-addressing-power-and-privilege-in-psychedelic-medicine/

Hippensteele, A. (2023, June 9). *FDA approves MDMA for clinical trial use investigating schizophrenia.* Pharmacy Times. https://www.pharmacytimes.com/view/fda-approves-mdma-for-clinical-trial-use-investigating-schizophrenia

Ho, J. T., Preller, K. H., & Lenggenhager, B. (2020). Neuropharmacological modulation of the aberrant bodily self through psychedelics. *Neuroscience & Biobehavioral Reviews, 108*, 526–541.

Hodge, A. T., Sukpraprut-Braaten, S., Narlesky, M., & Strayhan, R. C. (2022). The use of psilocybin in the treatment of psychiatric disorders with attention to relative safety profile: a systematic review. *Journal of Psychoactive Drugs, 55*(1), 40–50.

Hollister, L. E., Shelton, J., & Krieger, G. (1969). A controlled comparison of lysergic acid diethylamide (LSD) and dextroamphetamine in alcoholics. *American Journal of Psychiatry, 125*(10), 1352–1357.

Holroyd, J., & Brodsky, A. (1977). Psychologists' attitudes and practices regarding erotic and nonerotic physical contact with patients. *American Psychologist, 32*, 843–849.

Holroyd, J. C., & Brodsky, A. (1980). Does touching patients lead to sexual intercourse? *Professional Psychology, 11*, 807–811.

Holub, E. A., & Lee, S. S. (1990). Therapists' use of nonerotic physical contact: Ethical concerns. *Professional Psychology: Research and Practice, 21*, 115–117.

Holze, F., Becker, A. M., Kolaczynska, K. E., Duthaler, U., & Liechti, M. E. (2023). Pharmacokinetics and pharmacodynamics of oral psilocybin administration in healthy participants. *Clinical Pharmacology & Therapeutics, 113*(4), 822–831.

Horton, D. M., Morrison, B., & Schmidt, J. (2021). Systematized review of psychotherapeutic components of psilocybin-assisted psychotherapy. *American Journal of Psychotherapy, 74*(4), 140–149.

Horton, J. A., Clance, P. R., Sterk-Elifson, C., & Emshoff, J. (1995). Touch in psychotherapy: A survey of patients' experiences. *Psychotherapy: Theory, Research, Practice, Training, 32*(3), 443–457.

Hunter, M., & Struve, J. (1997). The ethical use of touch in psychotherapy. Sage Publications.

Hvenegaard, M., Moeller, S. B., Poulsen, S., Gondan, M., Grafton, B., Austin, S. F., ... & Watkins, E. R. (2020). Group rumination-focused cognitive-behavioural therapy (CBT) v group CBT for depression: Phase II trial. *Psychological Medicine, 50*(1), 11–19.

Irvine, A., & Luke, D. (2022). Apophenia, absorption and anxiety: Evidence for individual differences in positive and negative experiences of hallucinogen persisting perceptual disorder. *Journal of Psychedelic Studies, 6*(2), 88–103.

Jacobs, E., Yaden, D. B., & Earp, B. D. (2023). Toward a broader psychedelic bioethics. *AJOB Neuroscience, 14*(2), 126–129.

James, W. (1902/2003). *The varieties of religious experience: A study in human nature.* Routledge.

Jardim, A. V., Jardim, D. V., Chaves, B. R., Steglich, M., Ot'alora G, M., Mithoefer, M. C., ... & Schenberg, E. E. (2020). 3, 4-methylenedioxymethamphetamine (MDMA)-assisted psychotherapy for victims of sexual abuse with severe post-traumatic stress disorder: an open label pilot study in Brazil. *Brazilian Journal of Psychiatry, 43*, 181–185.

Johns Hopkins Medicine Newsroom. (2021, October 18). *Johns Hopkins Medicine receives first federal grant for psychedelic treatment research in 50 years.* https://www.hopkinsmedicine.org/news/newsroom/news-releases/johns-hopkins-medicine-receives-first-federal-grant-for-psychedelic-treatment-research-in-50-years

Johnson, M. W. (2020). Consciousness, religion, and gurus: pitfalls of psychedelic medicine. *ACS Pharmacology & Translational Science, 4*(2), 578–581.

Johnson, M. W., Garcia-Romeu, A., Cosimano, M. P., & Griffiths, R. R. (2014). Pilot study of the 5-HT2AR agonist psilocybin in the treatment of tobacco addiction. *Journal of Psychopharmacology, 28*(11), 983–992.

Johnson, M. W., Hendricks, P. S., Barrett, F. S., & Griffiths, R. R. (2019). Classic psychedelics: An integrative review of epidemiology, therapeutics, mystical experience, and brain network function. *Pharmacology & Therapeutics, 197*, 83–102.

Johnson, M. W., Richards, W. A., & Griffiths, R. R. (2008). Human hallucinogen research: guidelines for safety. *Journal of Psychopharmacology, 22*(6), 603–620.

La Torre, J. T., Mahammadli, M., Faber, S. C., Greenway, K. T., & Williams, M. T. (2023). Expert Opinion on Psychedelic-Assisted Psychotherapy for People with Psychopathological Psychotic Experiences and Psychotic Disorders. *International Journal of Mental Health and Addiction*, 1–25.

Jourard, S. M., & Rubin, J. (1968). Physical contact and self-disclosure. *Journal of Humanistic Psychology, 7*, 38–48.

Jylkkä, J. (2021). Reconciling mystical experiences with naturalistic psychedelic science: Reply to Sanders and Zijlmans. *ACS Pharmacology & Translational Science, 4*(4), 1468–1470.

Kaelen, M., Giribaldi, B., Raine, J., Evans, L., Timmermann, C., Rodriguez, N., ... & Carhart-Harris, R. (2018). The hidden therapist: Evidence for a central role of music in psychedelic therapy. *Psychopharmacology, 235*(2), 505–519.

Kangaslampi, S. (2023). Association between mystical-type experiences under psychedelics and improvements in well-being or mental health: A comprehensive review of the evidence. *Journal of Psychedelic Studies, 7*(1), 18–28.

Katz, R. (2017). *Indigenous healing psychology: Honoring the wisdom of the first peoples.* Simon and Schuster.

Katzman, J. (2018, September 8). *Rapid depression remission and the "therapeutic bends" with ketamine-assisted psychotherapy.* Psychedelics Today. https://psychedelicsto day.com/2018/09/08/rapid-depression-remission-therapeutic-bends-ketamine-assisted-psychotherapy/

Keiman, D. (2023, May 23). *Challenges of psychedelic medicines: Integrating challenging experiences* [video]. YouTube/Psychedelic Society of the Netherlands. https://www.youtube.com/watch?v=rpbjdtx6Fpo&t=113s

Kelly, J. R., Gillan, C. M., Prenderville, J., Kelly, C., Harkin, A., Clarke, G., & O'Keane, V. (2021). Psychedelic therapy's transdiagnostic effects: A research domain criteria (RDOC) perspective. *Frontiers in Psychiatry, 12*, 800072.

Kertay, L., & Reviere, S. L. (1993). The use of touch in psychotherapy: Theoretical and ethical considerations. *Psychotherapy: Theory, Research, Practice, Training, 30*(1), 32–40.

Kettner, H., Rosas, F. E., Timmermann, C., Kärtner, L., Carhart-Harris, R. L., & Roseman, L. (2021). Psychedelic communitas: intersubjective experience during psychedelic group sessions predicts enduring changes in psychological wellbeing and social connectedness. *Frontiers in Pharmacology, 12*, 623985.

King, F. (2023). *Psychedelics and the modern medical world* [video]. YouTube/UAB Psychedelic Studies Forum. https://www.youtube.com/watch?v=5RRRUHczrLc

Ko, K., Knight, G., Rucker, J. J., & Cleare, A. J. (2022). Psychedelics, mystical experience, and therapeutic efficacy: a systematic review. *Frontiers in Psychiatry*, *13*, 917199.

Koenig, H. G. (2009). Research on religion, spirituality, and mental health: A review. *Canadian Journal of Psychiatry*, *54*, 283–291

Krebs, T. S., & Johansen, P. Ø. (2012). Lysergic acid diethylamide (LSD) for alcoholism: meta-analysis of randomized controlled trials. *Journal of Psychopharmacology*, *26*(7), 994–1002.

Kurland, A., Savage, C., Pahnke, W. N., Grof, S., & Olsson, J. E. (1971). LSD in the treatment of alcoholics. *Pharmacopsychiatry*, *4*(02), 83–94.

Kurtom, M., Henning, A., & Espiridion, E. D. (2019). Hallucinogen-persisting perception disorder in a 21-year-old man. *Cureus*, *11*(2), e4077.

Lafrance, A., Loizaga-Velder, A., Fletcher, J., Renelli, M., Files, N., & Tupper, K. W. (2017). Nourishing the spirit: Exploratory research on ayahuasca experiences along the continuum of recovery from eating disorders. *Journal of Psychoactive Drugs*, *49*(5), 427–435.

Lafrance, A., Strahan, E., Bird, B. M., St. Pierre, M., & Walsh, Z. (2021). Classic psychedelic use and mechanisms of mental health: Exploring the mediating roles of spirituality and emotion processing on symptoms of anxiety, depressed mood, and disordered eating in a community sample. *Journal of Humanistic Psychology*, *137*(6), https://doi.org/10.1177/00221678211048049

Lamb, D. H., & Catanzaro, S. J. (1998). Sexual and nonsexual boundary violations involving psychologists, clients, supervisees, and students: Implications for professional practice. *Professional Psychology: Research and Practice*, *29*(5), 498–503.

La Torre, J. T., Mahammadli, M., Greenway, K., & Williams, M. (2022, January 25). *Expert opinion on psychedelic-assisted psychotherapy for people with psychotic symptoms*. Research Square. https://doi.org/10.21203/rs.3.rs-1241397/v1

Leary, T., Litwin, G. H., & Metzner, R. (1963). Reactions to psilocybjn administered in a supportive environment. *Journal of Nervous and Mental Disease*, *137*(6), 561–573.

Leaviss, J., & Uttley, L. (2015). Psychotherapeutic benefits of compassion-focused therapy: An early systematic review. *Psychological Medicine*, *45*(5), 927–945. doi:10.1017/S0033291714002141.

Leite, M. (2021, February 12). *Researchers demand reparations to Mazatecs for mushroom "spirit."* Chacruna. https://chacruna.net/researchers_demand_reparations_m azatecs/

Lekas, H. M., Pahl, K., & Fuller Lewis, C. (2020). Rethinking cultural competence: Shifting to cultural humility. *Health Services Insights*, *2020*, 13.

Leonard, J. B., Anderson, B., & Klein-Schwartz, W. (2018). Does getting high hurt? Characterization of cases of LSD and psilocybin-containing mushroom exposures to national poison centers between 2000 and 2016. *Journal of Psychopharmacology*, *32*(12), 1286–1294.

Leptourgos, P., Fortier-Davy, M., Carhart-Harris, R., Corlett, P. R., Dupuis, D., Halberstadt, A. L., ... & Jardri, R. (2020). Hallucinations under psychedelics and in the schizophrenia spectrum: an interdisciplinary and multiscale comparison. *Schizophrenia Bulletin*, *46*(6), 1396–1408.

Linehan, M. (2014). *DBT Skills training manual*. Guilford Publications.

Lovato, R. (2022, October 13–16). *The gentrification of consciousness*. Horizons Conference, New York, NY, United States.

Luke, D. (2023, April 20–22). *Fear & trembling in lost vagueness: The challenging psyche-delic experiences project* [video] YouTube/Breaking Convention. https://www.yout ube.com/watch?v=R_IfpY2hqzg

Lutkajtis, A., & Evans, J. (2023). Psychedelic integration challenges: Participant experiences after a psilocybin truffle retreat in the Netherlands. *Journal of Psychedelic Studies, 6*(3), 211–221.

MacLean, K. A., Johnson, M. W., & Griffiths, R. R. (2012). Mystical experiences occasioned by the hallucinogen psilocybin lead to increases in the personality do-main of openness. *Journal of Psychopharmacology, 25*(11), 1453–1461. https://doi. org/10.1177/0269881111420188

Mahmood, D., Alenezi, S. K., Anwar, M. J., Azam, F., Qureshi, K. A., & Jaremko, M. (2022). New paradigms of old psychedelics in schizophrenia. *Pharmaceuticals, 15*(5), 640.

Malan, D., & Coughlin Della Selva, P. (2007). *Lives transformed: A revolutionary method of dynamic psychotherapy* (rev. ed.). Karnac books.

Malcolm, B., & Thomas, K. (2022). Serotonin toxicity of serotonergic psychedelics. *Psychopharmacology, 239*(6), 1881–1891.

Malone, T. C., Mennenga, S. E., Guss, J., Podrebarac, S. K., Owens, L. T., Bossis, A. P., ... & Ross, S. (2018). Individual experiences in four cancer patients following psilocybin-assisted psychotherapy. *Frontiers in Pharmacology, 9*, 256.

MAPS. (2021, May 12). *MAPS wins appeal and authorization to study MDMA in healthy volunteer therapists.* MAPS.org. https://maps.org/news/media/maps-wins-appeal-and-authorization-to-study-mdma-in-healthy-volunteer-therapists/

MAPS. (2019). MAPS MDMA-assisted psychotherapy code of ethics. *MAPS Bulletin, 29*(1), 24–27.

Marcus, O. (2022). "Everybody's creating it along the way": ethical tensions among globalized ayahuasca shamanisms and therapeutic integration practices. *Interdisciplinary Science Reviews.* https://doi.org/10.1080/03080188.2022.2075201

Marrocu, A., Kettner, H., Weiss, B., Zeifman, R., Erritzoe, D., & Carhart-Harris, R. (2023). Psychiatric risks for worsened mental health after psychedelic use. *PsyArXiv.* https:// doi.org/10.31234/osf.io/2e34t

Martin, A. J. (1964). LSD analysis. *International Journal of Social Psychiatry, 10*(3), 165–169.

Masters, R. E. L., & Houston, J. (1966). *The varieties of psychedelic experience.* Holt, Rinehart & Winston.

Mastinu, A., Anyanwu, M., Carone, M., Abate, G., Bonini, S. A., Peron, G., ... & Memo, M. (2023). The bright side of psychedelics: latest advances and challenges in neuro-pharmacology. *International Journal of Molecular Sciences, 24*(2), 1329.

Mathai, D. S., Roberts, D. E., Nayak, S. M., Sepeda, N. D., Lehrner, A., Johnson, M., ... Garcia-Romeu, A. (2023, October 14). Shame, guilt and psychedelic experi-ence: Results from a prospective, longitudinal survey of real-world psilocybin use. https://doi.org/10.31234/osf.io/hm6jn

McAlpine, R., Blackburne, G., & Kamboj, S. (2023). *Development and psychometric val-idation of a novel scale for measuring "psychedelic preparedness".* Psyarxiv. https:// psyarxiv.com/gw9jp/download?format=pdf

McCullough, L., Magill, M. (2009). Affect-focused short-term dynamic therapy. In R. A. Levy & J. S. Ablon (Eds.), *Handbook of Evidence-Based Psychodynamic Psychotherapy.*

Current Clinical Psychiatry (pp. 249–277). Humana Press. https://doi.org/10.1007/978-1-59745-444-5_11

McNamee, S., Devenot, N., & Buisson, M. (2023). Studying harms is key to improving psychedelic-assisted therapy: Participants call for changes to research landscape. *JAMA Psychiatry, 80*(5), 411–412.

Meckel, F. (2019). Guidelines in applying psychedelic therapies. In M. Winkelman & B. Sessa (Eds.), *Advances in Psychedelic Medicine: State-of-the-Art Therapeutic Applications* (pp. 253–273). Praeger/ABC-CLIO.

McMillan, R. M. (2022). Psychedelic injustice: should bioethics tune in to the voices of psychedelic-using communities?. *Medical Humanities, 48*(3), 269–272.

Michaels, T. I., Purdon, J., Collins, A., & Williams, M. T. (2018). Inclusion of people of color in psychedelic-assisted psychotherapy: A review of the literature. *BMC Psychiatry, 18*(1), 1–14.

Miller, W. R. (2004). *Spiritual evocation: Guidelines for spiritual direction in drug abuse treatment.* Unpublished manuscript.

Miller, W. R., C'de Baca, J., Matthews, D. B., & Wilbourne, P. L. (2001). *Personal values card sort.* https://motivationalinterviewing.org/sites/default/files/valuescardsort_0.pdf

Miller, W. R., Forcehimes, A., O'Leary, M., & LaNoue, M. D. (2008). Spiritual direction in addiction treatment: Two clinical trials. *Journal of Substance Abuse Treatment, 35*(4), 434–442. doi:10.1016/j.jsat.2008.02.004

Miller, W. R., & Rollnick, S. (2013). *Motivational interviewing: Helping people change (applications of motivational interviewing).* Guilford Press.

Mintz, E. E. (1969). On the rationale of touch in psychotherapy. *Psychotherapy: Theory, Research & Practice, 6*(4), 232–234.

Mitchell JM, Bogenschutz M, Lilienstein A, Harrison C, Kleiman S, Parker-Guilbert K, ... Doblin R. (2021). MDMA-assisted therapy for severe PTSD: a randomized, double-blind, placebo-controlled phase 3 study. *Nature Medicine 27*(6):1025–1033. https://doi.org/10.1038/s41591-021-01336-3

Mithoefer, M. (2018). *MAPS-sponsored research at the 2017 annual meeting of the international society for traumatic stress studies: Signs of breaking through resistance.* MAPS Bulletin. https://maps.org/news/bulletin/michael-mithoefer-spring-2018/

Mithoefer, M. C., Mithoefer, A. T., Feduccia, A. A., Jerome, L., Wagner, M., Wymer, J., Holland, J., Hamilton, S., Yazar-Klosinski, B., Emerson, A., Doblin, R. (2018). 3,4-Methylenedioxymethamphetamine (MDMA)-assisted psychotherapy for post-traumatic stress disorder in military veterans, firefighters, and police officers: A randomised, double-blind, dose-response, phase 2 clinical trial. *The Lancet Psychiatry, 5*(6), 486–497.

Mithoefer, M. C., Mithoefer, A., Jerome, L., Ruse, J., Doblin, R., Gibson, E., Ot'alora G., M., & Sola, E. (2017). *A manual for MDMA-assisted psychotherapy in the treatment of post-traumatic stress disorder.* https://www.maps.org/research-archive/mdma/MDMA-Assisted-Psychotherapy-Treatment-Manual-Version7-19Aug15-FINAL.pdf

Mithoefer, M. C., Wagner, M., Mithoefer, A., Jerome, L., & Doblin, R. (2011). The safety and efficacy of ±3,4-methylenedioxymethamphetamine-assisted psychotherapy in subjects with chronic, treatment-resistant posttraumatic stress disorder: the first randomized controlled pilot study. *Journal of Psychopharmacology, 25*(4), 439–452.

Monson, C. M., Wagner, A. C., Mithoefer, A. T., Liebman, R. E., Feduccia, A. A., Jerome, L., ... & Mithoefer, M. C. (2020). MDMA-facilitated cognitive-behavioural conjoint therapy for posttraumatic stress disorder: an uncontrolled trial. *European Journal of Psychotraumatology*, *11*(1), 1840123.

Morales, J., Quan, E., Arshed, A., & Jordan, A. (2022). Racial disparities in access to psychedelic treatments and inclusion in research trials. *Psychiatric Annals*, *52*(12), 494–499.

Moreno, F., Wiegand, C., Taitano, E., & Delgado, P. (2006). Safety, tolerability, and efficacy of psilocybin in 9 patients with obsessive-compulsive disorder. *Journal of Clinical Psychiatry*, *67*, 1735–1740.

Morton, E., Sakai, K., Ashtari, A., Pleet, M., Michalak, E. E., & Woolley, J. (2023). Risks and benefits of psilocybin use in people with bipolar disorder: An international web-based survey on experiences of "magic mushroom" consumption. *Journal of Psychopharmacology*, *37*(1), 49–60.

Müller, F., Mühlhauser, M., Holze, F., Lang, U. E., Walter, M., Liechti, M. E., & Borgwardt, S. (2020). Treatment of a complex personality disorder using repeated doses of LSD: A case report on significant improvements in the absence of acute drug effects. *Frontiers in Psychiatry*, *11*, 573953.

Murphy, R., Kettner, H., Zeifman, R., Giribaldi, B., Kartner, L., Martell, J., . . . & Carhart-Harris, R. (2022). Therapeutic alliance and rapport modulate responses to psilocybin assisted therapy for depression. *Frontiers in Pharmacology*, *12*, 788155.

Muthukumaraswamy, S., Forsyth, A., & Sumner, R. L. (2022). The challenges ahead for psychedelic "medicine". *The Australian and New Zealand Journal of Psychiatry*, *56*(11), 1378–1383. https://doi.org/10.1177/00048674221081763

Muthukumaraswamy, S. D., Forsyth, A., & Lumley, T. (2021). Blinding and expectancy confounds in psychedelic randomized controlled trials. *Expert Review of Clinical Pharmacology*, *14*(9), 1133–1152.

Nayak, S. M., & Griffiths, R. R. (2022). A single belief-changing psychedelic experience is associated with increased attribution of consciousness to living and non-living entities. *Frontiers in Psychology*, *13*, 852248.

Neff, J., Holmes, S. M., Knight, K. R., Strong, S., Thompson-Lastad, A., McGuinness, C., ... & Nelson, N. (2020). Structural competency: curriculum for medical students, residents, and interprofessional teams on the structural factors that produce health disparities. *MedEdPORTAL*, *16*, 10888. https://doi.org/10.15766/mep_2 374-8265.10888

Negrin, D. (2020, June 9). *Colonial shadows in the psychedelic renaissance*. Chacruna. https://chacruna.net/colonial-shadows-in-the-psychedelic-renaissance/

Nichols, D. (1986). Differences between the mechanism of action of MDMA, MBDB, and the classic hallucinogens. Identification of a new therapeutic class: Entactogens. *Journal of Psychoactive Drugs*, *18*(4), 305–313.

Nichols, D. E. (2004). Hallucinogens. *Pharmacology & Therapeutics*, *101*(2), 131–181.

Niedenthal, P. M., Barsalou, L. W., Winkielman, P., Krauth-Gruber, S., & Ric, F. (2005). Embodiment in attitudes, social perception, and emotion. *Personality and Social Psychology Review*, *9*(3), 184–211.

Nielson, E. M. (2021). Psychedelics as a training experience for psychedelic therapists: Drawing on history to inform current practice. *Journal of Humanistic Psychology*, https://doi.org/10.1177/00221678211021204.

Nielson, E. M., & Guss, J. (2018). The influence of therapists' first-hand experience with psychedelics on psychedelic-assisted psychotherapy research and therapist training. *Journal of Psychedelic Studies*, *2*(2), 64–73.

Nielson, E. M., May, D. G., Forcehimes, A. A., & Bogenschutz, M. P. (2018). The psychedelic debriefing in alcohol dependence treatment: Illustrating key change phenomena through qualitative content analysis of clinical sessions. *Frontiers in Pharmacology*, *9*, 132. https://doi.org/10.3389/fphar.2018.00132

Nierenberg, M. A. (1972). Self-help first: A critical evaluation of "The family therapist's own family." *International Journal of Psychiatry*, *10*(1), 34–41.

Nolen-Hoeksema, S., McBride, A., & Larson, J. (1997). Rumination and psychological distress among bereaved partners. *Journal of Personality and Social Psychology*, *72*, 855–862.

Noorani, T. (2020). Making psychedelics into medicines: The politics and paradoxes of medicalization. *Journal of Psychedelic Studies*, *4*(1), 34–39. https://doi.org/10.1556/2054.2019.018

Noorani, T., Bedi, G., & Muthukumaraswamy, S. (2023). Dark loops: contagion effects, consistency and chemosocial matrices in psychedelic-assisted therapy trials. *Psychological Medicine*, *53*(13), 5892–5901.

Noorani, T., Garcia-Romeu, A., Swift, T. C., Griffiths, R. R., & Johnson, M. W. (2018). Psychedelic therapy for smoking cessation: Qualitative analysis of participant accounts. *Journal of Psychopharmacology*, *32*(7), 756–769.

Northrup, L. M. (2019, October). *Dynamics of sexual harm: Understanding the psychology of violation in healing relationships*. Presented at the Horizons Conference, New York.

Nour, M. M., Evans, L., & Carhart-Harris, R. L. (2016). Psychedelics, personality and political perspectives. *Journal of Psychoactive Drugs*, *49*(3), 182–191.

Nygart, V. A., Pommerencke, L. M., Haijen, E., Kettner, H., Kaelen, M., Mortensen, E. L., ... & Erritzoe, D. (2022). Antidepressant effects of a psychedelic experience in a large prospective naturalistic sample. *Journal of Psychopharmacology*, *36*(8), 932–942.

Oehen, P., Traber, R., Widmer, V., & Schnyder, U. (2013). A randomized, controlled pilot study of MDMA (±3, 4-methylenedioxymethamphetamine)-assisted psychotherapy for treatment of resistant, chronic post-traumatic stress disorder (PTSD). *Journal of Psychopharmacology*, *27*(1), 40–52.

Ogden, P., & Fisher, J. (2015). *Sensorimotor psychotherapy: Interventions for trauma and attachment (Norton series on interpersonal neurobiology)*. WW Norton & Company.

Oram, M. (2014). *The trials of psychedelic medicine: LSD psychotherapy, clinical science, and pharmaceutical regulation in the United States, 1949–1976* [Ph.D. thesis, University of Sydney]. Sydney eScholarship Repository. https://ses.library.usyd.edu.au/handle/2123/10511

Osborn, K. A. R., Ulvenes, P. G., Wampold, B. E., & McCullough, L. (2015). Creating change through focusing on affect: Affect phobia therapy. In N. C. Thoma, & D. McKay (Eds.), *Working with emotion in cognitive-behavioral therapy: Techniques for clinical practice* (pp. 146–171). The Guilford Press.

Ot'alora G, M., Grigsby, J., Poulter, B., Van Derveer III, J. W., Giron, S. G., Jerome, L., ... & Doblin, R. (2018). 3, 4-Methylenedioxymethamphetamine-assisted psychotherapy for treatment of chronic posttraumatic stress disorder: a randomized phase 2 controlled trial. *Journal of Psychopharmacology*, *32*(12), 1295–1307.

Ozcubukcu, A. (2022, March 9). *The gold standard for psychedelic-assisted therapy? Exploring the use of acceptance and commitment therapy (ACT)*. Clerkenwell Health Blog. https://www.clerkenwellhealth.com/blog-articles/gold-standard-for-psychede lic-assisted-therapy-act

Palhano-Fontes, F., Barreto, D., Onias, H., Andrade, K. C., Novaes, M. M., Pessoa, J. A., ... & Araújo, D. B. (2019). Rapid antidepressant effects of the psychedelic ayahuasca in treatment-resistant depression: a randomized placebo-controlled trial. *Psychological Medicine, 49*(4), 655–663.

Palitsky, R., Kaplan, D. M., Peacock, C., Zarrabi, A. J., Maples-Keller, J. L., Grant, G. H., ... & Raison, C. L. (2023). Importance of integrating spiritual, existential, religious, and theological components in psychedelic-assisted therapies. *JAMA Psychiatry, 80*(7), 743–749.

Papadopoulos, N. L. R., & Röhricht, F. (2014). An investigation into the application and processes of manualized group body psychotherapy for depressive disorder in a clinical trial. *Body, Movement and Dance in Psychotherapy, 9*(3), 167–180.

Partridge, C. H. (2018). *High culture: drugs, mysticism, and the pursuit of transcendence in the modern world*. Oxford University Press.

Passie, T. (2018). The early use of MDMA ("Ecstasy") in psychotherapy (1977–1985). *Drug Science, Policy, and Law, 4*, 1–19.

Passie, T., Loizaga Velder, A., Danforth, A., Grob, C. C., Greer, G., ... & Guss, J. (2023). *A proposal for a model training curriculum for substance-assisted psychotherapy (SAP)* [Manuscript in preparation].

Passie, T., Schlickting, M., & Bolle, R. (2022). *Psycholytic therapy*. Synergetic Press.

PatientNB (2022). A patient's perspective on the healing potential of psilocybin. In A. B. Belser, C. Cavnar, & B. C. Labate (Eds.), *Queering psychedelics: From oppression to liberation in psychedelic medicine* (pp. 129–132). Synergetic Press.

Pattison, T. E. (1973). Effects of touch on self-exploration and the therapeutic relationship. *Journal of Consulting and Clinical Psychology, 40*, 170–175.

Perception Restoration Foundation. (2021). *Frequently asked questions*. Perception Restoration Foundation. https://www.perception.foundation/faq

Perkins, D., Schubert, V., Simonová, H., Tófoli, L. F., Bouso, J. C., Horák, M., ... & Sarris, J. (2021). Influence of context and setting on the mental health and wellbeing outcomes of ayahuasca drinkers: results of a large international survey. *Frontiers in Pharmacology, 12*, 623979.

Peterson, A., Largent, E. A., Lynch, H. F., Karlawish, J., & Sisti, D. (2022). Journeying to Ixtlan: Ethics of psychedelic medicine and research for Alzheimer's disease and related dementias. *AJOB Neuroscience, 14*(2), 107–123.

Phelps, J. (2017). Developing guidelines and competencies for the training of psychedelic therapists. *Journal of Humanistic Psychology, 57*(5), 450–487.

Phelps, J. (2022, September 22–24). *10 values and skills of the ethical psychedelic therapist*. Interdisciplinary Conference on Psychedelic Research, Haarlem, The Netherlands.

Phillips, J. A., & Nugent, C. N. (2014). Suicide and the Great Recession of 2007–2009: The role of economic factors in the 50 US states. *Social Science & Medicine, 116*, 22–31.

Podrebarac, S. K., O'Donnell, K. C., Mennenga, S. E., Owens, L. T., Malone, T. C., Duane, J. H., & Bogenschutz, M. P. (2021). Spiritual experiences in psychedelic-assisted psychotherapy: Case reports of communion with the divine, the departed, and saints in research using psilocybin for the treatment of alcohol dependence. *Spirituality in Clinical Practice, 8*(3), 177–187. https://doi.org/10.1037/scp0000242

Pokorny, T., Preller, K. H., Kometer, M., Dziobek, I., & Vollenweider, F. X. (2017). Effect of psilocybin on empathy and moral decision-making. *International Journal of Neuropsychopharmacology, 20*(9), 747–757. https://doi.org/10.1093/ijnp/pyx047

Pokorny, T., Preller, K. H., Kraehenmann, R., & Vollenweider, F. X. (2016). Modulatory effect of the 5-HT1A agonist buspirone and the mixed non-hallucinogenic 5-HT1A/2A agonist ergotamine on psilocybin-induced psychedelic experience. *European Neuropsychopharmacology, 26*(4), 756–766.

Pollan, M. (2015, February 9). The trip treatment. *The New Yorker*, 9.

Pots, W., & Chakhssi, F. (2022). Psilocybin-assisted compassion focused therapy for depression. *Frontiers in Psychology, 13*, 812930.

Prideaux, E. (2023a, February 23). HPPD, "Flashbacks", and the problem of psychedelic anxiety. Psychedelic Support. https://psychedelic.support/resources/hppd-flashbacks-and-the-problem-of-psychedelic-anxiety/

Prideaux, E. (2023b, February 13). *Living with hallucinogen persisting perception disorder (HPPD)*. Ecstatic Integration. https://www.ecstaticintegration.org/p/living-with-hallucinogen-persisting

Prideaux, E. (2023c, May 23). *Challenges of psychedelic medicines: Should we be talking more about HPPD?* [video]. YouTube/Psychedelic Society of the Netherlands. https://www.youtube.com/watch?v=jj6xruYIjF8

Prilleltensky, I. (1994). *The morals and politics of psychology: Psychological discourse and the status quo*. State University of New York Press.

Proudman, D., Greenberg, P., & Nellesen, D. (2021). The growing burden of major depressive disorders (MDD): implications for researchers and policy makers. *PharmacoEconomics, 39*, 619–625.

Ragnhildstveit, A., Roscoe, J., Bass, L. C., Averill, C. L., Abdallah, C. G., & Averill, L. A. (2023). The potential of ketamine for posttraumatic stress disorder: a review of clinical evidence. *Therapeutic Advances in Psychopharmacology, 13*, 20451253231154125.

Reiff, C. M., Richman, E. E., Nemeroff, C. B., Carpenter, L. L., Widge, A. S., Rodriguez, C. I., ... & Work Group on Biomarkers and Novel Treatments, a Division of the American Psychiatric Association Council of Research. (2020). Psychedelics and psychedelic-assisted psychotherapy. *American Journal of Psychiatry, 177*(5), 391–410.

Richards, W. A. (2015). *Sacred knowledge: Psychedelics and religious experiences*. Columbia University Press.

Rønberg, M. T. (2019). Depression: Out-of-tune embodiment, loss of bodily resonance, and body work. *Medical Anthropology, 38*(4), 399–411.

Roseman, L., Haijen, E., Idialu-Ikato, K., Kaelen, M., Watts, R., & Carhart-Harris, R. (2019). Emotional breakthrough and psychedelics: validation of the emotional breakthrough inventory. *Journal of Psychopharmacology, 33*(9), 1076–1087.

Roseman, L., Nutt, D. J., Carhart-Harris, R.L. (2018). Quality of acute psychedelic experience predicts therapeutic efficacy of psilocybin for treatment-resistant depression. *Frontiers in Pharmacology, 8*, 974. doi:10.3389/fphar.2017.00974

Ross, S., Agin-Liebes, G., Lo, S., Zeifman, R. J., Ghazal, L., Benville, J., ... & Mennenga, S. E. (2021). Acute and sustained reductions in loss of meaning and suicidal ideation following psilocybin-assisted psychotherapy for psychiatric and existential distress in life-threatening cancer. *ACS Pharmacology & Translational Science, 4*(2), 553–562.

Ross, S., Bossis, A., Guss, J., Agin-Liebes, G., Malone, T., Cohen, B., ... & Schmidt, B. L. (2016). Rapid and sustained symptom reduction following psilocybin treatment for anxiety and depression in patients with life-threatening cancer: a randomized controlled trial. *Journal of Psychopharmacology, 30*(12), 1165–1180.

Rucker, J. J. H., Jelen, L. A., Flynn, S., Frowde, K. D., & Young, A. H. (2016). Psychedelics in the treatment of unipolar mood disorders: A systematic review. *Journal of Psychopharmacology, 30*(12), 1220–1229. https://doi.org/10.1177/026988111 6679368

Rucker, J. J., Iliff, J., & Nutt, D. J. (2018). Psychiatry & the psychedelic drugs. Past, present & future. *Neuropharmacology, 142,* 200–218.

Rucker, J. J., Marwood, L., Ajantaival, R. L. J., Bird, C., Eriksson, H., Harrison, J., ... & Young, A. H. (2022). The effects of psilocybin on cognitive and emotional functions in healthy participants: Results from a phase 1, randomised, placebo-controlled trial involving simultaneous psilocybin administration and preparation. *Journal of Psychopharmacology, 36*(1), 114–125.

Rupp, M. (2017, June 21). *The psychedelic experience.* Sapien Soup. https://sapiensoup. com/psychedelic-experience

Rush, B., Marcus, O., Ron Shore, M. P. A., Cunningham, L., & Rideout, K. (2022). Psychedelic medicine: A rapid review of therapeutic applications and implications for future research. Homeward Research Institute. http://hriresearch.s3.amazonaws. com/uploads/2022/11/Psychedelic-Medicine-Report-Final-v5.pdf

Russ, S. L., Carhart-Harris, R. L., Maruyama, G., & Elliott, M. S. (2019). Replication and extension of a model predicting response to psilocybin. *Psychopharmacology, 236,* 3221–3230.

Sanches, R. F., de Lima Osório, F., Dos Santos, R. G., Macedo, L. R., Maia-de-Oliveira, J. P., Wichert-Ana, L., ... & Hallak, J. E. (2016). Antidepressant effects of a single dose of ayahuasca in patients with recurrent depression: a SPECT study. *Journal of Clinical Psychopharmacology, 36*(1), 77–81.

Sanders, J. W., & Zijlmans, J. (2021). Moving past mysticism in psychedelic science. *ACS Pharmacology & Translational Science, 4*(3), 1253–1255.

Saunders, D., Svob, C., Pan, L., Abraham, E., Posner, J., Weissman, M., & Wickramaratne, P. (2021). Differential association of spirituality and religiosity with rumination: Implications for the treatment of depression. *Journal of Nervous and Mental Disease, 209*(5), 370–377.

Schlag, A. K., Aday, J., Salam, I., Neill, J. C., & Nutt, D. J. (2022). Adverse effects of psychedelics: From anecdotes and misinformation to systematic science. *Journal of Psychopharmacology, 36*(3), 258–272.

Schmid, Y., Enzler, F., Gasser, P., Grouzmann, E., Preller, K. H., Vollenweider, F. X., ... & Liechti, M. E. (2015). Acute effects of lysergic acid diethylamide in healthy subjects. *Biological Psychiatry, 78*(8), 544–553.

Schneier, F. R., Feusner, J., Wheaton, M. G., Gomez, G. J., Cornejo, G., Naraindas, A. M., & Hellerstein, D. J. (2023). Pilot study of single-dose psilocybin for serotonin reuptake inhibitor-resistant body dysmorphic disorder. *Journal of Psychiatric Research, 161,* 364–370.

Schultes, R. E., Hofmann, A., & Rätsch, C. (2001). *Plants of the Gods: Their sacred, healing, and hallucinogenic powers*. Healing Arts Press.

Schwartzman, C. M., & Muir, H. J. (2019). Personal psychotherapy for the psychotherapist in training. *Psychotherapy Bulletin, 54*(4), 15–21.

Segal, Z.V., Williams, J.M., & Teasdale, J.D. (2012). *Mindfulness-based cognitive therapy for depression: A new approach to relapse prevention*. Guilford Press.

Sessa, B., & Fischer, F. M. (2015). Underground MDMA-, LSD-and 2-CB-assisted individual and group psychotherapy in Zurich: Outcomes, implications and commentary. *Drug Science, Policy and Law, 2*, 2050324515578080.

Sessa, B., Higbed, L., O'Brien, S., Durant, C., Sakal, C., Titheradge, D., ... & Nutt, D. J. (2021). First study of safety and tolerability of 3, 4-methylenedioxymethamphetamine-assisted psychotherapy in patients with alcohol use disorder. *Journal of Psychopharmacology, 35*(4), 375–383.

Shankin, D. (2023, February). *6 ways that working with art and creativity can support psychedelic integration*. [Post] LinkedIn. https://www.linkedin.com/feed/update/urn:li:activity:7031426073095467009?updateEntityUrn=urn%3Ali%3Afs_feedUpdate%3A%28V2%2Curn%3Ali%3Aactivity%3A7031426073095467009%29

Sharma, S. (2021, October 11). *On sacred reciprocity: Giving back to our indigenous predecessors in the psychedelic movement*. Psychedelic Spotlight. https://psychedelicspotlight.com/indigenous-peoples-day-sacred-reciprocity-predecessors-psychedelic-movement/

Shnayder, S., Ameli, R., Sinaii, N., Berger, A., & Agrawal, M. (2023). Psilocybin-assisted therapy improves psycho-social-spiritual well-being in cancer patients. *Journal of Affective Disorders, 323*, 592–597.

Sjoberg, B. M., & Hollister, L. E. (1965). The effects of psychotomimetic drugs on primary suggestibility. *Psychopharmacologia, 8*(4), 251–262.

Sloshower, J., Guss, J., Krause, R., Wallace, R. M., Williams, M. T., Reed, S., & Skinta, M. D. (2020). Psilocybin-assisted therapy of major depressive disorder using acceptance and commitment therapy as a therapeutic frame. *Journal of Contextual Behavioral Science, 15*, 12–19.

Sloshower, J., Skosnik, P. D., Safi-Aghdam, H., Pathania, S., Syed, S., Pittman, B., D'Souza, D. C. (2023). Psilocybin-assisted therapy for major depressive disorder: An exploratory placebo-controlled, fixed-order trial. *Journal of Psychopharmacology, 37*(7), 698–706.

Smith, D. T., Faber, S. C., Buchanan, N. T., Foster, D., & Green, L. (2022). The need for psychedelic-assisted therapy in the Black community and the burdens of its provision. *Frontiers in Psychiatry, 12*, 774736.

Smith, E. W. L., Clance, P. R., & Imes, S. (Ed.). (1998). *Touch in psychotherapy: Theory, research, and practice*. Guilford Press.

Smith, W. R., & Sisti, D. (2021). Ethics and ego dissolution: the case of psilocybin. *Journal of Medical Ethics, 47*(12), 807–814.

Söderberg, J. (2023). The psychedelic renaissance. *Prometheus, 38*(4), 385–398.

St. Aime, F. (in press). *Unlearning as a liberatory and anti-oppressive psychotherapeutic practice*. Routledge.

Stauffer, C. S., Brown, M. R., Adams, D., Cassity, M., & Sevelius, J. (2022). MDMA-assisted psychotherapy: Inclusion of transgender and gender diverse people in the frontiers of PTSD treatment trials. *Frontiers in Psychiatry, 13*, 932605.

Stockwell, S. R., & Dye, A. (1980). Effects of counselor touch on counseling outcome. *Journal of Counseling Psychology, 27,* 443–446.

Stolaroff, M. (2004). *The secret chief revealed: Conversations with a pioneer of the underground therapy movement.* MAPS Press.

Strauss, D., de la Salle, S., Sloshower, J., & Williams, M. T. (2022). Research abuses against people of colour and other vulnerable groups in early psychedelic research. *Journal of Medical Ethics, 48*(10), 728–737.

Strickland, J. C., Garcia-Romeu, A., & Johnson, M. W. (2020). Set and setting: A randomized study of different musical genres in supporting psychedelic therapy. *ACS Pharmacology & Translational Science, 4*(2), 472–478.

Studerus, E., Gamma, A., & Vollenweider, F. X. (2010). Psychometric evaluation of the altered states of consciousness rating scale (OAV). *PloS One, 5*(8), e12412.

Substance Abuse and Mental Health Services Administration (2014). *A treatment improvement protocol: Trauma-informed care in behavioral health services, Tip 57.* U.S. Department of Health and Human Services. https://store.samhsa.gov/sites/default/files/sma14-4816.pdf

Substance Abuse and Mental Health Services Administration. (2020) *National survey on drug use and health (NSDUH).* Substance Abuse and Mental Health Services Administration.

Swift, T. C., Belser, A. B., Agin-Liebes, G., Devenot, N., Terrana, S., Friedman, H. L., ... & Ross, S. (2017). Cancer at the dinner table: Experiences of psilocybin-assisted psychotherapy for the treatment of cancer-related distress. *Journal of Humanistic Psychology, 57*(5), 488–519. https://doi.org/10.1177/0022167817715966

Swift, T. C., Petersen, R., Belser, A. B., Bossis, A. P., Garcia, A., & Griffiths, R. (2023). *The reflections of diverse religious leaders following administration of psilocybin-facilitated experience: A phenomenological analysis* [Manuscript in preparation].

Swoon. (2019, October 12). Unearthing the Medea: The intersection of art & psychedelic assisted therapy [video]. YouTube/Horizons: Perspectives on Psychedelics. https://www.youtube.com/watch?v=-_9RZWHrrbw

Taylor, C. T., Lyubomirsky, S., & Stein, M. B. (2017). Upregulating the positive affect system in anxiety and depression: Outcomes of a positive activity intervention. *Depression and Anxiety, 34*(3), 267–280.

Taylor, K. (in press). *The peer consultation group handbook: InnerEthics ethical awareness tools for facilitators of psychedelic sessions and other extra-ordinary states of consciousness.* Hanford Mead.

Taylor, K. (2017). *The ethics of caring: Finding right relationship with clients.* Hanford Mead.

Thal, S. B., Bright, S. J., Sharbanee, J. M., Wenge, T., & Skeffington, P. M. (2021). Current perspective on the therapeutic preset for substance-assisted psychotherapy. *Frontiers in Psychology, 12,* 617224.

Thrul, J., & Garcia-Romeu, A. (2021). Whitewashing psychedelics: racial equity in the emerging field of psychedelic-assisted mental health research and treatment. *Drugs: Education, Prevention and Policy, 28*(3), 211–214.

Timmermann, C., Kettner, H., Letheby, C., Roseman, L., Rosas, F. E., & Carhart-Harris, R. L. (2021). Psychedelics alter metaphysical beliefs. *Scientific Reports, 11*(1), 1–13.

Van der Kolk, B. (2014). *The body keeps the score: Mind, brain and body in the transformation of trauma.* Penguin UK.

van der Kolk, B. A., Wang, J., Yehuda, R., Coker, A., Bedrosian, L., Mithoefer, M., ... & Doblin, R. (2023). *The Effects of MDMA assisted therapy of PTSD on self-experience.* medRxiv, https://www.medrxiv.org/content/10.1101/2023.01.03.23284143v1.

van Elk, M., & Fried, E. I. (2023). *History repeating: A roadmap to address common problems in psychedelic science.* PsyArXiv Preprints. https://doi.org/10.31234/osf.io/ak6gx

van Elk, M., & Yaden, D. B. (2022). Pharmacological, neural, and psychological mechanisms underlying psychedelics: A critical review. *Neuroscience & Biobehavioral Reviews, 140,* 104793.

von Rotz, R., Schindowski, E. M., Jungwirth, J., Schuldt, A., Rieser, N. M., Zahoranszky, K., ... & Vollenweider, F. X. (2022). Single-dose psilocybin-assisted therapy in major depressive disorder: A placebo-controlled, double-blind randomized clinical trial. *eClinicalMedicine, 56,* 101809.

Wagner, A., Mithoefer, M., & Doblin, R. (2019). Bringing psychedelics and entactogens into mainstream pharmaceuticals: A focus on MDMA. *Advances in Psychedelic Medicine, 3,* 336–357.

Walsh, R. (2003). Entheogens: True or false?. *International Journal of Transpersonal Studies, 22*(1), 3.

Walsh, Z., Mollaahmetoglu, O. M., Rootman, J., Golsof, S., Keeler, J., Marsh, B., ... & Morgan, C. J. (2022). Ketamine for the treatment of mental health and substance use disorders: comprehensive systematic review. *BJPsych Open, 8*(1), e19.

Watkins, E. R. (2016). *Rumination-focused cognitive behavioral therapy for depression.* Guilford press.

Watts, R. (2021). *Psilocybin for depression: The ACE model manual.* https://osf.io/preprints/psyarxiv/5x2bu/

Watts, R. (2022, February 28). *Can magic mushrooms unlock depression? What I've learned in the five years since my TEDx talk.* Medium. https://medium.com/@DrRosalindWatts/can-magic-mushrooms-unlock-depression-what-ive-learned-in-the-5-years-since-my-tedx-talk-767c83963134

Watts, R., Day, C., Krzanowski, J., Nutt, D., & Carhart-Harris, R. (2017). Patients' accounts of increased "connectedness" and "acceptance" after psilocybin for treatment-resistant depression. *Journal of Humanistic Psychology, 57*(5), 520–564.

Watts, R., & Luoma, J. B. (2020). The use of the psychological flexibility model to support psychedelic assisted therapy. *Journal of Contextual Behavioral Science, 15,* 92–102.

Weiss, B., Miller, J. D., Carter, N. T., & Keith Campbell, W. (2021). Examining changes in personality following shamanic ceremonial use of ayahuasca. *Scientific Reports, 11*(1), 1–15.

Weiss, B., Wingert, A., Erritzoe, D., & Campbell, W. K. (2023). Prevalence and therapeutic impact of adverse life event reexperiencing under ceremonial ayahuasca. *Scientific Reports, 13*(1), 9438.

Weiss, H., Johanson, G., & Monda, L. (2015). *Hakomi mindfulness-centered somatic psychotherapy: A comprehensive guide to theory and practice.* WW Norton & Company.

Williams, M. T., Reed, S., & Aggarwal, R. (2020). Culturally informed research design issues in a study for MDMA-assisted psychotherapy for posttraumatic stress disorder. *Journal of Psychedelic Studies, 4*(1), 40–50. https://doi.org/10.1556/2054.2019.016

Williams, M. T., Reed, S., & George, J. (2021). Culture and psychedelic psycho-therapy: Ethnic and racial themes from three Black women therapists. *Journal of Psychedelic Studies, 4*(3), 125–138.

Williams, K., Romero, O. S. G., Braunstein, M., & Brant, S. (2022). Indigenous philosophies and the "psychedelic renaissance". *Anthropology of Consciousness, 33*(2), 506–527.

Wilson, K. G., & Groom, J. (2002). *The valued living questionnaire.* https://www.div12.org/wp-content/uploads/2015/06/Valued-Living-Questionnaire.pdf

Winkelman, M. (2019). Introduction: Evidence for entheogen use in prehistory and world religions. *Journal of Psychedelic Studies, 3*(2), 43–62.

Winstock, A., Barratt, M., Ferris, J., & Maier, L. (2017). *Global drug survey.* GDS Core Research Team. https://www.globaldrugsurvey.com/wp-content/themes/globaldrugsurvey/results/GDS2017_key-findings-report_final.pdf

Wolf, G., Singh, S. Blakolmer, K., Lerer, L., Lifschytz, T., Heresco-Levy, U., ... & Lerer, B. (2022). Could psychedelic drugs have a role in the treatment of schizophrenia? Rationale and strategy for safe implementation. *Molecular Psychiatry, 28*, 44–58. https://doi.org/10.1038/s41380-022-01832-z

Wolff, M. (2023, August 21-September 3). *Psychedelic therapy is psychotherapy — Connecting the dots between two fields that belong together* [Conference presentation]. INSIGHT: Berlin, Germany. https://www.youtube.com/watch?v=8DyyeWI9Mq4

Wolff, M., Evens, R., Mertens, L. J., Koslowski, M., Betzler, F., Gründer, G., & Jungaberle, H. (2020). Learning to let go: A cognitive-behavioral model of how psychedelic therapy promotes acceptance. *Frontiers in Psychiatry, 11*, 5. https://doi-org.avoserv2.library.fordham.edu/10.3389/fpsyt.2020.00005

Wolfson, P. E., Andries, J., Feduccia, A. A., Jerome, L., Wang, J. B., Williams, E., ... & Doblin, R. (2020). MDMA-assisted psychotherapy for treatment of anxiety and other psychological distress related to life-threatening illnesses: a randomized pilot study. *Scientific Reports, 10*(1), 1–15.

Woolfe, S. (2023). *Using metta meditation to deal with depression.* Invisible Illness. Retrieved from https://medium.com/invisible-illness/using-metta-meditation-to-deal-with-depression-8a28d4e12b00

Yaden, D. B., Earp, D., Graziosi, M., Friedman-Wheeler, D., Luoma, J. B., & Johnson, M. W. (2022). Psychedelics and psychotherapy: cognitive-behavioral approaches as default. *Frontiers in Psychology, 13*, 1604.

Yu, Y., Matlin, S. L., Crusto, C. A., Hunter, B., & Tebes, J. K. (2022). Double stigma and help-seeking barriers among Blacks with a behavioral health disorder. *Psychiatric Rehabilitation Journal, 45*(2), 183–191.

Zeifman, R. J., & Wagner, A. C. (2020). Exploring the case for research on incorporating psychedelics within interventions for borderline personality disorder. *Journal of Contextual Behavioral Science, 15*, 1–11.

For the benefit of digital users, indexed terms that span two pages (e.g., 52–53) may, on occasion, appear on only one of those pages.

Tables, figures, and boxes are indicated by *t*, *f*, and *b* following the page number